CULTURES OF HEALING

This volume brings together for the first time an updated collection of articles exploring poverty, poor relief, illness, and health care as they intersected in Western Europe, the Mediterranean and the Middle East, during a 'long' Middle Ages. It offers a thorough and wide-ranging investigation into the institution of the hospital and the development of medicine and charity, with focuses on the history of music therapy and the history of ideas and perceptions fundamental to psychoanalysis.

The collection is both sequel and complement to Horden's earlier volume of collected studies, *Hospitals and Healing from Antiquity to the Later Middle Ages* (2008). It will be welcomed by all those interested in the premodern history of healing and welfare for its breadth of scope and scholarly depth.

Peregrine Horden is Professor of Medieval History at Royal Holloway, University of London. He is co-author, with Nicholas Purcell, of *The Corrupting Sea* (2000) and of both its forthcoming successor and a collection of supplementary studies entitled *The Boundless Sea*. He is also writing a global history of hospitals.

VARIORUM COLLECTED STUDIES SERIES

For more information about this series, please visit: https://www.routledge.
com/history/series/VARIORUMCS

CULTURES OF HEALING

Medieval and After

Collected Studies

Peregrine Horden

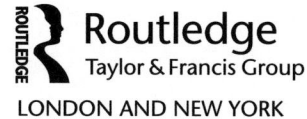

Routledge
Taylor & Francis Group

LONDON AND NEW YORK

First published 2019
by Routledge

2 Park Square, Milton Park, Abingdon, Oxfordshire OX14 4RN
52 Vanderbilt Avenue, New York, NY 10017

*Routledge is an imprint of the Taylor & Francis Group, an informa
business*

First issued in paperback 2020

British Library Cataloguing-in-Publication Data
A catalogue record for this book is available from the British
Library

Library of Congress Cataloging-in-Publication Data
Names: Horden, Peregrine, author.
Title: Cultures of healing : medieval and after / Peregrine Horden.
Description: Milton Park, Abingdon, Oxon ; New York, NY :
Routledge, 2019. |
Series: Variorum collected studies series | Includes bibliographical
references and index.
Identifiers: LCCN 2018040531 | ISBN 9781472456144 (hardback) |
ISBN 9780429023590 (e-book)
Subjects: LCSH: Medicine, Medieval. | Hospitals, Medieval.
Classification: LCC R141 .H66 2019 | DDC 610.9/02—dc23
LC record available at https://lccn.loc.gov/2018040531

ISBN: 978-1-4724-5614-4 (hbk)
ISBN: 978-0-367-66172-4 (pbk)

Typeset in Times New Roman
by codeMantra

VARIORUM COLLECTED STUDIES SERIES CS1073

CONTENTS

CONTENTS

CONTENTS

PREFACE

The studies collected here explore the domains of poverty and poor relief, and illness and health care, as they overlap or intersect in western Europe, the Mediterranean and the Middle East, during a 'long' Middle Ages. A more descriptive, if scarcely commercial, title might be: 'Healing and care of the sick and needy in the context of political, social, cultural and religious history, from Late Antiquity, through the Middle Ages, and into more recent centuries where there are topics illuminated by a medieval perspective'.

'Cultures of Healing': the 'healing' in the actual title thus has to be taken in a very broad sense. It embraces the attempted 'social healing' of charity, Jewish, Christian, and Islamic (Chapters 1–5, 8, 9, 13); the healing of body, mind, and soul variously practised by priests, doctors, and others; the auto-therapy of ordinary people with no special credentials or experience (2–7, 12, 13). The 'cultures' in the actual title stands for all the relevant contexts (political, social, and so on) in which the kinds of healing studied were embedded and in terms of which they must be understood. It is meant to evoke an open, anthropological conception of culture, not one confined to cultivated elites (e.g. 4 and 19). In many ways what I do is standard social history of charity and medicine. I have always resisted the reduction of everything to discourse or social construction, and do not think Foucault had all the answers. A recent 'turn' in the study of health and disease away from the constructivist towards the 'hard data' of ancient DNA and the like suggests that a synthesis of several different types of evidence and approach, textual and archaeological, in the history of healing remains desirable, and may even be moving from the rear- to the vanguard. That is what I have tried to practise. I am drawn to the histories of charity and medicine because both require transects through society, potentially involving every social group, every kind of subject, every type of data.

'Medieval and After': the study of both charity and medicine also can benefit from a view over the long term, whether the focus is Hippocratic medicine, the paradigm of which was not finally dissolved until well into the nineteenth century, or religious charity with its roots in the Bible or the Qur'an. Questions of continuity or discontinuity, novelty or tradition, are important and can be tackled only by trampling down chronological boundaries. That is why it is often useful for a medievalist to move later. As a historian of medicine who loves music, I ventured into the history of music therapy, which I first came across in medieval Islamic hospitals before turning to study several of its more recent forms. Doing that took me from antiquity and the Middle Ages to the sixteenth to late twentieth centuries (14–16).[1] I am emphatically not tracing some grand transition from medieval to modern, partly because I do not know what 'modernity' is, and partly because of its inherent teleology. So much theorizing of modernity implies that history is a one-way street, and a comparativist historian who looks across several centuries or periods needs to move in more than a single direction. I once strayed into the history of Freud and psychoanalysis (18), treating it as a part of the intellectual history of the last century, a culture of healing if ever there was one. But reading in that area not only joined up with topics in the history of psychotherapy that I had come to under the music therapy heading (16); it helped me approach questions prompted by evidence of early medieval monasticism (17). More generally, though I do not argue the case in what follows, I have found in psychoanalysis – with its dynamic system of invisible entities, technical rhetoric, immunity to critique and counter-example, assumed explanatory power, and crucial complicity between therapist and patient – a very helpful analogy for the successes of medieval Galenic medicine.

This collection complements and overlaps with my earlier *Hospitals and Healing from Antiquity to the Later Middle Ages* (2008). The hospital, an institution in which healing, charity, and politics meet, remains a preoccupation here, viewed both over the long term and in close-up, as I worry away at its origins and early diffusion, at the medicine that has been dispensed within it, and at its effects on the poor and sick and on society as a whole (2–5, 8, 9, 11). Other forms and sources of charity are adduced for comparison and in one case, as a contribution to the history of the medieval parish, they are given a study of their own (13). A variety of healers appear: not only learned doctors but also nurses, saints in their shrines, alchemists prolonging life, magicians (e.g. 4, 6, 12). Likewise, a variety of sources and explanations of illness or perceived abnormality, including sexual and mental abnormality: humours, demons, families, sinfulness (and the Freudian id) (4–6, 18). There is also a range of medicines, from the usual sort of drugs to soothing music and vulture's giblets (14–16, 7). The geographical focus is western Eurasia, but there are brief excursions to America (1, 16). And I plan, elsewhere, to pursue the history of 'the first hospitals', in a monograph of that title, on a global scale.[2]

I have arranged the chapters as far as possible by period covered, rather than by theme, putting fourth-century hospitals first, after an opening panorama, and ending with the recent ethnography of demons.

The old-style Variorum offered photographic reprints, the listing of addenda and corrigenda being the only means of updating. The new style of text derives from the author's computer, and that presents both temptation and challenge. The challenge is that the original computer file, assuming one can find it, never exactly matches what was eventually published. The temptation, since corrections can now be made anywhere in the text, is to start extensive rewriting – to which there might be no end. I have resisted temptation (this one at least) and not rewritten on that scale. The principle has been to respect the integrity of the original form and argument of each paper. Thus, two previously unpublished papers from a few years ago have been checked and the references have been updated, but they have not been recast (6 and 17). Three contributions, as indicated in their opening notes, have been carved out of larger originals but not otherwise fundamentally changed (1, 15, 16). Overlaps between papers, as I tackle the same problem at different times and from different angles, have not been removed: I wanted each paper to be self-sufficient. I have, however, allowed myself very minor alterations, correction of local errors, and omission of a few topical references that date a piece, and I have inserted proper notes in place of brief in-text cross-references to other parts of the volumes in which some chapters first appeared. I have not updated existing endnotes systematically (especially with such a fast-developing profession as contemporary music therapy), but I have added a few more recent references in square brackets. Where fuller discussion of the newer literature of the subject seemed called for, I have written a separate Postscript (7, 13, 15, 18). Much of the labour has focused on getting the computer file to match what is in print. But occasionally I have reversed the well-intentioned ministrations of editors and copy-editors and restored a slightly longer, slightly different original – the director's cut.

Oxford   Peregrine Horden
August 2018

Notes

1 See now also P. Horden, 'Ottomans, Neo-Ottomans and Invented Tradition in Hospital Music Therapy', in L. Clark and E. Danbury (eds), *'A Verray Parfit Praktisour': Essays presented to Carole Rawcliffe* (Woodbridge: Boydell, 2017), pp. 175–183.
2 For an analogous attempt at a global, comparative history (and anthropology) of humours, see Peregrine Horden and Elisabeth Hsu (eds), *The Body in Balance: Humoral Medicines in Practice* (New York: Berghahn, 2013).

ACKNOWLEDGEMENTS

The author and publishers wish to thank the following for permission to reprint articles in this collection:

Ashgate Publishing (5, 14, 15, 16); Bristol Classical Press (18); Cambridge University Press (4); De Gruyter Oldenbourg (8, 12); the editor of *Eikasmòs* (10, 11); Koninklijke Brill NV (19); Massachusetts Institute of Technology and the editors of the *Journal of Interdisciplinary History* (3); Oxford University Press (2, 7); Paul Watkins Publishing (Shaun Tyas) (13); Peter Lang AG, Internationaler Verlag der Wissenschaften (1, 9).

The author thanks Michael Greenwood, John Henderson, Alessandro Pastore, and John Smedley for their support, Humaira Erfan-Ahmed and Leen Van Broeck for indispensable help with the preparation the text, and Sarah Barrett for meticulous copy-editing.

The research for these articles was variously supported by All Souls College, Oxford; Royal Holloway University of London; and the Wellcome Trust.

1

THE WORLD OF THE HOSPITAL

Comparisons and continuities

I A cross-roads of hospital history?

Vienna around the year 1780.[1] Anyone with a time machine and a desire to gain some vantage point on the long-term history of hospitals, but allowed just one period and place to visit, could make a far worse choice of venue. In this city with a population of over a quarter of a million people, some 1,000 hospital beds were available for the care of the sick and needy. They were distributed across a range of institutions that varied greatly in size and services. But most exemplified a tradition of Catholic charity that would have been instantly recognisable back in the Middle Ages. Under the Church's aegis, though subsidised – inadequately – by the government, they offered shelter and nursing to poor immigrants, the homeless, the elderly, and the needy sick. There was the Bürgerspital, the oldest in the city, with 200 beds, founded in the thirteenth century. There was the Bäckenhäusel, which had been established as a lazaretto or plague house in 1656, a year in which the Viennese suffered very badly from plague. And there was the Great Poorhouse, dating from 1693. Reports of high institutional mortality, in these and a few other lesser establishments, did nothing to diminish their reputations as gateways to death. By the 1780s one-third of hospital patients were reckoned to have contracted the *morbus Viennensis*, the 'Viennese disease' of pulmonary tuberculosis.

At the more salubrious end of the spectrum, a few private institutions such as the seventy-bed Spanish hospital could attract paying middle-class patients, and a monastic hospital in the city even set aside rooms for the nobility. Nor was learned medicine lacking. Formal clinical medical instruction was already several decades old in Vienna in 1780. It had been formally instituted in 1753 by Gerard van Swieten, the Empress Maria Theresa's personal physician and a disciple of Hermann Boerhaave, whose ward round was observed by his students in Leyden's municipal hospital from the gallery of a special ward.[2] This ward was the *collegium medico-practicum*, in which lay six male and six female patients each selected for some exemplary pathological condition. In Vienna another Boerhaave student, Anton de Haen, carried out what has been famed (mistakenly) as the first such bedside teaching.[3] It took place in two rooms of six beds each in the Bürgerspital, by the eighteenth century metamorphosed into a retirement home for the elderly. This contribution to university teaching was financed by the emperor, and was part of a sweeping curricular reform designed to produce a corps of well-trained professionals who would oversee, police-like, the public health and medical needs of the Austrian masses. Though a follower of Hippocrates, and thus guided by two thousand years of tradition in his clinical observations, de Haen also developed an interest in thermometry, and many of his colleagues were engaged in research that would, within decades, contribute to the dissolution of the Hippocratic paradigm.

In 1784, not only the teaching but the whole configuration of Vienna's hospital regime changed. Having seen the fire-ravaged and decrepit Hôtel-Dieu in Paris while visiting his sister Marie Antoinette in 1777, Joseph II decided to centralise hospital care and to confine it to the sick, emulating (as he hoped) the best and avoiding the worst of the French model.[4] Poor relief was clumsily devolved to parishes and fraternities. Foreign beggars were expelled. The assets of twelve existing Viennese hospitals were 'nationalised'. The massive old alms house was turned into the two thousand-bed Allgemeines Krankenhaus or General Hospital, although it still sheltered the poor as well as providing medicine for the sick.

In accordance with Enlightenment rationalism, the general hospital was neatly divided into four medical and two surgical sections, one venereal section, and one for contagious diseases. There was a lying-in facility, a tower for the insane, and an establishment for foundlings. Some space in private rooms was reserved for patients with means. The emphasis lay on using secular medicine to help the sick recover. The hospital had a staff of some fifteen university-educated physicians, an equal number of surgeons, and 140 lay attendants. Yet even though no altars were to be seen, two resident Catholic priests toured the wards daily, administering the sacraments. By 1800, after some vicissitudes, the hospital had added its own medical library. Stables were converted into isolation wards. A surgical amphitheatre was constructed so that operations would no longer be performed on the wards; and there was a new mortuary in which physicians and senior students dissected their own deceased patients. Since 1785, there had also been a subordinate military hospital, the *Josephinum*.

Some of these reforms and developments were attributable to Johann Peter Frank, author of the *System of a Complete Medical Police*.[5] His totalitarian ambitions for the health of the masses appealed to Joseph II's 'enlightened despotism'. The emperor's successor but one, Francis II, appointed Frank director of the General Hospital in 1795, his mission being in part to combat the enormous risk of cross-infection run by patients in such a large establishment.

What first strikes the time traveller about the hospitals of late Enlightenment Vienna is their sheer variety and the range of functions that they performed, even when rationalised by despotic emperors and medical 'policemen'. The poor – whether indigenous or immigrant – the aged, the pregnant, the insane, the syphilitic are all embraced by them, alongside the acutely and chronically sick. The environment in which some attempt is made to meet their needs is an 'over-determined' one (the Freudian analogy surely permissible in this of all cities). That is, it is subject to pressures from every conceivable direction – demographic, financial, governmental, and ideological as well as medical. It has to be interpreted within the widest context of Viennese history.

Aspects of this hospital scene apparently point to the future. In the general hospital there is a clear shift from almshouse to house of the sick: the new purpose is to promote recovery rather than to offer palliative care. This hospital is no longer primarily an agent of poor relief. University-trained physicians are present, if not in proportionally very large numbers. There is a degree of secularisation: in the absence of altars, the liturgical round becomes far less prominent than the ward round.

'Fast forward' only a few decades and it is in the maternity wards of the same general hospital that, in 1848, Ignaz Semmelweiss will make the observations and deductions that herald modern – biologically effective – antisepsis. Such antisepsis is one of the essential preconditions of the hospital as we have known it in the later twentieth and early twenty-first centuries: the hospital that is accepted, and indeed preferred, as the place of treatment for serious conditions by all socio-economic groups, not only the poor. In Enlightenment Vienna, there were already better-off patients paying for privacy and superior medical attention, and their history is a good deal older than that. Frank was combating the cross-infections that would keep many away from hospital wards.

Also pointing to what we take to be modernity is the use of the wards and the autopsy room by physicians or surgeons for medical education and enquiry. We are at an early chapter – though by no means the first, as Boerhaave shows, without even looking back to the real beginnings in the Renaissance – in a story that will lead to the conception of the hospital as situated at the 'cutting edge' of medical technology and research.[6] In such a hospital, so its critics have contended, patients almost cease to be persons and become more like specimens. Removed from their normal surroundings, they can be treated in ways that ignore those surroundings precisely because the physician is now focusing on disease entities, undistracted by the 'whole person'. That reductionism, which only in relatively recent times has shown any sign of being reversed in favour of paying attention to patient 'narratives', originates in clinical education and its conceptual or physical alignment of cases that are medically, rather than socially, similar.

Such education was centuries old in Joseph II's Vienna, and is one respect in which the example of the city's hospital seems to point us back in time as well as forwards. Another respect is the emperor's desire for centralisation under governmental control. This is really a phenomenon that historians label 'early modern' or even 'Renaissance' rather than 'Enlightenment'.[7] In many ways it was old-fashioned in France when Joseph visited his sister and inspected the massive and not very salubrious Hôtel-Dieu. Large hospitals had long been seen by reformers to generate at least as much disease as they cured. In France, where the general hospitals were most numerous and prominent, their mission to house and discipline the disorderly poor actually had the effect of enhancing the medical, curative function of other smaller hospitals, to whom they passed suitable cases.

The old hospitals still functioning in Joseph II's time not surprisingly take us deepest into the past of hospital history. Here was exemplified a tradition of Catholic charity that, if a millennium younger than the Hippocratic medicine with which it could be associated, was still of considerable antiquity. The earliest of Vienna's surviving hospitals had been a part of a great wave of foundations that spread right across western Europe in the 'high' Middle Ages of the twelfth to thirteenth centuries. The lack of 'true' medical attention, the low discharge rate, and the corresponding patient mortality were always likely to be exaggerated by later 'reformers' of the sixteenth to eighteenth centuries, blackening the objects of their reform to an extent that later historians can easily accept too uncritically. The least we can say, by way of counter-argument, is that there were notable havens in which the best and most expensive of contemporary medicine was available free to patients. And it was not only in Protestant northern Europe that an emphasis on ensuring the patient a safe passage to the other world was counterbalanced by a this-worldly concern to get a sick or injured labourer quickly back to work. That aim had for example been demonstrated much earlier in some of the hospitals of Italian Renaissance cities. Still, surveying European hospitals over several centuries preceding the reign of Joseph II makes three conclusions unavoidable. First, hospitals were essentially institutions of charity in which the primary criteria of admission were as likely to be economic and social as they were to be medical. Second, secular medicine was almost always subordinate to the therapy of the sacraments in Catholic countries, or to the ethical imperatives of a godly community in Protestant ones. Finally, those who could afford to stay at home for treatment or poor relief nearly always did so. It was only when hospitals, under financial pressure, took in better-off pensioners offering lifetime security in return for benefactions that the choice between hospital and home became more evenly balanced.

II A view of the long term in hospital history

Taking Vienna c.1780 as a 'moment' in hospital history alerts us to many components in the generally accepted outlines of the subject.[8] I shall now retrace those outlines, adding some minor modifications without, I hope, distorting the received view, and giving proportionate space to the medieval

4

and early modern period instead of cantering briskly through them as a mere warm-up to 'modernity'. More substantial reservations and additions will be set out in the next section.

Hospitals were originally Christian charitable foundations for the overnight care of transients or immigrants, the local poor also lacking in the support networks that transients would have left behind, and the sick who could not pay for treatment.[9] They had, as we shall see later, a few forerunners in pagan antiquity, but they were essentially an architectural expression of the Christian charitable imperative. They began to be founded by rulers, leading churchmen, and wealthy pious individuals after the 'establishment' of the Christian Church by Constantine in the early fourth century. These *xenodocheia* (houses for strangers, as they were originally called) spread rapidly across the Byzantine empire and, more slowly, around the Mediterranean, to France, Italy, and Spain. Some, especially in major pilgrimage centres, were quite large. Some, again in the largest cities, were highly 'medicalised' in that they had wards for specific diseases or conditions, and physicians and surgeons on their staff. Others specialised in the care of the poor, the elderly, the blind, and so on.

In general, early medieval hospitals increase in size and complexity, and probably also in numbers, as one traverses Eurasia in an easterly direction. Thus western European hospitals were, on the whole, more hospice-like, offering the ultimate therapy of the sacraments, less intent on returning patients to the community than in easing chronic need and the effects of aging – or of leprosy. The biggest Byzantine hospitals displayed a more obvious emphasis on secular medicine. When the 'hospital idea' was exported from Byzantium to Islam, primarily through the intermediary of Christian communities in Islamic lands, in the ninth and tenth centuries, hospitals attained what it is tempting to conceive as a new stage in their development. Islamic hospitals were not so overwhelmingly charitable, catering more prominently for well-to-do patients. They offered medical treatment by court physicians. They were, indeed, centres of medical learning and teaching. And many of them introduced a relatively novel element: they housed the insane – treating them perhaps harshly, but in a medical manner, as sick rather than possessed.

The hospital spread eastwards, across Asia, principally with Islam (as did Islamic medicine) rather than with Christian missionaries. Thus one major chapter in hospital history is the story of Islamic foundations, a story that stretches with few interruptions from tenth-century Baghdad to parts of India and Sri Lanka in the present day. But the next major phase of European hospital history begins in the twelfth century.[10] In Byzantine Constantinople, medicalisation seemingly reached its apogee in the Pantocrator hospital (attached to a monastery) in which there were almost more physicians and support staff than patients. In the Crusader states the Knights Hospitaller's hospital of St John in Jerusalem stands out as, by western standards, a medically intensive establishment, and as one which showed its charitable ethos in a pronounced and individual way, by proclaiming the 'Lordship of the Poor' – whom the Knights of St John were to serve as if the poor underlings were really their 'feudal' superiors.[11] More generally, across the Crusaders' home territories in western Europe, hospitals were founded for the poor and, among the sick, especially for the leprous. Yet this was not because paupers and lepers were becoming proportionately more numerous, but because the prayers of such unfortunates were increasingly recognised as a sure means of helping donors' souls through purgatorial fire. The Catholic doctrine of purgatory may not have solidified until the thirteenth century, but its ingredients were already clearly recognised long before.

In parts of northern Europe, the wave of foundations that began in the twelfth century had lost impetus by the time of the Black Death. Fewer hospitals were founded. In England, for example, the almshouse, with its distinct if conjoined dwellings for the respectable elderly, became the favoured type of foundation. Many existing hospitals also mutated into retirement homes, into chantries (offering liturgy rather than charity), or into colleges of priests.

Naturally there were exceptions to this general picture, mostly to be found in the larger cities. Paris, with its Hôtel-Dieu, is one of them. No medieval English hospital could measure up to its size or the number of its medical personnel. The main contrast to the northern pattern is, however, to be found in southern Europe, to some extent in Spain,[12] but especially in the Italian city-states of the later Middle Ages and Renaissance. The hospitals of Renaissance Florence in the fifteenth and sixteenth centuries were, for example, widely admired and often the objects of emulation, as in the case of Santa Maria Nuova, which became the model for the Savoy Hospital in London. In their combination of a continuing religious ethos – altars in view of the patients, the literal centrality of the sacraments to daily life – with lay, sometimes civic, control, they show how difficult it is to carve hospital history up into periods. For they straddle the end of the Middle Ages and the beginnings of the early modern period. And, right back in the fourteenth century, they already anticipate what are usually taken to be early modern features of hospitals in major cities: lay control, centralisation, learned physicians in attendance, pharmacies attached, rapid turnover of patients (no gateways to death here, although women patients did stay for longer than men). It is in Italy too that we encounter the first specialised hospitals in Europe to have been founded in any numbers since the *leprosaria* of the twelfth and thirteenth centuries: large foundling hospitals like the famous Innocenti in Florence and, later, hospitals for victims of the era's two greatest scourges, plague and the Great Pox.[13]

A degree of continuity across the supposed medieval/early modern divide is evident not only in Catholic Europe but even in England. The dissolution of almost all hospitals at the Henrician Reformation, as well as monasteries, obviously marked a break in hospital history. But many hospitals were quite rapidly refounded and new ones added – not just in London (as is commonly observed), but in provincial cities such as Norwich.[14] These hospitals of the later sixteenth century broke with English traditions only in one respect, which aligns them more with their continental coevals. They, or the bigger ones at least, had attendant physicians; they were attuned to ideas about the potential of hospitals that had been aired in Italy over two centuries previously.

As we move closer in time to the Viennese example with which we began, we return to developments already sketched. The French model has usually been taken as defining the next distinct phase. In this, a division arose. On the one hand, there were the general hospitals that provided some medical care, but served primarily as catch-all establishments for the supposed work-shy, vagrants, gypsies, religious dissidents, prostitutes, beggars, the disabled, and the insane. On the other hand, there were the older *hôtels-Dieu* that, with the aforementioned social groups interned elsewhere, could concentrate more on acute and curable sickness.[15] But it should be remembered that the *hôpital général* was not peculiar to France. It was in some respects an elaboration of that English sixteenth-century invention and export, the workhouse. Further, the apparently clear distinction between it and the *hôtel-Dieu* is muddied by all the other kinds of hospital that continued to develop alongside them, in France and elsewhere in Europe. These included lying-in hospitals, hostels for vagabonds, houses for the reform of prostitutes, 'conservatories' for the moral education of orphans, and, not least, the military hospital, 'a kind of laboratory for experimentation in medical services within a hospital setting'.[16]

At the opposite extreme from the governmental schemes manifested in large general hospitals, we find the 'voluntary hospitals'. These establishments began to appear in England in the 1720s, and are often treated as another distinct chapter in hospital history. They are projected against a background from which hospitals had mostly disappeared, which makes them seem a novel departure. And they are presented as peculiarly English when in fact they had continental counterparts or imitations, in Germany, Switzerland, and elsewhere. Seen in the *longue durée* of hospital history their peculiarity is less in the fact that they were, at least to begin with, controlled by their leading (financially most beneficent) 'voluntary' subscribers than in the particular way in which this control was exercised. Hospital benefactors had been determining the nature of institutions to which they lent their support since the earliest Christian foundations of the fourth century. They had set the criteria of admission in generic terms, and doubtless exercised influence over the selection of individual patients on occasion. What was new in the eighteenth century was the regularising of this connection between patron and patient, such that the purchase of a subscription at a particular level brought corresponding privileges in the nomination of inmates.[17]

Power to the patrons is one strident theme in hospital history of the eighteenth century – and many preceding centuries. The equivalent for the nineteenth century and since is conventionally: power to the physicians, and to the surgeons; and then power to the professional administrators. The centuries do not divide neatly, of course; and developments since the late eighteenth century are so many and various that they defeat all brief generalisation. The two largest and clearest phenomena of the nineteenth and early twentieth centuries are surely these. First, the enormous expansion of patient demand for hospital services (crudely estimated as a tenfold increase across the nineteenth century in Britain)[18] and the concomitant increase in the number of hospital beds (over fourfold in England and Wales between 1861 and 1938).[19] Second, the growing status of hospital medicine and surgery, such that by about 1920 they had achieved the dominance that we take to be the defining feature of the modern hospital. General hospitals consumed more resources and offered a greater range of services than any other type of health care provider. So it was c.1800–c.1920, so it has been ever since.[20]

To elaborate only on the second phenomenon: from the later eighteenth century, doctors on the whole supplanted governors in the determination of hospital admissions, staff appointments, and overall policy. For the first time in history, hospital medicine was different in kind from non-hospital medicine, and not just a simplified, cheaper, version of a medical 'vernacular'. New techniques and instruments – the electro-cardiograph in the nineteenth century, the iron lung and dialysis machine in the twentieth – were either developed in hospitals or were used in them as nowhere else. The medicine with which they were involved was based conceptually in pathological anatomy – as revealed in the post mortem and refined in the hospital laboratory. With effective antisepsis and anaesthesia, the hospital became by the early twentieth century the almost exclusive locus of surgery too. The criteria for admission were now chiefly medical rather than socioeconomic. In England, as the Poor Law hospitals of the later nineteenth century removed pauper patients from the voluntary hospitals, so the latter became far more acceptable to paying patients than they had ever been before – either middle-class fee-payers or the working poor who contributed to some insurance scheme. Design was changing too – the pavilion style advocated by Florence Nightingale being adopted in response to concerns about the hospital environment and the need for fresh air and cleanliness. (Such concerns were hardly new and clearly affected hospital architecture in, for instance, Renaissance Florence, but on the basis of a very different – humoral – medical theory.) Reference to Nightingale is a reminder, if any were needed, to add to the overall picture the changing image of the hospital nurse between 1830 and c.1918 – from *relatively* unskilled carer to respectable educated professional – even though the image does a serious injustice to the longer-term background of women in nursing orders who provided hospital food and basic medication and surgery in eighteenth-century France,[21] not to mention earlier generations of women who had been dispensing remedies in hospitals since the Middle Ages.[22]

Enhanced specialisation is the final major feature of nineteenth to twentieth century hospitals to be noted: hospitals for teaching; eye, skin, and fever hospitals; and above all that characteristically nineteenth-century phenomenon, the lunatic asylum. The insane had a long if patchy history of being admitted to general hospitals in Europe since the later Middle Ages (earlier in some places, especially in Islamic lands, but even in the late antique Mediterranean world).[23] Small private asylums proliferated in the second half of the eighteenth century, but the large, dedicated asylum and the whole social and legal culture of 'asylumdom' is a nineteenth-century development lasting until the decarceration movement of the 1960s. By the mid-nineteenth century, in parallel to the centrality of the hospital to general medicine, 'the asylum was endorsed as the sole, officially approved response to the problems posed by mental illness'.[24]

Perhaps the most recent phase to date in hospital history should be assigned a beginning in the 1960s. What distinguishes the twentieth century may prove to be less the formation of the British National Health Service or the elaboration of national or individual insurance schemes in other countries, but the sharply rising costs of the capital- and technology-intensive hospital medicine, of which such schemes are only particular expressions. The critique of hospitals that emerged in the 1960s and that has continued to be voiced in the twenty-first century seemingly marks the end of a relatively brief, quite positive, phase in hospital history. There had been 'anti-hospital' movements before, in later medieval England perhaps, as patrons favoured other types of foundation, and at the close of the late eighteenth century for example;[25] and the hospital had often (although not nearly as often as modern historians used to maintain) been stigmatised as a locus of pauperism, infection, and death. Yet it has experienced no downturn in its general reputation quite as dramatic as that registered by the biomedical 'high-tech' hospital in the later twentieth century. After many decades of growing popularity, hospitals are now a focus of those anxieties about bureaucratic, corporate modern medicine, its costs and allegedly skewed priorities, and the nosocomial infections that it passes to those whom it should be curing – anxieties that enhance the attraction of alternative therapies. Hospitals are likely victims of further cost-reducing decentralisation: the devolving of services to outpatient clinics and primary health care providers. It is not hard to foresee a time when the power and cheapness of computer-run medical technology could nullify the economies of scale and concentration that have been the rationale for hospitals' existence since the time of Joseph II, if not from the very beginning. As the late Roy Porter wrote in one of his last books:

> Whether, for its part, the general medicine of the future needs, or can afford, the ever-expanding hospital complex remains unclear. Today's huge general hospitals may soon seem medicine's dinosaurs. Will they go the way of the lunatic asylums?[26]

III Minding the gaps

Such is one possible view of the long term in hospital history, from the fourth century to the twenty-first. It adds a few local twists and comments of its own, but essentially is meant to convey a broadly uncontroversial narrative. It is, of course, nevertheless seriously deficient, and not just in the ways that inevitably attend summaries of over 1,500 years of history in a few paragraphs.

Some of the deficiencies are glaring. First, the story has been mainly European. I have not so far mentioned hospitals in North America.[27] The earliest such hospital is the Pennsylvania Hospital (1751), followed by the New York Hospital (1791) and then, after a pause, the Massachusetts General (1821). These were modelled on the English voluntary hospitals, and, in simplified outline, the story of American hospitals is that of European hospitals – telescoped in the initial stages, varied in subsequent ones, but still overall clearly recognisable. The wealthy physicians who specialised in diseases of the rich nonetheless used poor patients to burnish their expertise, and these patients lay in the hospitals philanthropically financed by the physicians' rich patients.

The multiplication of institutions that in Europe began in the twelfth century came late to North America even when allowance is made for its having started only in 1751. A survey of 1873 revealed no more than 120 general hospitals in the entire country. The Civil War, with its one million hospital cases in the North alone, seemingly produced no major lasting changes to hospital provision. At the end of the war the military hospitals were closed and most of the soldiers still needing treatment were packed off to their families. It required the unprecedented immigration, urbanisation, and industrialisation of the century's closing decades to produce a significant expansion of hospital establishment. By 1909 there were over 4,300 hospitals with 420,000 beds, but it had been only relatively recently (after *c.*1880) that middle-class patients could be enticed to occupy any of them.

There is obviously much more to American hospital history – and not only since 1900. In keeping with the Eurocentricity of most hospital history written in English, America is so far only North America, and only since 1751. Yet there is wider history, both earlier and contemporary, that remains to be written in detail: colonial hospitals, exported from Old Spain to New Spain, for instance, as instruments of attempted control, conversion, acculturation, the containment of epidemics – and even medical experimentation.[28] There was a hospital on the Spanish Caribbean island of Santo Domingo from the very early sixteenth century, and one opened in what would become Mexico City soon after the subjugation of the Aztecs. It was followed in the 1530s by the first establishment exclusively for indigenous people. By the beginning of the seventeenth century there were some 128 hospitals in New Spain. Later that century, in New France, supposedly even the rich settlers availed themselves of hospital services.

This colonial hospital history of course extends to Asia and, later, Africa.[29] In Asia it again begins in the early sixteenth century. The Portuguese founded a hospital in Goa – for their own soldiers and seamen – soon after the creation of the colony in 1510. In the comparatively brief period during which Japan was open to foreigners, 1549–1639, the Portuguese were responsible for the first western-style hospital at the other end of Asia.[30] Such a history is but one aspect of the 'globalisation' of the hospital, the earlier phases of which were outlined above. Filling out the picture in this way does not go far enough, however. The narrative presented in section II above was not only European. It was also Christian. It takes the beginnings of Christian hospitals in the fourth century CE as the beginnings of hospital history *tout court*. That does some injustice to the various settings in which historians of the ancient world have, mostly without convincing result, tried to detect the pagan equivalent of the Christian hospital: in the courtyards of healing shrines in which the sick camped out for days at a time hoping for a therapeutic dream; in doctors' private clinics; and, above all, in the *valetudinaria* (literally, recovery homes; seldom medicalised; and few in number) in which some sick or injured soldiers and slaves were for a short time, during the 'high' Roman Empire, nursed back to health.[31]

Beginning – as we did – with Christianity may do another, and perhaps greater, injustice to the Jewish contribution. Jewish hospitals are first clearly attested in the sixth century CE. But both their medical development and the extent to which they inspired or imitated Christian hospitals remains unclear. It may be that, within synagogue complexes, a room or rooms had been set aside, hospital-like, for lodging transients a long time before the sixth century. And there was at least one first-century CE hospital-cum-guesthouse to cope with the great influx to the Jerusalem Temple. The history of the Jewish hospital deserves to be rescued from the margins and set alongside that of, on the one hand, the Christian hospital and, on the other, the mutation of the clearly Christian-inspired hospital idea characteristic of hospital founders in Islam.

Three religions of Abraham; three intertwined histories of hospital 'diasporas'. Even recognising that does not take us quite far enough. Hinduism, Buddhism, and Jainism each have their hospital histories – charitable in emphasis, and to that extent rather like the Judaeo-Christian type; but in the case of Jainism also producing the unusual feature (unusual in pre-modern times) of the hospital for sick animals.

This wider history of Asian hospitals brings out interesting, though presumably coincidental, similarities between East and West. It is not just that the groups to whom hospital charity is extended are similar – the sick poor, those unable to work, widows, orphans and so on. Chronological parallels are also detectable. In the early fifth century CE, for example, a Chinese Buddhist pilgrim touring India recorded:

> The cities and towns of this country are the greatest of all in the Middle Kingdom. The inhabitants are rich and prosperous, and vie with one another in the practice of benevolence and righteousness [...] The heads of the Vaiśya [merchant] families in them [all the kingdoms of north India] establish in the cities houses for dispensing charity and medicine. All the poor and destitute in the country, orphans, widowers, and childless men, maimed people and cripples, and all who are diseased, go to those houses, and are provided with every kind of help, and doctors examine their diseases. They get the food and medicines which their cases require, and are made to feel at ease; and when they are better, they go away of themselves.[32]

This has been called an account of a 'civic hospital system'.[33] It may not quite be that, but it prompts interesting comparisons with the hospitals contemporaneously being founded in the Byzantine empire.

The Middle Ages reveal other parallels. The medieval wave of European foundations beginning in the twelfth century is echoed in the government-sponsored poorhouses and hospitals being set up in northern Sung China.[34] A little later, at the time this western wave was cresting, around 1200 CE Jayarvarman VII of the Cambodian kingdom of Angkor was founding or restoring 102 hospitals across his kingdom. Some details of their intended organisation can be derived from inscriptions, for instance the stele of Say-feng, close to Vientiane in Laos, and among the northernmost points of the Angkorian kingdom. To quote an authoritative summary:

> The text of this inscription mentions the persons employed by the hospital: nursing staff and servants. The hospital is open to the four castes. Two doctors are to attend to each caste; they are assisted by a man and two women 'with a right to lodging'. The personnel also includes: 'two dispensers responsible for the distribution of remedies, receiving the measures of rice. Two cooks, with a right to fuel and water, who have to tend the flowers and the lawn, and to clean the temple [...] fourteen hospital warders, entrusted with the administration of the remedies [...] two women to grind the rice.' As the hospital is a religious foundation, 'two sacrificers and one astrologer, all three pious, are to be named by the Superior of the royal monastery. Every year each of them shall be provided

with the following: three coats and three lengths of cloth, fifteen pairs of garments, three pewter vases.' In addition they were to receive paddy, wax and pepper. The sick are to be fed with 'the rice forming part of the oblation to the deities [fixed] at one bushel a day' and with the remains of the sacrifices. The text next gives a long list of the medicaments placed by the king at the disposition of the sick: honey, sesame, clarified butter, a mixture of pepper, cumin and rottleria tinctoria, musk, asafoetida, camphor, sugar, 'aquatic animals', turpentine, sandalwood, coriander, cardamum, ginger, kakola, origano, mustard seed, senna, curcuma aromatica of two kinds etc.[35]

To mention only one other, final, example: in nineteenth to twenty-first century India, hospitals dispensing either Ayurvedic medicine, or *Unani tibb* – the 'Greek medicine' brought to India by Islam – have been erected, if not alongside, then not far from those dispensing western biomedicine.[36] Of course, the different medical systems have not remained uncontaminated by one another; in particular, Ayurveda and *Unani tibb* have accommodated aspects of their therapeutics to biomedicine. But the globalising of biomedicine has hardly produced a uniformly modern medical landscape, whether in hospitals or in medicine generally.

IV Against grand narrative

Hospital history is large and complicated – far more so than conventional Christocentric, Eurocentric accounts suggest. Not surprisingly, historians who seek an Olympian view try to divide this history up into phases or stages; I have done the same in the opening sections.

Several classifications are currently on offer, all essentially similar. Back in 1936 Henry Sigerist sensibly divided hospital history into three broad stages.[37] The first saw the institutional care of the sick arising in the medical facilities incidentally offered by poor houses, guest houses and (implausible as it now seems) prisons. The second stage began in the thirteenth century, when hospitals emerged as medical institutions for the indigent and dependent. The third, and so far final, stage began in the mid-nineteenth century when the 'progress of medicine and surgery' induced the emergence of the modern hospital – the hospital that we, in the 2000s, know and (sometimes) love.

Much more recently than Sigerist, Guenter Risse, who in a very helpful monograph favours a series of case studies over a continuous narrative, nonetheless essays a summary typology.[38] Overall he sees hospitals as symbols of community, deliverers of social welfare, and mechanisms for coping with suffering, illness, and death. The hospital is first, originally, a 'house of mercy'; then in the later Middle Ages (also the start of Sigerist's phase two) a 'house of segregation'; then in the Renaissance a 'house of rehabilitation'. In the eighteenth century the hospital becomes a 'house of care', as doctors come to dominate (in ways sketched above). From the 1880s it is a 'house of surgery', because of antisepsis, and for the first time it is used on a significant scale by the middle classes. For the last century or so, it has been a 'house of science'.

Risse's typology is elegant and memorable – and subtly qualified in all the appropriate ways. It may be preferable to proceeding by conventional historical periods (medieval, early modern, Enlightenment, and so on); as does Lindsay Granshaw, whose final division and longest section in her excellent survey article is, however, somewhat crudely, 'early modern and modern'.[39] But the problem with all these various ways of dividing up the hospital's past is not their artificiality or over-simplicity. All chronological schemes over-simplify, and are to be judged only by the heuristic value of the generalisations that result from them. The problem, rather, is in the way that the particular historiographical schemes that hospitals have attracted are all skewed towards a modernity defined by medicalisation. The background assumption is that true hospitals are medicalised – with medicalisation defined basically in terms of the presence of doctors and surgeons and, at a more sophisticated level, of the degree of authority that they wield, over the patients and over the institution as a whole. For Sigerist, that process began in the thirteenth century. For Risse, as for many others, it belongs above all to the nineteenth century and since. Whatever its particular inflection, the underlying idea is that there has been a great 'before' and 'after' in hospital history; some pivotal period in which charity gives way to medicine, care to cure, stigma to pride, the mortuary to the recovery room, the poor to the middle classes.

Why do we tend to think like this? Why do we look so persistently for the 'genesis of the modern', assessing over 1,500 years of hospital history on a yardstick calibrated for the last two centuries? The economic history of Europe since antiquity is not (or not usually) conceived solely as a search for the origins of industrial capitalism, nor the history of transport as a frustratingly long build-up to the railway and the steamship. Yet the historiography of hospitals is more often than not written with an eye on the present, or at least on the modern. Sometimes this is an effect of the rhetoric of hospital reformers over the past two centuries: reformers have tended to exaggerate the difference of 'before' from 'after', as if they are always engaged in dragging their particular hospitals from medieval darkness into modern light.

Historians have occasionally been seduced by this rhetoric from the past. But they have also generated theories of their own. The sociologist Nicholas Jewson strikingly identified the 'disappearance of the sick man' (and woman) in hospitals around the turn of the nineteenth century. A system of hospital medicine founded in a holistic view of the individual patient and his or her environment gave way to a reductive clinical emphasis on diseased parts; the individual person was disregarded (an accusation normally reserved for, and perhaps unduly influenced by, later twentieth-century medicine).[40]

The most famous proponent of a 'big bang' theory of the origins of the modern hospital is of course Michel Foucault. His identification of the French Revolution as the brief but explosive period of 'the birth of the clinic' has proved so influential that historians have to continue rehearsing it even though few of them now accept it. Indeed, his account perhaps continues to enjoy currency precisely because it offers a clear theory to attack so that a more 'smoothed out' view of hospital medicine in the eighteenth and early nineteenth centuries can be substituted without having to arrive at some alternative conception of the period. This 'smoother' historiography finds medicalisation (when it happened at all) to have been a far more complex phenomenon than Foucauldians have alleged, yielding perhaps surprising agents of change:

> Probably the most medical process in [French] hospitals in the seventeenth century was the diffusing of nursing communities. Far from such women being – as is often simplistically alleged – the bearers of a religiously inspired anti-medicine, careful study of the contracts they passed with hospitals reveals nursing communities as a prime agent of hospital medicalization.[41]

Or again:

> to a considerable extent, we may see in military hospitals one of the prime sites in which the hospital patient qua patient was constructed over the eighteenth century, long in advance of the 'birth of the clinic' in the 1790s. Their overtly functional orientation made it more likely that their inmates were more truly sick than might be the case in civilian hospitals.[42]

The modern medicalisation of the hospital – however we define 'modernity' and 'medicalisation' – is undeniably important. But it does not have to skew the overall history of hospitals – an outline into which specialists insert their particular contributions – to quite the extent that it mostly has up to now. It may be that, for the first millennium of its history, indeed for longer than that, the modal hospital – the commonest form of hospital – was charitable, funded for the poor and offering the therapy of religion, a regulated environment, and a proper diet, rather than the attentions of secular physicians. That first millennium must be viewed in its own light, rather than that cast by the period since 1900.

Alongside the modal European hospital, we must also place others that make up the rest of the global population. The modal hospital of the early

Byzantine empire was grounded in the therapy of the sacraments, even though right from the documented beginning of Byzantine hospitals some foundations had doctors attached. The modal Islamic hospital of say the eleventh century, like the modal Cambodian hospital of the twelfth, was on the other hand highly medicalised, to judge simply by medical manpower. Considering Renaissance Florence, the highly medicalised, seemingly modern, though still essentially religious, Santa Maria Nuova may distort our overall picture. But the modal Florentine hospital of the fifteenth century remained what it had been in the twelfth – small, without medical staff, and providing overnight accommodation to pilgrims and poor travellers rather than treating large numbers of sick people.

As we move later in period so the mode becomes more elusive. We saw at the start, with the example of Josephine Vienna, and later when we returned to the Enlightenment in England and France, that towards 1800 the hospital population was still extremely diverse, old and novel elements kaleidoscopically interconnected. And the twentieth century? It might seem obvious that the modal hospital has been the one at the forefront of medical technology and intervention. But that may be true only on a circular definition – that all genuine hospitals are medicalised to that degree. If we add to the list of hospital types the hospices for palliative care of the terminally ill that have multiplied since the 1970s, and other similar institutions that would have been counted as hospitals in any period before c.1800, then the mode may not be so certain. Abandon the outright privileging of western biomedicine; add in the global 'population' of famine relief centres, Ayurvedic hospitals, private hospitals owned and run by individual physicians (as in twentieth-century Japan), small temporary clinics offering only basic medication, leper sanctuaries – and the most common form of hospital in the world since 1900 may not be the technological showcase we thought it was.

V Hospital historiography

Of the making of hospital histories there is no end. The modal study has been to a great extent local, institutional, somewhat introspective, perhaps celebratory – a story of physicians and local activists, of progress. Yet since the 1970s a 'new' hospital historiography has also developed. It is comparative (not looking at just one institution at a time) and in the broadest sense sociological or contextual. That is, it studies hospitals in their social, cultural, and religious as well as their medical setting, recognising that there is always much more to a hospital than its doctors.

An excellent sample of this more recent approach – now not so new, of course, but still not the numerically dominant form of historical writing on the subject – is the collection edited by Lindsay Granshaw and Roy Porter, *The Hospital in History* (1989).[43] Theirs is a volume of enormous chronological scope, ranging from about 1100 to 1980. And, although six of its ten chapters deal with Britain, there are papers covering Italy, Germany, and the USA. The volume decisively breaks the traditional paradigm of hospital history written as if from the doctor's point of view. It offers a much more inclusive interpretation of the hospital in society based on an admirably broad variety of source material, not least visual evidence.[44] The functions of the hospital are shown to change over time, and an unprecedentedly wide range of institutions is considered, including children's hospitals. The volume also places a new emphasis on the vital relationship between hospitals, their founders and patrons, and the wider socio-political context, thus providing a valuable tool for reinterpreting the narrow, institutional vision of the hospital in history. The experience of patients before, during, and even after hospitalisation is brought into the picture. Another advance is to produce a more nuanced conception of the relationship between hospitals and their staff of administrators and nurses.

And yet, for all its sophistication, in the background of most of the contributions to Granshaw and Porter can be detected the Foucauldian master narrative of hospital history – a narrative predicated on the centrality to hospital history of the presence or absence of doctors and focused on the question of when they appeared on the scene so as to inaugurate modernity.[45] The overall trend of identifying some great transition from care to cure was, for the contributors to this volume, contradicted only by the history of cancer hospices. They were the exception proving the rule (even though some cancer hospices prescribe not only palliative treatment but also therapy based on pain relief).[46]

Since the publication of the Granshaw–Porter volume in 1989, there has, predictably, been a cascade of studies in hospital history. The catalogue of the Wellcome Library, to look no further, records a continuous and ample stream of publications in English alone. Many of these are substantial contributions, but they are still often chronologically restricted; others are local and introspective in scope and celebratory in tone;[47] others continue to chew over old debates.[48] Few collections in English have rivalled Granshaw and Porter in breadth.[49]

In what follows, rather than attempt to report comprehensively on this massive yet, on the whole, fragmented literature, I shall try to assess some broad trends in the historiography of the 2000s.[50]

VI The impact of hospitals

In contrast to the approach of Granshaw and Porter, there should be a deliberate decision to get away from medicalisation as the leitmotif. Instead we can expand their liberating multi-disciplinary perspective still further – to convey some of the most recent and innovative approaches in the wider field of the social history of medicine, not privileging any one aspect or period, so as to arrive at a rounded view of the hospital in society. Medicine and doctors certainly will appear, but as only one facet of changing varieties of therapy rather than as the defining moment in the arrival of modernity. Indeed the hospital's health-promoting role is seen within a much wider context than that of doctors, whether in relation to physicians of the soul (priests) or singers of the liturgy or the nursing staff or, more broadly, to the built and natural environments as stimulants to recovery.[51] Eric Gruber von Arni's discussion of the two major military hospitals for sick and maimed soldiers in seventeenth-century London, the Savoy and Ely House, serves as a good example of what conventional accounts of medicalisation so often downplay.[52] Emphasis was placed on increasing patients' mobility, with (for example) special wooden limbs being made. Ely House had a 'hot house' for sweating 'pox' patients with mercury, and sufferers were also sent to Bath for spa-water treatment. Considerable attention was paid to the environment in each hospital so that wards were frequently fumigated with burning pitch, even though patients must have suffered from inadequate ventilation.

To avoid the teleology of looking for precocious signs of modernity, we must consider the hospital over the long term. But we must also range widely in space. Although I have in earlier sections of this introduction sketched a world-wide history of hospitals, the main focus has remained Mediterranean or European and is indeed envisaged as complementary to Mark Harrison's collection on 'the hospital beyond the west'. This adds the much-needed African and Asian dimensions to the subject.[53]

One of the themes to emerge from recent research is the range of institutions which called themselves 'hospital', whether for the sick poor or for other disadvantaged groups, from pilgrims to foundlings and sick children to abandoned women or the insane. (The last of these are not considered here but have their own mature historiography.)[54] Moreover, within the broad categories that recur, we find an enormous variety of function – from isolation to control, from treating the curable to comforting the incurable, from providing education[55] to returning patients to the community so that they could continue to make a useful contribution to society.

A related theme, already encountered in our opening historical sketch, is specialisation, as prominent during the Middle Ages and Renaissance as it is today. Thus Max Satchell has discussed rural *leprosaria* in medieval England and Flurin Condrau has looked at sanatoria for TB patients in Germany and Italy.[56] These papers are part of a wider recent trend to examine specialised institutions, not only *leprosaria* and military establishments but isolation hospitals (*lazzaretti* for plague victims, and the new hospitals which emerged in the sixteenth century in response to that other 'new' disease, the Great Pox).[57] Hospitals set up to cope with the epidemics of more recent times, such as polio and AIDS, also belong in this tradition. Indeed, each new epidemic underlines the broad institutional continuity of society's response, a main plank of which remains the isolation hospital, whether during the outbreak of plague in India in the mid-1990s or during the SARS epidemic in 2003.

Specialisation of function relates to another theme of recent historiography, the centralisation of resources and the development of 'systems' of care, whether (as we saw above) in Renaissance Italy or late eighteenth-century Vienna or in the move towards municipal medicine in Britain during the 1920s and 1930s and the foundation of the National Health Service after the Second World War.[58] The process whereby the political élite gradually took over the direction of hospitals was common to most European cities, but was even more pronounced in sixteenth-century Italy as an outcome of the gradual exclusion of the aristocracy from the governance of the state.[59] As for France, analysis of the social background of hospital rectors has shown that, in the minor centres, they were drawn from groups of leading citizens, while in major cities they were nobles.[60] It would, however, be a mistake to assume too monolithic a power structure. In his study of the *Hôtel-Dieu* in Beaune in the seventeenth century, Kevin Robbins shows how the administrative staff and nursing sisters mounted a spirited defence of the 'public honesty' of the hospital against the patronal family of the de Pernes, who had wanted to use their institution as a hotel.[61]

Centralisation had its limits at the 'macro' level too. Just as Foucault's 'birth of the clinic' is no longer identifiable in the way he suggested, so it is now generally accepted that his related thesis of the early modern state's power over charitable institutions, and in particular of its 'great confinement' of the poor in the seventeenth century, is to say the least exaggerated. The mechanisms through which charities and their inmates might be controlled were far more flexible.[62] Furthermore, the charitable and religious institutions of the Counter-Reformation were – as Brian Pullan has shown – separated from the world to help to convert the sick, the poor, prostitutes, and Jews to a life of salvation and virtue.[63] Indeed, it has been argued that 'spiritual salvation' was the main objective in the hospitalisation of such patients – a perspective to be set against Foucault's emphasis on the dangers of poverty and the insanitary conditions of the early modern city.[64]

Moral discipline was a more subtle form of the exercise of power over the bodies and souls of patients. It represented a means of enforcing religious conformity and a moral way of life that one finds equally in the hospitals of Elizabethan London, in Friuli, and in areas under the influence of the Ottoman empire.[65] This was the same kind of intrusive surveillance, as Nathan Wachtel has outlined, that penetrated into the cells of the prisons of the Inquisition, recording secretly and efficiently the glances, words, gestures, and the actions of the inmates.[66] From the political and moral standpoint, discipline was justified by reference to the campaign against licence, vice, disorder, and the desire for change that supposedly characterised the insolent masses. They were seen as contaminating, infecting, and offending the dignity and decorum of the city, since they did not observe rules and laws. They represented a danger to social stability and were therefore 'la plus dangereuse peste des Etats'.[67]

Government policy, then, as in other places and times, originated in a set of more or less noble motives, ranging from a desire to protect hospitals from impoverishment to exploitation of their resources to using them as a means to control the poor and sick when they were seen as threats to public order and health. And if institutional patrons in the shape of governments had mixed motivations, so did individual patrons seeking to establish and maintain hospitals. At the very centre of a number of the more recent studies dealing with earlier periods is the theology of almsgiving, which links the provision of charity with salvation. This was clearly the case in Byzantium, where the major 'monastic multiplex' in Constantinople was founded principally for the commemoration of the soul of the emperor. Indeed, so concerned with commemoration were medieval patrons that hospital statutes frequently gave more space to the details of masses than to the treatment of inmates. Carole Rawcliffe has argued that in late medieval England the larger hospitals were transformed into liturgical spaces for the Christian departed. Kevin Robbins also shows how the founder of the great hospital of Beaune, Chancellor Rolin, made sure that he continued to control his institution from the grave. He laid down that his coats-of-arms should be visible on all the buildings as a constant reminder of his presence and patronage. As for Italy, Matthew Sneider demonstrates that a significant proportion of the expenditure of the four most affluent hospitals of Bologna was devoted to commemorative masses and other religious activities.[68]

The role of religion in hospitals in medieval and early modern Europe went far beyond the provision of masses. The aim of the hospital was to cure the soul of the patient and not just the body. Indeed, the vital role of religion in the treatment of the sick has been underlined by a series of major studies, not least the books by Carole Rawcliffe on the hospitals of late medieval Norwich and John Henderson on the Renaissance hospitals of Florence.[69] Rawcliffe demonstrates the fundamental role of images in healing, from altarpieces to stained-glass windows and sculpture, stressing how the commissioning of major works such as Roger van der Weiden's *Last Judgement* or the Isenheim Altarpiece played a fundamental role not simply in commemorating the patron but also in the hospital's everyday life.[70]

Splendid altarpieces and sculptural or fresco cycles in hospital churches and wards, as well as important collections of relics, performed an essential role in promoting the profile of the hospital and thereby encouraging almsgiving. Indeed, the maintenance of a constant income was vital for the flourishing of any hospital. As we noted above, Georgian England saw a flowering of hospitals and infirmaries for the sick poor supported by voluntary subscriptions. By 1800 there were thirty general infirmaries outside London and seven in the capital. In the following century, London became the centre of a hospital boom generated by the growth of medical schools: by 1850 there were forty-five hospitals with 26,000 beds.

Such initiatives were clearly expensive. One way to finance them adopted in eighteenth-century England was to distribute to potential subscribers prints 'proper to shew to Gentlemen': prints of, for example, St Bartholomew's re-building programme under James Gibbs or the elevations and plans of St George's in London. Great Ormond Street was also a voluntary hospital, and its founder, the physician Charles West, mounted a sizeable campaign to raise cash. It is significant that at this time there were no children's hospitals in Britain, partly because the medical establishment opposed children's hospitals for fear of competition, and partly because physicians did not take children's ailments seriously. West therefore involved important people on the hospital's Board. They included Charles Dickens, who had done so much to raise contemporary awareness of the plight of poor children, and Queen Victoria herself, who was persuaded to become the patron. Also, following a tradition of gracious ladies distributing their bounty to the poor in hospitals (a tradition that goes back to late antiquity), West encouraged visits from society ladies and female journalists, who were to spread the good news that Great Ormond Street was a means of inculcating middle-class values into working-class families. The 'catechism' of cleanliness and godliness became a leitmotif in the moral improvement of both mothers and children. As Andrea Tanner has shown, these women's role was vital in day-to-day fundraising, including the year-round bazaars, collections, and tea parties, as well as in raising subscriptions towards the hospital and in urging London female 'society' to visit the wards as part of their social round. Most significant was Queen Victoria's support; she was a regular visitor, and on one occasion sent hundreds of toys from a German toy factory that she had visited.[71]

The physical structure of the hospital is another recurrent topic of the more recent scholarship.[72] Few scholars, however, have followed the example of Thompson and Goldin's classic study of 1975, which traced the developing structure of the hospital in western Europe across the centuries.[73] Indeed, a theme which emerges from their book is the extent to which the physical form of the hospital was adapted to changing contexts and circumstances and yet also how far architectural models were imitated across time and space. A classic example of that imitation is provided by cruciform ward design, which became standard in some of the major Renaissance hospitals of central and northern Italy and was copied in other parts of both the Mediterranean (Spain and Portugal) and northern Europe.[74]

A common assumption of many hospital historians is that form followed function. Once we move away from the narrow vision of the 'medicalisation model', it becomes increasingly apparent that every hospital building responds to a variety of interrelated pressures, including those of patrons, governments, and patients as well as other interest groups. As Annmarie Adams reminds us, 'medical change does not necessarily inspire new architectural forms', even in recent years.[75] Rather, hospital architecture is more culturally than medically determined. Hospitals in nineteenth-century

Canada looked like Scottish castles, and interwar and postmodern hospitals like luxury hotels and shopping malls, while modern hospitals tend to resemble office buildings. Both the exterior elevations of hospitals and their disposition of space have responded not just to demands of medical science, but also to the grandiose concerns of patrons, as in the splendid example of Greenwich Hospital.

None of this is to deny that form was ever related to function. But it is important to distinguish between exterior and interior. Frequently the appreciation of the literate classes, these gentlemen on their Grand Tours of Europe, was excited above all by the outward design; such observers were less concerned with the interior. It was rather the role of master masons, architects, and medical authorities to consider how space should be used. There was, for example, a long-held belief in the need to promote airiness for the dispersal of the noxious fumes of disease. This can be discovered just as much in writers of the Italian Renaissance, like Marsilio Ficino, as in the designers of voluntary hospitals in the eighteenth century or of the pavilion style of the age of Nightingale. St Bartholomew's Hospital in London, for example, was planned with four detached wings around a square, large windows in the wards, and separate isolation facilities for contagious disease such as smallpox.

Up to this point, we have followed the lead of much of the literature in the field and examined the hospital principally as an urban phenomenon. Just as it is necessary, however, to ensure that the hospital is not detached from the wider social and political patronage networks of the city, so in some cases it is equally essential not to divorce it from the rural context. Indeed, in his study of English hospitals between 1100 and 1300, already cited, Max Satchell concludes that one in five of them can be defined as 'rural' (although it should be stressed that in this period England was indeed a rural 'backwater' in comparison with Italy). With the advantage of the *longue durée*, we can trace the origins of the whole hospital movement in Western Europe to the countryside. Some of the earliest Middle Eastern hospitals were attached to rural or suburban monasteries. Their medieval European successors have left visible reminders of the scale and importance of these monasteries' infirmaries, such as the vast wards of Ourscamps and Tonerre, while some of the numerous pilgrim hospices on the routes to Compostella or Rome expanded in time into substantial hospitals.

Some hospitals in the smaller urban centres and villages seem to have declined in the early modern period, partly because they were seen as centres of local solidarity and resistance to central authority. An example of this has been seen above at Beaune, but was also more generally true of France in the sixteenth to seventeenth centuries, as Daniel Hickey has shown.[76] Yet curiously, as so often in hospital history, the trend came to be reversed. The reversal happened in the nineteenth century, at least in northern Italy and southeast England, as Sergio Onger and Steve Cherry have shown.[77] Onger's study of health facilities in the Brescian territory reveals that there were a number of factors involved in the creation of new rural hospitals and the reduction of those in the main conglomerations. They were established to cope with the spread of disease, both endemic pellagra, the main cause of hospitalisation until the end of the nineteenth century, and epidemic typhus and cholera. It was also believed that new hospitals lent prestige to local communities and promoted social harmony in a period when the country-side was undergoing great economic change. The Brescian example confirms the general contention of this chapter that changes in hospital history can be understood only in relation to wider factors which often have little to do with medicine, and which undermine any teleological narrative.[78]

Finally, under this rural heading, we should invoke an English initiative in health care, the cottage hospital. Because of the high levels of poverty, those at the bottom of the social pile would have been unable to pay for professional medical treatment unless they were fortunate enough to belong to friendly societies or workers' clubs. Cottage hospitals were particularly significant for rural areas because they addressed local needs. These hospitals were run by GPs, who performed simple operations in them and, along with competent nursing staff, offered patients the necessary periods of recuperation that they would have been unlikely to enjoy in larger city hospitals.

Whether in urban or rural contexts, the one constant of all these hospitals was the patient. So far in this discussion he or she has remained obscure, the object of patrons, administrators, priests, doctors, and nurses, rather than self-determining. Largely due to the influence of Roy Porter, much has been done to redress this long-standing imbalance in the historiography and restore the viewpoint of the patient to the historian's purview. The publication of a number of studies of patients in early modern Europe based on analysis of letter collections, diaries, and trial records is part of a wider scholarly trend to explore the narratives of everyday events.[79] Rarely, however, does this type of evidence survive from the hand of the *hospital* patient. He or she normally remains silent since, before the nineteenth century, surviving documentation relating to patients tends to consist only of entry and death registers. These, as will be seen below, provide invaluable information on demographic events and social background, but little on the patient's personal experience of the hospital.

Petitions are one type of source that does allow us to come closer to understanding when and why the sick wanted to be hospitalised, as is demonstrated by Louise Gray's study of those seeking admission to a hospital in rural southern Germany in the seventeenth and eighteenth centuries.[80] Even though the 'voice' of the poor was mediated through the hand of the scribes who actually wrote the petitions, accompanying witness statements from priests, administrators, and doctors did confirm the veracity of their claims. These patients were, however, unusual in that they suffered from chronic conditions, excluded from the average general hospital. The petitions reveal that men and women applied to the hospital as a last resort, for their sickness had made it impossible for them to survive by any other means. Some of them, however, declared their willingness to work in the hospital, and they were given light tasks, such as cutting wood for the kitchen and harvesting fruit. Indeed, work was encouraged since it was seen as combating idleness and diabolical temptation; only prisoners and the bedridden were exempt. Emphasis on work was also an important aspect of the British treatment of TB patients in the nineteenth century. Flurin Condrau describes such treatment as 'graduated labour therapy' for the working class; the aim was to return the patient to his job.[81] That this did not always happen is attested by the early twentieth-century case of the young worker Moritz Bromme, who kept an autobiography of his repeated visits to the sanatorium. Though each time he was discharged as 'cured', the necessity to support a family of four children meant that he had to return to his factory job, only to get worse again and to have to return to what his foreman described as the 'cougher's castle'. Bromm recorded a growing scepticism of the therapy offered him.

We should not generalise too readily. Sometimes the hospital was indeed a last resort, as Gray shows. On other occasions, as Sandra Cavallo's work on early modern Turin has demonstrated, it was a strategic resource of the family or individual in managing what we might call the patient's career – a resource to be drawn on in some phases of illness or economic need, and by no means necessarily the final phases.[82] This is also reflected at Great Ormond Street. Parents were not simply passive and unthinking recipients of charity. It was not unknown for them to remove their offspring early because of perceived poor treatment or the unhappiness of their children, whom they were rarely allowed to see. Thus 800 patients were removed by families between 1852 and 1899, often against medical advice. That behaviour reminds us of the power of the family to reject or accept hospital treatment, contradicting a prevalent view of the London poor as helpless and unable to evaluate the medicine provided by professionals. Such manifestations of patient power further undermine Foucault's twin conceptions of a great confinement and the power of the clinical 'gaze'.

Physicians' diagnoses and their disease terminology nonetheless underlay the selection of patients for some of the more specialised hospitals. Did the term 'incurable' mean the same in the sixteenth century as in the eighteenth? Did the terms 'healed' or 'cured' change over time? The condition 'cured' was often taken to mean that an individual was again fit to work. Through her examination of the petitions of the poor, Gray also shows that disease categories and labels could even change from day to day and according to the person who was recording them. Condrau points out that, although some sanatoria claimed high success rates, in fact 50 per cent of those who left as 'cured' died within five years of discharge.

Levels of mortality have long been a major concern for hospitals: they affect their public reputation and ultimately the willingness of both private and public sponsors to continue financial support. Mortality was especially a preoccupation for anybody running a foundling home, given the general recognition throughout pre-industrial Europe that up to a third of all babies born would die in infancy. The constant tension between available finance and required services has been brought out by Alysa Levene in her discussion of the famous Innocenti hospital in Florence, which in the eighteenth century saw both an expansion in its facilities for orphans and an increase in the rate of abandonment.[83] Given that wet-nurses were the most expensive part of the operation – despite their notoriously low pay – various experiments were introduced to save money. A cheaper alternative adopted in the 1740s was to feed infants with cows' milk. Indeed this was also recommended by the famous Florentine medical reformer, Antonio Cocchi. But the practice was abandoned because, as had been discovered elsewhere, it led to an increase in infant mortality.[84] This was also the effect of a second innovation, an attempt to reduce the number of wet-nurses employed. Their supply was always prone to shortage, particularly in the summer, when agricultural labour proved a more profitable alternative. However, as Levene concludes, the only solution to ensuring the long-term survival of infants was to place them promptly with external wet-nurses.

An overarching theme of some of the more recent historiography on the subject is the imperative of examining the hospital within a wider context to understand its impact, whether in terms of its effects on the local population or of its major role in the local economy as a purchaser of goods or an investor in property or banks.[85] The importance of the hospital as a local employer has also begun to be examined. That extends the analysis of its charitable role to include employing the able-bodied poor, as exemplified by the 'corrodians' of many medieval hospitals, who entered into a lifetime contract; board, lodging, and care in sickness was provided in return for their labour and property. All this leads to a reconsideration of the relationship between formal (institutional) and informal (domestic) systems of support. And that in turn raises wider questions about the changing relationship between in-patients and out-patients, seen in the context of demographic regimes and social and family structures.[86]

Superficially, it might be possible to conclude that there was a certain uniformity of experience over the period examined here, from late antiquity to the present day. This stems partly from the very nature of the subject: we are examining a single institution (or a 'family resemblance group' of institutions). Yet, another way of interpreting the phenomenon is that the traditional Whiggish vision of hospital history has been abandoned. In other words, we are not seeing here a form of progressive development towards the triumph of modern biomedicine in hospitals. Rather, the very repetition

25

of the same themes in different periods points to a long series of reactions to previous forms of 'indoor' solutions to the problems of poverty and sickness, though these reactions in their turn might lead to the imitation of past models, just as post-modern hospitals contain architectural elements of earlier designs. But even when earlier models or those imported from other countries were being adopted, the process led to transmutation, whether in terms of hospital regulations, therapies, or design. As the English Baroque may have been inspired by Italian architecture but was altered in its transplantation to England, so the Savoy Hospital and the London Foundling Hospital were different from their original models, the Florentine hospitals of Santa Maria Nuova and the Innocenti.

In the post-postmodern age in which we now live, globalisation is everything. For the old hospital history, the subject is narrowly conceived. For the 'new' hospital history, which goes back to Granshaw and Porter and their fellow scholars, the world must be the limit.

Notes

1 What follows is an essay in overview and interpretation. References are therefore minimal, offering only some background and guidance through controversies. [This chapter was originally co-written with John Henderson and Alessandro Pastore. With their kind permission, I have reproduced substantially unchanged the main historical sections for which I was primarily responsible, that is, sections I–V; and I have compressed section VI by my co-editors while adding full references to some of the other contributions in the collection that this chapter introduces, *The Impact of Hospitals*. That volume was published by Peter Lang for the International Network for the History of Hospitals, and more recent work on hospital history can at least be sampled through its latest outputs, such as C. Bonfield, J. Reinarz, and T. Huguet-Termes (eds), *Hospitals and Communities, 1100–1960*, and L. Abreu and S. Sheard (eds), *Hospital Life: Theory and Practice from the Medieval to the Modern* (both Oxford, 2013). I have not made the attempt to update systematically the references that follow. I will, however, allow one exception and highlight *From Western Medicine to Global Medicine: The Hospital beyond the West*, cited in n. 29 below, which covers the nineteenth and twentieth centuries and which in scope is an indispensable complement to the present survey.] For the section that follows, see G. B. Risse, 'Before the Clinic Was "Born": Methodological Perspectives in Hospital History', in N. Finzsch and R. Jütte (eds), *Institutions of Confinement: Hospitals, Asylums, and Prisons in Western Europe and North America, 1500–1950* (Cambridge, 1996), pp. 75–96, at 87–91 (to which I am heavily indebted); Risse, *Mending Bodies, Saving Souls: A History of Hospitals* (New York, 1999), pp. 257–88; A. Cunningham and R. French (eds), *The Medical Enlightenment of the Eighteenth Century* (Cambridge, 1990); P. P. Bernard, 'The Limits of Absolutism: Joseph II and the Allgemeines Krankenhaus', *Eighteenth-Century Studies*, 9 (1975–6), pp. 193–215; D. Jetter, *Wien von den Anfängen bis um 1900*, Geschichte des Hospitals vol. 5 (Wiesbaden, 1982); B. Pohl-Resl, *Rechnen mit der Ewigkeit: das Wiener Bürgerspital im Mittelalter* (Vienna, 1996). I do not know of a monograph for Austria comparable to M. Lindemann, *Health and Healing in Eighteenth-Century Germany* (Baltimore, MD, 1997).

2 Though see T. H. Broman, *The Transformation of German Academic Medicine 1750–1820* (Cambridge, 1996), pp. 59–63, for some qualifications of the conventional narrative.

3 The introduction of clinical hospital teaching is now normally attributed to Giambattista da Monte; see J. J. Bylebyl, 'The School of Padua: Humanistic Medicine in the Sixteenth Century', in C. Webster (ed.), *Health, Medicine and Mortality in the Sixteenth Century* (Cambridge, 1979), p. 348.

4 See Risse, 'Before the Clinic', pp. 92–3, for medical and surgical education in the Hôtel-Dieu at the time.

5 *System einer vollständigen medicinischen Polizey*, 4 vols (Mannheim, 1780–88), trans. E. Vilim from 3rd revised edn as *A System of Complete Medical Police* (Baltimore, MD, 1976).

6 See n. 3.

7 See A. Pastore, *Le regole dei corpi: medicina e disciplina nell'Italia moderna* (Bologna, 2006).

8 The best brief overview is still L. Granshaw, 'The Hospital', in W. F. Bynum and R. Porter (eds), *Companion Encyclopedia of the History of Medicine* (London, 1993), pp. 1180–1203. The various monographs of D. Jetter contain much valuable detail. See e.g. his *Das europäische Hospital: von der Spätantike bis 1800* (Cologne, 1986) and *Grundzüge der Krankenhausgeschichte, 1800–1900* (Darmstadt, 1977).

9 For what follows, see P. Horden, 'The Earliest Hospitals in Byzantium, Western Europe, and Islam', in M. Cohen (ed.), *Journal of Interdisciplinary History*, special issue, 'Poverty and Charity: Judaism, Christianity, Islam', 35 (2005), pp. 361–89 [reprinted in the present collection]; T. S. Miller, *The Birth of the Hospital in the Byzantine Empire*, 2nd edn (Baltimore, MD, 1977).

10 For western European overviews, see J. Imbert, *Les hôpitaux en droit canonique* (Paris, 1947); M. Mollat, *The Poor in the Middle Ages* (New Haven, CT, 1978); B. Bowers (ed.), *The Medieval Hospital and Medical Practice* (Aldershot, 2007).

11 P. Mitchell, *Medicine in the Crusades: Warfare, Wounds and the Medieval Surgeon* (Cambridge, 2004), ch. 2, and the new interpretation and survey of F.-O. Touati, 'La terre sainte: un laboratoire hospitalier au Moyen Age?', in N. Bulst and K.-H. Spiess (eds), *Sozialgeschichte Mittelalterlicher Hospitäler* (Ostfildern, 2007), pp. 169–211.

12 J. W. Brodman, *Charity and Welfare: Hospitals and the Poor in Medieval Catalonia* (Philadelphia, 1998), pp. 94–8.

13 J. Henderson, *The Renaissance Hospital: Healing the Body and Healing the Soul* (New Haven, CT, 2006); J. Arrizabalaga, J. Henderson, and R. French, *The Great Pox: The French Disease in Renaissance Europe* (New Haven, CT, 1997).

14 C. Rawcliffe, *Medicine for the Soul: The Life, Death and Resurrection of an English Medieval Hospital* (Stroud, 1999).

15 See T. J. McHugh, 'Establishing Medical Men at the Paris Hôtel-Dieu, 1500–1715', *Social History of Medicine*, 19 (2006), pp. 209–24.

16 C. Jones, 'The Construction of the Hospital Patient in Early Modern France', in Finzsch and Jütte, *Institutions of Confinement*, p. 68; L. Brockliss and C. Jones, *The Medical World of Early Modern France* (Oxford, 1997), pp. 689–700.

17 For brief synthesis and further references, see S. De Renzi, 'Policies of Health: Disease, Poverty and Hospitals', in P. Elmer (ed.), *The Healing Arts: Health, Disease and Society in Europe 1500–1800* (Manchester, 2004), pp. 150–60.

18 Granshaw, 'The Hospital', p. 1195.

19 H. Marland, 'The Changing Role of the Hospital, 1800–1900', in D. Brunton (ed.), *Medicine Transformed: Health, Disease and Society in Europe 1800–1930* (Manchester, 2004), p. 239.

20 For what follows, convenient syntheses are: U. Tröhler and C.-R. Prüll, 'The Rise of the Modern Hospital', in I. Loudon (ed.), *Western Medicine: An Illustrated History* (Oxford and New York, 1997), pp. 160–75; L. Granshaw, 'The Rise of the Modern Hospital in Britain', in A. Wear (ed.), *Medicine in Society: Historical Essays* (Cambridge, 1992), pp. 197–218. See also the very useful sections on hospitals in W. F. Bynum et al., *The Western Medical Tradition 1800 to 2000* (Cambridge, 2006), pp. 53–64, 84–5, 150–62, 269–81, 349–52, 439–50.

21 Brockliss and Jones, *Medical World*, pp. 269–72, 686; M. Rhodes, 'Women in Medicine: Doctors and Nurses, 1850–1920', in Brunton, *Medicine Transformed*, pp. 164–76; C. Jones, *The Charitable Imperative: Hospitals and Nursing in Ancien Regime and Revolutionary France* (London, 1989); S. Broomhall, *Women's Medical Work in Early Modern France* (Manchester, 2004).

22 See e.g. the discussion in Henderson, *The Renaissance Hospital*, ch. 6, and C. Rawcliffe, 'Hospital Nurses and their Work', in R. Britnell (ed.), *Daily Life in the Middle Ages* (Stroud, 1998), pp. 43–64.

23 M.W. Dols, *Majnūn: The Madman in Medieval Islamic Society* (Oxford, 1992), pp. 112–57; H. C. E. Midelfort, *A History of Madness in Sixteenth-Century Germany* (Stanford, CA, 1999).

24 A. Scull, 'A Convenient Place to Get Rid of Inconvenient People: The Victorian Lunatic Asylum', in A. D. King (ed.), *Buildings and Society* (London, 1980), p. 38, cited by J. Andrews, 'The Rise of the Asylum in Britain', in Brunton, *Medicine Transformed*, p. 301.

25 Brockliss and Jones, *Medical World*, p. 677.

26 R. Porter, *Blood and Guts: A Short History of Medicine* (London, 2002), p. 152.

27 For what follows, see further M. J. Vogel, 'The Transformation of the American Hospital', in Finzsch and Jütte, *Institutions of Confinement*, pp. 39–54; M. J. Vogel, *The Invention of the Modern Hospital: Boston, 1870–1930* (Chicago, 1980); J. H. Warner and J. A. Tighe (eds), *Major Problems in the History of American Medicine and Public Health* (Boston, 2001); C. E. Rosenberg, *The Care of Strangers: The Rise of America's Hospital System* (New York, 1987); D. Rosner, *A Once Charitable Enterprise: Hospitals and Health Care in Brooklyn and New York, 1885–1915* (Cambridge, 1982); R. Stevens, *In Sickness and in Wealth: American Hospitals in the Twentieth Century* (Baltimore, MD, 1999).

28 R. L. Numbers (ed.), *Medicine in the New World: New Spain, New France, and New England* (Knoxville, 1987); G. Risse, 'Shelter and Care for Natives and Colonists: Hospitals in Sixteenth-Century New Spain', in S. Varey, R. Chabrán, and D. B. Weiner (eds), *Searching the Secrets of Nature: The Life and Works of Dr. Francisco Hernández* (Stanford, CA, 2000), pp. 65–81 (a reference I owe to Andrew Wear).

29 [See M. Harrison, M. Jones and H. Sweet (eds), *From Western Medicine to Global Medicine: The Hospital beyond the West* (New Delhi, 2009), the 'Introduction' to which was kindly sent to me by Mark Harrison in advance of publication.]

30 J. Van Alphen and A. Aris (eds), *Oriental Medicine: An Illustrated Guide to the Asian Arts of Healing* (Boston, 1995), p.234.

31 Horden, 'Earliest Hospitals', with bibliography for this and what follows.

32 J. Legge, *A Record of Buddhistic Kingdoms, being an Account by the Chinese Monk Fâ-Hien of his Travels in India and Ceylon (AD 399–414) [...]*(Oxford, 1966, repr. New York, 1965), cited by D. Wujastyk, *The Roots of Ayurveda*, rev. edn (London, 2003), p. xv.

33 Ibid.

34 H. Scogin, 'Poor Relief in Northern Sung China', *Oriens Extremus*, 25 (1978), pp. 30–46, a reference I owe to Peter Brown.

35 M. Giteau, *The Civilization of Angkor* (New York, 1976), p. 234, drawing on G. Cœdès, 'La stèle de Ta-Prohm', reprinted in his *Articles sur le pays Khmer*, vol. 2 (Paris, 1992), pp. 11–49.

36 G. N. A. Attewell, *Refiguring Unani Tibb: Plural Healing in Late Colonial India* (Hyderabad, 2007).

37 H. Sigerist, 'An Outline of the Development of the Hospital', *Bulletin of the History of Medicine*, 4 (1936), pp. 573–81.

38 Risse, *Mending Bodies, Saving Souls.*

39 Granshaw, 'The Hospital'.

40 N. Jewson, 'The Disappearance of the Sick Man from Medical Cosmology 1770–1870', *Sociology*, 10 (1976), pp. 225–44.

41 C. Jones, 'The Construction of the Hospital Patient in Early Modern France', in Finzsch and Jütte, *Institutions of Confinements*, p. 66.

42 Ibid. 69.

43 L. Granshaw and R. Porter (eds), *The Hospital in History* (London, 1989).

44 For the older historiography, see the review article on a sample of it by J. Guy, 'Of the Writing of Hospital Histories There Is No End', *Bulletin of the History of Medicine*, 59 (1985), pp. 415–43.

45 Granshaw and Porter (eds), *Hospital in History*, pp. 1–2, 24, 29, 51, 94, 110, 123, 150, 182, 221, 243.

46 Ibid. 221–41.

47 M. Garbellotti, 'Ospedali e storia nell'Italia moderna: percorsi di ricerca', *Medicina e storia*, 3 (2003), pp. 116–17.

48 Cf. J. Frangos, *From Housing the Poor to Healing the Sick: The Changing Institution of Paris Hospitals under the Old Regime and Revolution* (Madison, WI, 1997); O. Keel, *L'avènement de la médecine clinique moderne en Europe, 1750–1815: politiques, institutions et savoirs* (Montreal, 2001).

49 See e.g. Finzsch and Jütte, *Institutions of Confinement*; Y. Kawakita, S. Sakai, and Y. Otsuka (eds), *History of Hospitals: The Evolution of Health Care Facilities. Proceedings of the 11th International Symposium on the Comparative History of Medicine East and West* (Osaka, 1989), which does look back to the Middle Ages, but is essentially a (very welcome) comparison of modern Japanese and modern western hospitals; J. Barry and C. Jones (eds), *Medicine and Charity before the Welfare State* (London, 1991), not wholly, of course, about hospitals.

50 [With particular reference to Henderson, Horden, and Pastore (eds), *The Impact of Hospitals 300–2000* (hereafter *Impact*), which this chapter originally introduced.]

51 Cf. S. Cherry, *Medical Services and the Hospitals in Britain 1860–1939* (Cambridge, 1996).

52 E. Gruber Von Arni, '"Tempora mutantur et nos mutamur in illis": The Experience of Sick and Wounded Soldiers during the English Civil Wars and Interregnum, 1642–60', in *Impact*, pp. 317–40.

53 Harrison et al., *From Western Medicine to Global Medicine.*

54 Andrews, 'The Rise of the Asylum' surveys the major literature. It is enough to mention the names of Andrew Scull, Roy Porter, and Andrews himself. See e.g. R. Porter and D. Wright (eds), *The Confinement of the Insane: International Perspectives, 1800–1965* (Cambridge, 2003).

55 See e.g. S. C. Lawrence, *Charitable Knowledge: Hospital Pupils and Practitioners in Eighteenth-Century London* (Cambridge, 1996); K. Waddington, *Medical Education at St Bartholomew's Hospital, 1123–1995* (Woodbridge, 2003).

56 M. Satchell, 'Towards a Landscape History of the Rural Hospital in England, 1100–1300', *Impact*, pp. 237–56; F. Condrau, 'The Institutional Career of Tuberculosis: Social Policy, Medical Institutions and Patients before World War II', *Impact*, pp. 341–71.

57 On leprosy, see esp. C. Rawcliffe, *Leprosy in Medieval England* (Woodbridge, 2006), with F.-O. Touati, *Maladie et société au Moyen Âge: la lèpre, les lépreux et les léproseries dans la province ecclésiastique de Sens jusqu'au milieu du XIVe siècle* (Brussels, 1998). For an outline of the evolution of *lazzaretti* for plague, see C. M. Cipolla, *Public Health and the Medical Profession in the Renaissance* (Cambridge, 1976), ch. 1; on isolation hospitals for the Great Pox, see Henderson in Arrizabalaga et al., *The Great Pox*, chs 2, 7, and 8; R. Jütte, 'Syphilis and Confinement: Hospitals in Early Modern Germany', in Finzsch and Jütte, *Institutions of Confinement*, pp. 97–115; K. P. Siena, *Venereal Disease, Hospitals and the Urban Poor: London's 'Foul Wards', 1600–1800* (Rochester, 2004).

58 On state funding and care in Britain, see J. Mohan and M. Gorsky, *Don't Look Back? Voluntary and Charitable Finance of Hospitals in Britain, Past and Present* (London, 2001), and M. Gorsky, *Patterns of Philanthropy: Charity and Society in Nineteenth-Century Bristol* (Woodbridge, 1999).

59 M. Berengo, *L'Europa delle città: il volto della società urbana tra medioevo ed età moderna* (Turin, 1999), pp. 609, 611.

60 J.-P. Gutton (ed.), *Les administrateurs d'hôpitaux dans la France d'Ancien Régime* (Lyon, 1999).

61 K. C. Robbins, 'Patrimony, Trust, and Trusteeship: The Practice and Control of Burgundian Philanthropy at Beaune's Hôtel-Dieu, c. 1630', *Impact*, pp. 77–92.

62 C. Jones and R. Porter, 'Introduction', in C. Jones and R. Porter (eds), *Reassessing Foucault: Power, Medicine and the Body* (London, 1998), p. 4; R. Jütte, *Poverty and Deviance in Early Modern Europe* (Cambridge, 1996).

63 B. Pullan, 'The Old Catholicism, the New Catholicism, and the Poor', in G. Politi, M. Rosa, and F. Della Peruta (eds), *Timore e carità: i poveri nell'Italia moderna* (Cremona, 1982), pp. 17–18.

64 Risse, *Mending Bodies, Saving Souls*, pp. 218–19, though for the counterexample of Venice, which during the course of the sixteenth century gradually developed an integrated charitable system in response to poverty in general and to sickness in particular, see R. Palmer, 'L'assistenza medica nella Venezia cinquecentesca', in B. Aikema and D. Meijers (eds), *Nel regno dei poveri: arte e storia dei grandi ospedali Veneziani in età moderna, 1474–1797* (Venice, 1989), pp. 35–42.

65 I. W. Archer, *The Pursuit of Stability: Social Relations in Elizabethan London* (Cambridge, 1991), pp. 154–5; A. Pastore, 'Introduction', in *Sanità e società: Friuli-Venezia Giulia, secoli XVI–XX* (Udine, 1986), pp. 17–18.

66 N. Wachtel, *La foi du souvenir: labyrinthes marranes* (Paris, 2001).

67 Cited in A.-M. Piuz, 'Pauvres et pauvreté dans les sociétés pré-industrielles', *Revue suisse d'histoire*, 23 (1973), p. 547.

68 Horden, 'Alms and the Man' (reprinted as Ch. 9 below); C. Rawcliffe, '"A Word from Our Sponsor": Advertising the Patron in the Medieval Hospital', *Impact*, pp. 167–93; Robbins, 'Patrimony, Trust'; M. T. Sneider, 'The Treasury of the Poor: Hospital Finance in Sixteenth- and Seventeenth-Century Bologna', *Impact*, pp. 93–115.

69 Rawcliffe, *Medicine for the Soul*; P. Horden, 'Religion as Medicine: Music in Medieval Hospitals', in P. Biller and J. Ziegler (eds), *Religion and Medicine in the Middle Ages* (Woodbridge, 2001), pp. 135–53; idem, 'A Non-Natural Environment: Medicine without Doctors and the Medieval European Hospital', in Bowers, *The Medieval Hospital*, pp. 133–45; Henderson, *The Renaissance Hospital*.

70 See also A. Hayum, *The Isenheim Altarpiece: God's Medicine and the Painter's Vision* (Princeton, NJ, 1989).

71 A. Tanner, 'Too Many Mothers? Female Roles in a Metropolitan Victorian Children's Hospital', *Impact*, pp. 135–64.

72 See e.g. C. Stevenson, *Medicine and Magnificence: British Hospital and Asylum Architecture, 1660–1815* (New Haven, CT, 2000); J. Taylor, *The Architect and the Pavilion Hospital: Dialogue and Design Creativity in England, 1850–1914* (Leicester, 1997); Aikema and Meijers, *Nel regno dei poveri*.

73 J. D. Thompson and G. Goldin, *The Hospital: A Social and Architectural History* (New Haven, CT, 1975). See also Jetter, *Das europäische Hospital*; H. Richardson (ed.), *English Hospitals 1660–1948* (London, 1998). For the medieval and early modern periods, see esp. F.-O. Touati (ed.), *Archéologie et architecture hospitalières de l'antiquité tardive à l'aube des temps modernes* (Paris, 2004).

74 Henderson, The Renaissance Hospital.

75 A. Adams, '"That Was Then, This Is Now": Hospital Architecture in the Age(s) of Revolution, 1970–2001', *Impact*, pp. 219–34.

76 D. Hickey, *Local Hospitals in Ancien Régime France: Rationalization, Resistance, Renewal, 1530–1789* (Montreal, 1997), esp. pp. 200–203. See also, on early modern Italian hospitals in small centres and rural areas, M. Garbellotti, *Le risorse dei poveri: carità e tutela della salute nel principato vescovile di Trento in età moderna* (Bologna, 2007).

77 S. Onger, 'The Formation of the Hospital Network in the Brescian Region between the Eighteenth and Twentieth Centuries', *Impact*, pp. 257–73; S. Cherry '"Keeping Your Hand In" and Holding On: General Practitioners and Rural Hospitals in Nineteenth- and Twentieth-Century East Anglia', *Impact*, pp. 275–93.

78 P. Frascani, 'L'ospedale moderno in Europa e Stati Uniti: riflessioni sulla recente storiografia', *Società e storia*, 52 (1991), p. 405.

79 Cf. R. Porter, 'The Patient's View: Doing History from Below', *Theory and Society*, 14 (1985), pp. 175–98, and R. Porter (ed.), *Patients and Practitioners: Lay Perceptions of Medicine in Preindustrial Society* (Cambridge, 1985); more recently, G. Pomata, *Contracting a Cure: Patients, Healers and the Law in Early Modern Bologna* (Baltimore, MD, 1998). For one of the few studies of the life of hospital patients, see M. Louis-Courvoisier, *Soigner et consoler: la vie quotidienne dans un hôpital à la fin de l'Ancien Regime, Genève, 1750–1820* (Geneva, 2000). More generally, see J. S. Amelang, *The Flight of Icarus: Artisan Autobiography in Early Modern Europe* (Stanford, CA, 1998), and O. Niccoli, *Storie di ogni giorno in una città del Seicento* (Rome, 2000).

80 L. Gray, 'Hospitals and the Lives of the Chronically Sick: Coping with Illness in the Narratives of the Rural Poor in Early Modern Germany', *Impact*, pp. 297–315.

81 Condrau, 'The Institutional Career of Tuberculosis'.

82 S. Cavallo, 'Family Obligations and Inequalities in Access to Care in Northern Italy, Seventeenth to Eighteenth Centuries', in P. Horden and R. Smith (eds), *The Locus of Care: Families, Communities, Institutions and the Provision of Welfare since Antiquity* (London, 1988), pp. 90–110; P. Horden, 'Family History and Hospital History in the Middle Ages', in E. Sonnino (ed.), *Living in the City (14th–20th Centuries)* (Rome, 2004), pp. 255–82.

83 A. Levene, 'Saving the Innocents: Nursing Foundlings in Florence and London in the Eighteenth Century', *Impact*, pp. 375–93.

84 A. Cocchi, *Relazione dello Spedale di Santa Maria Nuova di Firenze*, ed. M. Mannelli Goggioli and R. Pasta (Florence, 2000).

85 O. Faure, *Genèse de l'hôpital moderne: les hospices civils de Lyon de 1802 à 1845* (Lyon, 1982), p. 8; see also K. Waddington, *Charity and the London Hospitals, 1850–98* (Woodbridge, 2000).

86 On this theme, see Horden and Smith, *The Locus of Care*; Horden, 'Family History and Hospital History'; M. Dupree, 'Family Care and Hospital Care: The Sick Poor in Nineteenth-Century Glasgow', *Social History of Medicine*, 6 (1993), pp. 195–211. For a similar approach to the care of the mentally ill, see P. Bartlett and D. Wright (eds), *Outside the Walls of the Asylum: The History of Care in the Community 1750–2000* (London, 1999).

2

POVERTY, CHARITY, AND THE INVENTION OF THE HOSPITAL

Are we harming anyone in building lodgings [*katagogia*] for strangers, for those who visit us while on a journey and for those who require some care [*therapeias*] because of sickness, and when we extend to them the necessary comforts, such as [male] nurses [*nosokomountas*], those who give medical assistance [*iatrouontas*], beasts of burden, and escorts? All these must apply the skills needed for life and those that have been devised for living decently; they must also have buildings suitable for their work, all of which are an honour to the place, and, as their reputation is credited to our governor, confer glory on him.[1]

I

The year is 371 or 372. Basil, the new bishop of Caesarea (modern Kayseri, Turkey), writes to the provincial governor Elias. From the letter's opening, we can infer that Elias has wanted to see the bishop and hear his answers to accusations made against him. Relations between Basil and Elias have, in any case, been strained. Basil's management of the local church and its endowment has now come under scrutiny, and claims have evidently been made that Roman government is being damaged. In writing to Elias, Basil concedes, with heavy irony, that his accusers may have a point. He has erected a magnificent church in a suburb of Caesarea with suitable accommodation for bishop and clergy and a guest suite for the governor. Admittedly, that may have been going too far. But who could possibly object to this charitable 'multiplex', with its appropriate personnel and infrastructure, all of which redounds to the governor's glory?

The background to this exchange is not altogether easy to reconstruct. We have to rely on carefully redacted letter collections (in which we have only half the correspondence); on sermons that are hard to date because they mix timeless verities with topicality and were selected for copying with a view to their future pastoral usefulness, not the needs of social historians; and on naturally laudatory accounts by Basil's brother, Gregory of Nyssa, and his friend, Gregory Nazianzen. The latter's funeral oration was reworked for publication after being delivered on the third anniversary of Basil's death in 379.[2] None of these writings displayed much duty to exact chronology or circumstantial detail. It seems, however, that Basil had served as chief adviser to his predecessor as bishop, Eusebius. With him, too, relations had become fraught, although Basil had recently assumed de facto leadership of the local church because Eusebius was elderly and ill.[3] This phase of Basil's career coincided with a period of food stress and epidemic disease that lasted several years into the 370s and so into Basil's early years as bishop. It would be remembered as very severe.[4]

Through sermons deploying all the rhetorical skills that he owed to his Athenian education, Basil induced the local wealthy elites to release onto the market their local grain hoards (from caves that are still such a feature of the area) rather than wait for the price to reach the stratosphere. He may have drawn on his own patrimony to purchase some of it. 'Open to the world the dark cave of mammon . . . the hungry are wasting away before your face.'[5] He also established a soup kitchen, or at least some organized distributions of soup and meat, working in it himself along with fellow clergy, perhaps supporting 'even' Jewish children (a striking detail in Gregory of Nyssa).[6] In this, Basil was following the precocious example of his grandparents' philanthropy in exile in the mountains of Pontus during a time of persecution and, indeed, more recently the philanthropy of his siblings.[7]

Despite the sharply expressed theological differences between them, his activities attracted the attention of the ageing emperor Valens (whose name Basil drops artfully in the letter quoted here). For Valens, Caesarea was important as a staging post en route to and from his capital in Antioch and as a source of munitions and horses. At some point, perhaps even before Basil became bishop in 370, the emperor donated land that provided space or revenue for his philanthropic initiatives.[8] Yet Basil still had to struggle for local control of the church with Valens and his 'vicar'. Perhaps he had not consulted the emperor about the specific use to which his donation would be put. Moreover, Basil's conversion of ad hoc famine relief measures into permanent structures for the overnight shelter of the needy remained controversial for some while. Witness the squabble that erupted between a later director of his hospital, Sacerdos, and the man who would succeed Basil as bishop.[9]

Basil's plans for this philanthropic complex were nothing if not ambitious. After his death, it could be lauded by Gregory Nazianzen as a 'new city' and came to bear its founder's own name, being known as the Basileias or some variant on that.[10] With its adjacent monastery and all the workshops, outbuildings, and accommodation, it may indeed have looked like a new city, a secondary conurbation outside the old city centre of Caesarea. It may even underlie the nucleus of modern Kayseri, although it is not clear from any other evidence, documentary or archaeological, when that was established.[11]

In this 'new city,' and in seeming abundance, lay 'the common treasury for those with possessions . . . even what people need to live on [implying that, for poorer donors too, their accumulated gifts are earning them a heavenly reward]; a place where disease is studied philosophically [*philosopheitai*: both Christian and medical wisdom?] . . . where compassion is held in genuine esteem.' It was 'the easiest way up to heaven', for donors as much as for terminally ill inmates.[12] Yet it is hard to tell what exactly the suburban complex comprised. Basil himself described the central charity as a *katagogion* (hostel or lodging house) and a *ptochotropheion* (literally, place where the indigent are looked after). He also refers in his shorter rule for monks to a *xenodocheion*, hospice for strangers, which is likely to be identical with, or at least very similar to, the main 'public' hospital, since Basil evinces concern for the sins of its inmates. This hospital seems to have had a chapel. There was also, less ambiguously, a separate establishment for lepers, some of them disfigured beyond recognition. And we can add to the list the orphans looked after in the monastery's school.[13]

On the other hand, we must not add any special medical facility. Basil knew some Galenic medicine.[14] Often in ill health himself, he may have consulted a variety of healers. He was too interested in, and impressed by, learned medicine to ignore its therapeutic potential. This is not a hospital in a modern sense, yet nor is it simply a hospice for the terminally ill, 'a stairway to heaven'. In his hospital, Basil offered inmates 'doctoring' as well as nursing: 'doctoring' rather than 'doctors'. In many ways that was, admittedly, a distinction without a difference. Basil's world lacked any form of professional medical accreditation, and the title 'doctor' could be earned only through clinical success. Still, the language suggests attendants in the hospital with a variety of skills rather than specialists.

Who were the beneficiaries of this care, this therapy? In the first place, they were the victims of prolonged 'food stress' – not famine in the sense of absolute shortage but as a failure of 'entitlement', since the rich had grain stored in their barns that they were reluctant to release until Basil's preaching.[15] An account of a later famine in Edessa (modern Urfa) may evoke some of the demographic circumstances: 'the infirm in the villages, along with the elderly and the young, women and children, and those racked by hunger . . . went into the cities to live by begging.'[16] At least some of their equivalents in Caesarea would have been sustained by hospital life in the Basileias.

Even when swollen by refugees, Caesarea was not a very large city. In 1500, the earliest date for which any statistics are available, it could boast only 2,287 tax-paying adults. In normal times, it may well not have generated many poor and needy people. Yet it lay in the middle of the horse-rearing countryside for which Cappadocia was famed, with no network of subordinate towns that could help absorb migrants in periods of crisis.[17] It was a major crossroads in Cappadocia's highways linking the capital and Syria, and would have seen a considerable number of transients, some of the 'strangers' to which Basil's hospital may well explicitly have catered.[18]

Little else can be said. The poor are amply present in the sermons and orations of these years: present in harrowing but stereotypical vignettes.[19] As individuals with life histories – or, indeed, with any personality – they are beneath notice. In the immediate aftermath of the food crisis, all sorts of people might have sought temporary relief at Basil's soup kitchen. But soon, what was becoming an exemplary institution may have accepted only exemplary patients: suitable paupers whose names were already on the bishop's approved list.[20] Basil called his hospital a *ptochotropheion*. *Ptochos* was a commonly used term for the absolutely indigent, dependent for survival on handouts or begging; the *ptochos* was to be contrasted with the *penes*, the 'labouring pauper' who had just about adequate resources in good times but not enough to survive a crisis unaided.[21] That might suggest the very poorest as the group targeted for admission. But Basil, like so many others, was inconsistent in his terminology. He stressed the importance of distinguishing the genuinely needy from avaricious scroungers. He generally advocated selectivity in his advice to monastic almoners.[22] In his sermons, he refers to *penetes* more often than to *ptochoi*, and in his shorter rule for monks, echoing Origen, he defines the *ptochos* as he who has fallen from wealth into need (the 'shame-faced' pauper of later ages) and is therefore less worthy than the *penes*, who has always been needy.[23]

We can therefore not be sure who was favoured in his hospital: Christians, primarily, rather than Jews or pagans; free men and women rather than slaves;[24] perhaps those in 'shallow' (or 'conjonctural') poverty needing temporary assistance (*penetes*). Overall, it is far from clear that the open-handedness of his famine relief measures was carried over into the governance of his hospital. It is in keeping with his austere, even grim programme that the town's lepers, at the extremity of need and sickness, are not mentioned in his surviving writings, and that, in his funeral oration, Gregory Nazianzen praises the Basileias for removing the appalling sight of them from the city's streets.[25] Basil emerges as perhaps having more in common than we might expect with a later, more conventional bishop of Caesarea, Firmus (d. 439). In one of his surviving letters, Firmus shows that he does not want the Basileias to be a haven for footloose peasants who have abandoned their landlords and their tax obligations.[26]

II

'Are we harming anyone?' Basil had asked. What indeed could be more innocent or straightforward than a hospital or hostel for the poor and sick erected in the suburbs? Centuries of Christian teaching, going back to

Christ's injunction to the rich man who would be perfect (Matthew 19:21) and encapsulated in the widely read 'sentence' of Sextus – 'God does not listen to the plea of one who does not himself listen to the plea of those in need'[27] – made it clear that assistance to those most affected by disaster or indigence benefited recipient and donor alike. It might now, in the 'hungry '70s', seem natural to give such assistance architectural expression.

A hospital in its basic and, in world-historical terms, most widespread form is a place, an area, designated for the overnight care of the needy.[28] Its ethos is nearly always charitable, and it is to be distinguished from 'outdoor' relief centres from which food or goods are distributed. The recipients of the hospital's services are therefore in some sense poor – but they are not necessarily sick. The definition of the modern hospital (from around 1850 onward) as essentially medical – as constituting a vanguard of medical expenditure and research – should not be applied to earlier periods, despite the obsession of many hospital historians with separating out from the rest the 'true' hospitals, those with attendant doctors, regardless of the period being studied.[29]

Still, the history of hospitals is far from straightforward, as the outline of Basil's activity on becoming the new bishop of Caesarea should have begun to show. It was less than a decade since the death of a pagan emperor, Julian – and who could be confident that he was the last of his type? There may have been a Christian majority in the population of Caesarea, but, if so, it was probably not an overwhelming one. Christian charity, especially in its most assertive, architectural form, had to earn approbation from several constituencies. These included the imperial court; the governor's office; the local notables, many of them pagan; admirers of the previous bishop, who does not seem to have done much for the poor; the 'middling sort' in city and suburbs, whose contributions were in aggregate very important to church finances (in particular to the stipends of the clergy);[30] and even the various categories of the poor themselves, not all of whom will have been entitled to benefit from Basil's foundation.

The politics of institutional charity in Caesarea in about 370 were shifting and complicated to a degree that we can never hope to recover from the surviving texts. We can, though, sense something of the risk that Basil was taking. The hospital would soon become part of the Christian Church's 'reformatting' of the ancient city, replacing a representation of society in terms of citizen and non-citizen with one resting on the polarity of rich and poor (in both city and countryside). Basil's philanthropic project was uncomfortably ambiguous. He was acting in some respects like a wealthy civic benefactor, using his personal means to establish an amenity that was above all a memorial to his wealth and generosity. He was an old-style euergetist, a 'nourisher' (*tropheus*) of his city.[31] The pagan tradition of civic public building and distributions had begun to atrophy in Asia Minor, as in other parts of the empire, during the third century.[32] Even so, enough of it presumably remained, in ideal if not in practice, to provide a template against which Basil's activities sat very awkwardly. His objective was radically new: a foundation that explicitly benefited the pauper, not the citizen. He was advertising his claims to civic leadership, as a 'lover of the poor' rather than a lover of his city.[33] It is no coincidence that the Basileias was soon echoed by smaller hospitals dotted across the Cappadocian countryside and over-seen by another fourth-century innovation, 'country bishops'.[34] Neither the old city nor its new suburb, but rather the poor wherever they were, defined the bishop's sphere of action.

III

This is looking ahead, to some wider ramifications of Basil's initiative. And looking ahead, though tempting, makes it hard to recapture (so familiar does the hospital seem) the sheer novelty of Basil's conception. Let us therefore go back and start at the very beginning of the story – or at least attempt to do so, since the evidence is fragmentary, mostly written some time after the actions described, and often sharply partisan.[35] It has been claimed that we should start in the 320s, with the infirmary (and perhaps the guest house) of what is usually taken as the first monastery, that of Pachomius at Tabennesi (north of Thebes in Egypt). Thus, it is argued, the 'place where the sick brothers lie' referred to in, for instance, the Bohairic (Coptic) *Life* of Pachomius should count as the first Christian hospital.[36] Those who redacted, or even framed, the various rules ('precepts') for Pachomian monks also hint at a designated place for the sick. But the evidence of the infirmary, like so much else in the Pachomian dossier, is uncertain. The biographers and redactors may on some points speak to us of developments after the founder's death in 346. And in any case, still more to the point, Pachomius was not establishing a 'public' hospital for the poor. Some paupers might have taken temporary refuge in the guest house, alongside those of greater means. But that is again not a facility with any broad ambition for the relief of the needy. Basil had visited Egypt in the mid-350s after his conversion to the ascetic life as a pilgrim collecting monastic experiences, but he would not have travelled as far south as the Pachomian monasteries; and like so many others in the later fourth century, he seems to have been largely ignorant of what Pachomius had achieved.[37]

For the first instance of a foundation that really seems to anticipate Basil's, we have to look a little later. We are now in the middle of the fourth century.

> The blessed Leontius, the bishop of Antioch in Syria, a man who was in all respects faithful . . . for the true faith [which others dubbed Arianism], who also had responsibility for the hospices [*xenodo-cheia*] for the care of strangers, appointed men who were devout in their concern for these, among whom were three men exceedingly zealous in piety.

So, in his entry for the year 350, writes the author of the *Chronicon Paschale* (Easter Chronicle), perhaps a clerical bureaucrat in the Great Church in Constantinople in the early seventh century, but dependent on local official chronologies as well as on the somewhat unreliable historian Philostorgius.[38] Leontius is mentioned to introduce the three men who help run the hospitals in Antioch; and they in turn appear in the narrative only because they miraculously convert a scornful Jew, who comes to work alongside them in one of those hospitals. We should not put too much emphasis on the date 350. Leontius was patriarch of Antioch from 344 to 358. The hospitals are not represented as his personal creation. But then, to the author of the *Chronicon Paschale*, writing over two and a half centuries later, they are a mere incidental detail, by his time a thoroughly familiar part of the ecclesiastical landscape. He is not interested in their specific origins. On the other hand, there was no reason for him to invent this rather slight incidental detail in the short narration of a miracle, which takes us (we may guess) back into the 340s. It is thus one of the very earliest creditable references that we have to Christian hospitals for the local poor or strangers.[39]

At about the same time in Constantinople, one Macedonius was, after a bloody and protracted struggle and the intervention of the emperor Constantius II, installed as bishop.[40] Some of the support that facilitated his installation apparently came from monasteries that he had already founded in the city. These monasteries were administered by a deacon called Marathonius, 'a zealous superintendent [*epitropos*] of the hospitals for the poor [*ptocheia*] and the monastic houses of men and women', according to the mid-fifth-century ecclesiastical historian Sozomen.[41] It is not clear that Macedonius the bishop himself founded hospitals; nor is it clear when those under the deacon Marathonius were established. But we do know that Marathonius, formerly a bureaucrat from the office of the praetorian prefect, was converted to the life of asceticism, monasteries, and charity by Eustathius of Sebaste, some time before 356, and presumably around the time that Macedonius was struggling to become bishop of Constantinople.[42]

Eustathius (*c.*300–*c.*380) was a powerful and controversial figure, but to us he is wrapped in some obscurity.[43] His father had been bishop of Sebaste (modern Sivas in Turkey) in Byzantine Armenia Minor. He was linked, by his many detractors, to the 'Arian' movement in Alexandria. In his middle years, he shuttled between Constantinople, Cappadocia, Armenia, and Pontus. In 339, and then again in 343, his following was condemned by provincial church councils for, in the words of Sozomen, founding 'a society of monks' and propounding 'a monastic philosophy'.[44] His supporters, at least as characterized by those who condemned them, were extremely ascetic, and also radical in their treatment of slaves and women. It was some refraction of their ideas that underlay the monasteries of Constantinople, the first monasteries in the city. Despite being anathematized by the Council of Gangra, Eustathius was chosen as bishop of Sebaste (his father's see) around 356. There, he founded a *ptochotropheion*. This could have been a soup kitchen, but is more likely, given the term's subsequent usage, not least by Basil, to have been a hospice for the poor, or hospital.[45] The connection between Basil and Eustathius is controversial. Basil had been influenced by him in the early stages of his ascetic career, but perhaps not since, and probably not as a philanthropist.

Next in chronological sequence, under the year 360 the *Chronicon Paschale* reports that Constantius was making provision for the hospitals of Constantinople, and this, too, seems to look forward to Basil and the imperial patronage that he would enjoy from Valens.[46]

A final piece of evidence to add to the dossier takes us outside the empire, to the other side of the Euphrates frontier and into the Christian kingdom of Armenia. Here, some time between 353 and 358, the Patriarch Nerses reportedly used grants of royal land to create a network of rural hospitals for the shelter and, indeed, the confinement of the poor, the sick, lepers, and paralytics, who might otherwise turn into troublesome beggars. The report dates from the later-fifth-century anonymous Armenian *Epic Histories* that have traditionally been attributed to P'austos Buzand (sometimes mistransliterated as Faustus of Byzantium).[47] By itself, neither the information nor its chronology would be very reliable. But the retrospective placing of the patriarch's initiative in the 350s fits well with the phase of hospital foundations to the west that we have just reviewed, and is not wholly implausible. Basil visited some part of Armenia in 373. There is also some indirect evidence that the Armenian hospitals reflected the example of hospitals both in Constantinople and also in Eustathius's much nearer episcopal see of Sebaste. The probability that radical ascetic ideas associated with Eustathius achieved some currency in the Armenian kingdom is signalled by the fact that the canons of the Council of Gangra anathematizing his adherents were translated into Armenian and incorporated into the Armenian Church's body of canon law.[48]

IV

Basil's is the early charitable development documented in contemporary or near-contemporary writing. (There is seemingly no archaeology of Caesarea to help us.) If we allow some later but credible evidence into the dossier – from up to the fifth century – then the background to his initiative is to be found only in immediately preceding decades. It does not come from much earlier than the 340s or 350s. That is, the short-term background is the only background. The hospital – a designated charitable arena for the overnight relief of the needy explicitly designated as such – turns out to be a quite recent invention in Basil's time. Emperors and monks and bishops seem to be the leading players. Especially if we here discount the Pachomian infirmary, many of them can be linked to the circle of Basil's erstwhile mentor,

Eustathius, and thus to a particular period of no more than thirty years and a particular set of places: Constantinople and a few cities in Asia Minor.

To make explicit the underlying point: the first hospitals were Christian; and they were mid-fourth-century. That entails several negatives. First, we are in the reign of Constantius II (337–361) and then, for Basil's enterprise in welfare, of Valens (364–378). We are not in the reign of Constantine, whose largesse to the Christian Church he 'established' was unprecedented in scale and included much charity, but no hospitals – or at least so it appears if we reject what, in this context, is late evidence, projecting onto the founding figure an image actually elaborated by his successors.[49]

A fortiori, we are not in pre-Constantinian times. In its first two centuries at least, early Christian charity was limited, discriminating in its reach, introverted. This is no place to defend that assertion fully.[50] We should simply note its important corollary: hospitals ('indoor' or overnight relief on an institutional scale) seem to have had no place in it. This charity is focused for the most part on distributions – outdoor relief – of money, food, and clothing. The infrastructure of house churches, characteristic of the first two Christian centuries and, to a considerable extent, of the third as well, probably could not support a room or building designated for overnight support. There is no sign of any such accommodation in the tiny early Christian complex at Dura Europos, and nor should we expect there to be.[51] The culture of early Christian charity was, indeed, in some respects the converse of the hospital: a culture of mobility, which comes down to us in letters of 'peace' or 'recommendation' carried by travellers who are of the faith.[52]

The accommodation required by such people was, or was meant to be, of limited duration, and to be offered mainly by the bishop. But a guest room is not, ideologically speaking, in terms of its public expression, a hospital – although it might have resembled one in a material sense. And when, in early Christian writings, we can catch sight of charity in action, the emphasis is always on the great outdoors of need dispersed across the city. Tertullian outlines the varieties of aid to which the common charitable pot was dedicated in the Carthaginian Church of his day (toward 200):[53] no 'indoor' relief, no overnight shelter, but support and burial for the poor and help for orphans and the elderly, the shipwrecked, and those condemned to the mines, exile, or imprisonment. Cyprian of Carthage is the best documented charitable bishop from the pre-Constantinian centuries, and even in the extreme circumstances of an epidemic, he does not seem to have provided a roof over the heads of any of the needy.[54] In the middle years of the third century, he was using poor relief – presumably any form of it at his ready disposal – to demonstrate and consolidate the Christian population under his bishopric. But there is no mention of a hospital in his surviving correspondence. From the middle of the third century again (251, to be exact) we have the well-known letter from the bishop of Rome, Cornelius, listing all those maintained by his church, from priests down to doorkeepers and 'more than 1500 widows and indigent people'.[55] But as well as noting the scale of his operation, in what was probably the largest Christian community in the empire at that time, we should also register what the list seemingly does not contain: no administrators, attendants, or inmates of a hospital, at least not as such. Roman indigents were more likely to have benefited from 'outdoor' relief. Distributions were the thing, such as that presumably intended to be made from the store of aristocratic cast-offs itemized in the early-fourth-century inventory of the church at Cirta, North Africa.[56] The Egyptian papyri in many respects take us as close we can get anywhere in the later Roman world to the everyday life of the church. It is significant that in the surviving fragments there is no mention of hospitals from much earlier than the sixth century.[57]

In all this, the only place of overnight relief was the bishop's house. General episcopal hospitality was urged in Pauline epistles,[58] and shelter of the destitute was attributed to bishops in a parable of *The Shepherd of Hermas*.[59] How was it manifested in practice?

> Coming home late one night, he found a poor woman lying in the street, so much exhausted that she could not walk: he took her upon his back, and carried her to his house, where he discovered that she was one of those wretched females who had fallen into the lowest state of vice, poverty and disease. Instead of harshly upbraiding her he had her taken care of with all tenderness for a long time, at a considerable expense, till she was restored to health.

This was no bishop, but Dr. Johnson as reported by Boswell.[60] It is quite hard to find late antique evidence of such hospitality in action. A letter preserved by Eusebius from the bishop of Corinth to Soter, the bishop of Rome, written in about 170, praises his paternal care for all visitors (not especially the poor).[61] Cyprian, from his exile, urges his priests to support strangers from his personal funds.[62]

V

So far, all the examples have been Christian; and indeed, the evidence, such as it is, in general suggests that the hospital of this period is a Christian invention of the fourth century. For support, we can look briefly at three other religio-cultural traditions: Zoroastrianism, paganism, and Judaism.

The first can be disposed of briefly. The relevance of Zoroastrianism is to those hospitals of Nerses in the kingdom of Armenia. In Nerses's time, the kingdom lay firmly within the orbit of Sasanid Iran, and part of it would soon be ruled directly by the Iranian shahs. Nerses was a 'protector of the poor' in a Christian, but also in an Iranian-Zoroastrian, tradition.[63] Yet, while Zoroastrian charity took many documented forms, several of which resemble Christian charity, the endowment of hospitals was apparently not among them. There are no known Iranian precedents for Nerses's charitable initiative. For inspiration, he might well therefore, as already surmised, have looked westward, into Roman Asia Minor.[64]

As for paganism, now is the moment to introduce one of the greatest tributes paid to Christian charity by one of Christianity's most resolute imperial opponents. In 362, having arrived at Ancyra (modern Ankara) en route to the Persian frontier, the emperor Julian famously wrote to Arsacius, the high priest of Galatia:[65]

> In every city establish frequent hospitals [*xenodocheia*] in order that strangers [migrant poor?] may benefit from our benevolence [*philanthropia*] . . . whoever is in need. . . . For it is disgraceful that, when no Jew ever has to beg and the impious Galilaeans [i.e., Christians] support not only their own poor but ours as well, our own people should seem destitute of support from us.

That passage is well known to specialists and frequently cited. Less often noticed is the striking range of institutions that the emperor is said (polemically, by Gregory Nazianzen) to want to found. They included not only hospitals for the needy, but inns, houses of virgins, 'sacred places' (*hagneuteria*), and academies – a strange refraction of the Judaeo-Christian exemplar.[66] Also less often noticed is the emperor's admiration (reported, it must again be conceded, only by Christians) for the Christian network of contacts and especially of episcopal hospitality represented by the practice of equipping the traveller with letters of recommendation. This, according to Sozomen, was the aspect of church organization that he chiefly admired.[67] But his own letter attests that what has brought him up short is the recent proliferation of hospitals in certain cities of the empire, especially in Syria and Armenia.

There was no pagan tradition on which Julian could draw. Temples may have offered shelter or distributions to pilgrims (who might be poor on arrival, if not on departure from home). But they did not do this as an explicit contribution to poor relief. Accommodation at healing shrines was there to facilitate prolonged attendance at the shrine. It was not part of the healing, and presumably it had to be paid for, if only in kind.[68]

For a relatively brief period, the Romans had occasionally built hospitals (*valetudinaria*) for slaves and soldiers: buildings within which the two categories of labourers who mattered most to the functioning of the empire might be repaired when broken down and then sent back to work.[69] Slave hospitals were favoured by some of the richest owners from the first century BCE to the end of the first century CE. That is, they came to be built when the supply of slaves through conquest had diminished, prices had risen, and it was worth maintaining those who could work and breed. When the empire's crucial labour force became *coloni*, tied to the land and living in quasi-peasant households, slave hospitals were no longer economical or indeed necessary.

The chronology of the rise and fall of military hospitals is later, but can be explained in similar structural-cum-economic terms. These hospitals date from the time of Augustus until around the middle of the third century CE. They correspond to the period when the army was often operating well beyond the frontier in areas largely bereft of friendly settlements where sick and wounded soldiers could be helpfully accommodated. When, in the third century, the army was reorganized and a local militia, supported where needed by a mobile field army, defended the frontier, the construction of fortress hospitals ceased. Sick soldiers were thereafter cared for by their families or in their tents – just as sick *coloni* were tended by their wives or relatives. The age of Roman hospitals was over. Even at its height, moreover, neither kind of hospital was at all widespread. The Roman writer known as Hyginus implied that a hospital was to be found in every fortress. Yet the archaeological evidence is slight – slighter than used to be thought because the identification of a number of proposed sites of *valetudinaria* has been questioned.[70] About the number and distribution of slave hospitals even less is known. These hospitals – to repeat – belong to a highly specific niche in Roman history. They reflect a calculation of the economies of scale to be made by the directed reconstitution of the workforce. Such a calculation is quite removed from late antique thinking about the poor, and will not be repeated until the later Middle Ages in Italy, when hospitals will once again attempt a rapid turnover of sick labourers.

Finally, the Jews. Were not Jewish hospitals the model for Christian ones?

> Theodotos, son of Vettenos the priest and *archisynagogos* . . . built the synagogue . . . and as a hostel with chambers and water installations for the accommodation of those who, coming from abroad, have need of it.

So runs a well-known inscription from first-century Jerusalem.[71] It has been claimed as marking the first Jewish medical hospital. But there is no reason to think that doctors attended those staying in it. Three aspects of the establishment should, rather, be stressed. First, as a 'hostel with chambers', it resembles the already-mentioned hostels that could be found near any major shrine in the ancient world. The Temple in Jerusalem was perhaps the largest temple of its time, and virtually the sole focus of Jewish pilgrimage. It undoubtedly attracted far more visitors than did most pagan shrines, which would come fully to life only once or twice a year for a great festival. Its facilities were presumably offered in a more charitable spirit than the pagan ones were. Still, it is no surprise that the Jerusalem synagogue of the first century CE, whether before or after the destruction of the Second Temple in the year 70, should cater to needy visitors. The second, more surprising feature is that there seems to have been no wider system of organized charity in Jerusalem at the time; individual initiatives such as that of Theodotos were crucial.[72] Third, there is little or no specific evidence of other such hospices attached to synagogues in the first three or four centuries CE – despite a number of rabbinic texts showing that travellers might be lodged within a synagogue precinct.[73] Clear archaeological, epigraphic, and documentary evidence is simply lacking. If lodging was to be had at synagogues, it was perhaps offered informally, ad hoc – as in the bishop's house. There was, apparently, no distinct, and distinctively named, hospital. The paradox of the Jerusalem hostel is, therefore, that it blends far better into a pagan than a Jewish context. And it looks forward to Christian hospitals of almost three centuries later rather than standing in a demonstrable tradition of its own. Perhaps not coincidentally, the one Jewish charitable institution of late antiquity that can be documented, albeit tentatively, is a soup kitchen rather than a hospital.[74]

With the exception, then, of the Roman *valetudinaria* – specialized in function, immensely different in character from later Christian hospitals, and long defunct by the time of the first Christian hospitals – there were probably no hospitals at all in the Mediterranean world or the Middle East before the reign of Constantius II. To that extent, the Christian hospitals of the fourth century really do mark a break with the past.

VI

How can we measure the success of this novel development? Julian is probably the first and most significant, if hostile, witness to its rapid impact. Granted, he was reacting to Jewish as well as to Christian charity. But it was perhaps only Christian hospitals that he could imitate. A sermon once attributed to John Chrysostom, and presumably of his time, refers to Christian *xenodocheia* as being evident throughout the inhabited world.[75] That was claiming too much. But it is arresting to find the learned Nilus of Ancyra (d. *c.*430) redeploying in his correspondence the older metaphor of Christ the physician as active in the 'hospital' of the world.[76] The idea had caught on, and it changed the way bishops responded to crisis. If we can trust the detail of Palladius on this, Ephrem the Syrian improvised a hospital in Edessa in a time of food shortage, arranging some 300 beds and covering for them in the city's porticoes. It is unlikely that a bishop would have responded in such a way a few decades earlier.[77] Ephrem's initiative would have been in 372–373, when Basil's hospital complex might not have been finished. By 398, there was at least one hospital in Constantinople besides the monastic foundations outlined earlier. On arrival as bishop, Chrysostom studied the church's accounts (a revealing detail in Palladius's *Life* – would they had survived), transferred to the hospital (*nosokomeion*) the surplus he found in those accounts, and later established other hospitals, installing in them monastic doctors, cooks, and attendants.[78] It was not, however, only in such major centers that the need was felt. Fifth-century Syrian canons decree that *xenodocheia* should be established in each town, and *plebia* (poor houses) are legislated about at the Council of Chalcedon.[79] Occasional inscriptions also reveal to us hospitals in quite minor or remote towns – well below the radar of chronicler or hagiographer.[80]

Most such hospitals will have been small. True, we read from time to time of multistory structures and hospitals of seventy or even two hundred beds.[81] To estimate the numbers of patients, we should also probably double the number of beds, as almost all but the most lavish medieval founders would do. Nor should we take the enumeration of beds for granted, when the more flexible (and space-saving?) provision of straw or pallets was always a possibility.[82] Yet the large places were exceptional. So was the hospital in Constantinople, glimpsed in the prism of seventh-century hagiography, that was big enough to have more than one ward and to offer surgery and specialist help for eye diseases.[83] Other foundations were big enough to segregate the patients by gender.

To conclude that most hospitals were small is not to reduce them to a single model. Although they were all supposed to come under episcopal supervision, hospitals were variously planned, founded, endowed, and supported by members of the imperial family, aristocrats, clerics, monks, and private lay families or individuals. We have already seen a variety of labels in the written evidence: *nosokomeia* explicitly for the sick, *xenodocheia* or *xenones* ostensibly for poor transients, *ptocheia* or *ptochotropheia* for the indigent, and leper houses. We can add lying-in hospitals, orphanages, old people's homes, and (mostly, after our period) a few houses for the blind and for repentant prostitutes. What we do not find, though it might have been expected, is any sign of a hospital explicitly for plague victims, although foundations of the later sixth century may indirectly reflect the pandemic's ravages: the 'plague of Justinian' is a nonevent in the world of hospitals, as it is in the medical world.[84]

This variety may tell us more about the ambitions of founders to distinguish their creations than about the specific needs of beneficiaries. The links between poverty, rootlessness, and ill health in premodern or modern developing societies are obvious enough. They blurred most of the boundaries that founders tried to maintain in the functions they set for their establishments. Perhaps less obvious are the equally resilient links between 'high' medicine and basic nursing and between secular and religious therapies – links that confound any attempt to separate medical establishments from the rest. In late ancient medical thinking, attention to the patient's psychology and environment – the provision of spiritual comfort, clean water, and wholesome food – *was* part of medicine. Christ, the physician of souls, stood behind, or rather above, the secular physician of bodies, and the two kinds of therapy complemented each other. Granted, a self-styled doctor might cost more than a lay attendant, and hospital benefactors will have taken this into account. But those founders who added *iatroi* to the personnel of their institutions were not necessarily raising them into a superior category of therapeutic excellence. The hospital, as a supposed 'revolution in the organization of medical care,' in fact had no discernible impact upon – indeed, is not mentioned in – the surviving medical writing of late antiquity.[85]

That is also why it is implausible to suggest that Justinian so highly esteemed the medicine available in hospitals that he somehow transferred (in an edict for which there is no direct evidence) the 'public physicians' (*archiatroi*) to the hospitals, ensuring the place of hospital medicine in the front line of medical teaching and practice for centuries to come. It was not like that. The medicine of the hospitals we are looking at blends into the wider scene, not only of basic medication and nursing but also of the charitable provision of rest and protection from the elements, vital for sick poor and healthy poor alike. Of course, hospital medicine was not everywhere the same. Those in the capital with doctors on call will have been the more sophisticated in their resources – pharmacopoeias, *instrumentaria* – culminating (perhaps) well after the end of our period in the hospital of the twelfth-century Pantocrator monastery. For the majority, I suggest, it is unhelpful to ask whether medicine was available to the inmates and who dispensed it.[86]

How many hospitals were there? Counting such places in Byzantium has a venerable history. It began in 1680 with Du Cange's *Constantinoplis Christiana*, which listed some 35 charitable foundations in the capital. Janin's more recent, but not wholly reliable, tabulation for Constantinople finds thirty-one hospitals (*xenones* and others) and 27 old people's homes.[87] The most recent gathering of material from the provinces, reaching forward to the ninth century, supplies a total of more than 160 charitable facilities, of which the most numerous are *xenodocheia* and *xenones* (71), *nosokomeia* (44), and *ptocheia* (21).[88] All such aggregates are to be greeted with caution. Some small hospitals will have eluded those who produced the extant documents; others – such, anyway, is the lesson of later hospital history – will rapidly have gone out of business. Still, these totals are likely to represent a considerable underestimate. The study of inscriptions and sealings will surely bring further instances to light. And already the Egyptian papyri are presenting a much more densely populated picture than other kinds of evidence could supply.

Overall, we seem to have some 75 references to hospitals in Egypt from about 550 to about 700, including those of Alexandria.[89] Most of these derive from papyri related to middle Egypt. A few village hospitals are evident, but the majority cluster in the capitals of three districts (*nomes*). One of these, Hermopolis, seems, in the first half of the seventh century, to have had as many as seven *nosokomeia* in operation at the same time.[90] Although such foundations all eventually fell to some degree under episcopal supervision, many of the hospitals attested in the papyri will have been small private affairs, and the papyri offer an incomparable (if inevitably very partial and fragmentary) ground-level view of their endowment and staffing. We learn of one hospital run, exceptionally, by a family of *archiatroi*, and another with a female administrator. We may at least entertain the possibility that other relatively small towns and villages across the empire (not to mention the metropolis) were as well supplied with charitable accommodation.

VII

If that were so, it would complicate the question of why hospitals were founded. The private Egyptian ones, which originally had little to do with bishops or monks, seem, with a few exceptions, to date from the sixth century onward and may therefore represent a second wave of foundations, in which the philanthropic projects of emperors, bishops, and monks of the fourth to fifth centuries were widely required and imitated.

Why were those earlier ones founded? We should at once admit a genuine role for compassion, the 'care of the poor' that is such a feature of the 'discourse' and practice of the period under review.[91] Of course, there was a degree of self-interest involved, too. The imitation *of* Christ in charitable acts was a form of giving *to* Christ and as such (the Gospels had demonstrated) was a considerable down payment on the 'purchase of paradise': Luke 11:41: 'give alms and all things will be clean unto you.' Both founders of charities and donors to them would hope to have earned the gratitude and prayers of the recipients of their generosity, and the prayers of the poor would benefit their souls in the afterlife more than those of almost anyone else. Founders could also enjoy wider secular renown among their contemporaries, especially if their association with a charity was publicized in its name.[92]

Explanation in this form is too general for hospitals, however. It could apply to a wider range of charitable practices and an extensive variety of charitable foundations, such as the soup kitchen or the distribution of clothing. We need greater precision, an explanation that captures the chronology, types, and distribution of the hospitals we have been looking at. These hospitals cannot – or cannot only – be seen as a normal expression of the charitable imperative; otherwise, we might have found them in pre-Constantinian times. To take an example from outside the Byzantine world that was probably not at all extreme: Augustine's episcopal complex at Hippo (Bone, in modern Algeria) in the early fifth century had 120 or so rooms. There was surely space there for the accommodation of some of the deserving needy (à la Dr. Johnson), and doubtless space was found. Yet it took the energy of a priest, Leporius, whom Augustine had ordained, to bring into being Hippo's first *xenodochium* (the Latinized Greek is telling). Of course, there will have been organizational tasks inherent in that process that now escape us – the assignment of rents and donations, the provision (perhaps) of beds and bedding on a greater scale than ad hoc hospitality demanded, the recruiting of attendants (perhaps even some with medical skills) and of an administrator. Still, the impression given is that to found a hospital is an ideological statement, rather than just the construction or designation of some rooms.[93]

The significance of ideology in the making of hospitals is one reason why an explanation of their proliferation in simple terms of demography will not quite work. The *xenodocheion* is a place for *xenoi*, strangers, migrants, the rootless. Leporius himself had been a refugee. One (probably) fifth-century story from Syria of an anonymous 'man of God' has him, as the scion of a senatorial family in Rome, taking ship and ending up in Edessa. There he lived a life of unremitting prayer and austerity among the indigent begging outside the church, an *aksnoyo*, a stranger, who, when ill, was placed in the 'place for strangers', the hospital.[94] Having read such narratives, we may be tempted to see the proliferation of hospitals as a reflex response to demographic change, especially migration. Certainly, particular crises could be a stimulus to action, as in Basil's case. Yet it is not clear that, in the fourth or fifth centuries, the countryside of the eastern Mediterranean was on the verge of Malthusian crisis, of a kind that might promote more than the usual influx of migrants to the bigger cities. There is no sign of general overpopulation. We find strong demographic growth and agricultural expansion, undeniably, but they express themselves in prosperous villages and farmsteads that were unlikely to have been generating enough casualties of the system to account, by themselves, for the development of new kinds of poor relief.[95]

The strangers of the 'place for strangers,' the *xenodocheion*, must be differently conceived. Man is a wanderer, Basil had asserted in a heated exchange with the prefect Modestus, 'confined to no place'.[96] All Christians are strangers (*xenoi*) and sojourners, in need of hospitality and accommodation, but not in a commercial, seedy inn or *pandocheion* – to which the hospital is perhaps a deliberate antithesis.[97] We thus need to turn from potential economic or social causes to explanations that have more to do with the Church and theology.

One such associates many of the very earliest hospitals, in fourth-century Constantinople and some cities of Asia Minor, with Arianism – that is, with a Christologically distinct 'party' of monks and bishops and a related type of asceticism that could have emphasized poor relief. The difficulty with this approach is that, outside the crude polemics of the self-appointed orthodox, Arianism did not yet exist as a particular affiliation in the middle of the fourth century. There was only a wide spectrum of views on the Christology at issue, and the only evidence of an association between their various proponents and a style of charity is the charity itself, so the argument is circular as well as reductive.[98]

More pertinent, and transcending all such supposed divisions among fourth-century clerics, is the way poor relief generally and hospitals in particular displayed the breadth of the Church's social concerns, its 'bracketing' of the whole free population (not slaves), its promotion of a new 'aesthetic of society' in which 'rich and poor' had replaced 'citizen and non-citizen' as the defining polarity.[99] The fourth-century Church benefited from valuable tax immunities. It needed a highly visible symbol of its deployment of the wealth generated not only by these immunities but also by massive imperial and aristocratic largesse, as well as by the small donations of ordinary believers. It needed some form of 'conspicuous expenditure'. The hospital highlighted the needy as the defining group in the new Christian representation of society. It legitimated the Church's wealth by showing that it was being channelled into purposes that no one could reasonably question.

This explanation applies best in cities, where episcopal leadership had to be asserted and maintained and where wealth was concentrated. But monasteries situated away from major episcopal centres could, however subliminally, deploy a related justification to their benefactors for their poor relief and care for guests. These, too, were a visible return for blessings received.[100] Of course, there were always balances to be struck. How much wealth should be put into charity as against other forms of generally approved expenditure? Should monks cripple their domestic economy through charity to passing vagrants, who might not even be Christian? Should bishops build churches rather than hospitals? Both churches and hospitals came, in law, to fall into the same category of 'divine' (*theioi*) or 'sacred houses' (*euageis oikoi*),[101] and we should not be swayed by the decoration of churches or the likely austerity of hospitals into separating them too starkly as expressions of piety. Nonetheless, hard choices often presented themselves. Finding a surplus in the accounts, Chrysostom opted for more hospitals. In the Syriac story of the 'man of God' in Edessa, the great monk-bishop Rabbula is presented as converting from 'other business' to charity after finding the empty grave of the anonymous holy man, who had died in hospital. 'He desisted from constructing many buildings.'[102] Admittedly, his purported reasoning had nothing to do with the involuntary poor. It was of greater concern that any indigent in the hospital might be a saint incognito: 'who knows whether there are many like this saint who delight in abasement, but are nobles to God in their souls, not recognized by the people.' Rabbula was indeed reputed, by his own biographer, to have shunned great building projects, to have transformed what was a hospital in name only into a well-endowed establishment with clean linen and soft beds, and to have created a hospital for women.[103] A hospital was thus, as we might put it, a step up from out-door distribution, an architectural expression of the welfare promotion of churches and monasteries. But it was also a step down, or perhaps sideways, from extravagant church-building.[104]

Decisions about the direction to take could be controversial. We have seen that in Basil's case. There must have been many other such disputes. When Chrysostom built a suburban leper hospital, the local landowners were reportedly angered because property values declined, as well as fearful of contagion.[105] Wherever they emerged, but especially in the civic context, hospitals reconfigured spaces, much more so than other forms of institutional charity, precisely because of their forcible combination of architecture and ideology. Part of the ideological context within which hospitals have to be understood is thus the Christian 'production of space'. That did not only involve churches and hospitals as spaces for poverty and its relief. It is no coincidence that the first stages of the history of Christian cemeteries for the poor matches, so far as we can tell from the limited evidence, the chronology of early hospitals. The poor gained their own space in death as they, or some of them, gained their own space in life.[106]

Rehearsing various possible explanations for the first hospitals, sight of the poor patients themselves has been somewhat lost. Apart from a handful of laudatory vignettes (e.g. Rabbula's bed linen), we can say little about the regular inmates or patients of hospitals. Who were they, economically, socially? How long did they stay? In what circumstances, death apart, did they leave? Gregory Nazianzen's advocacy of the hospital as a 'sweet stair-way to heaven' was hardly a demographic analysis of patient outcomes. How were these hospitals staffed, managed, and endowed? Again, stray glimpses of hospital directors apart, we cannot tell.[107] This is no accident. The church accounts that Chrysostom read, like the lists of paupers in receipt of alms that we know to have been compiled in this period, were of no interest to biographers or chroniclers. Holy ones masquerading as beggars were more to their taste. Not even the rubbish tips of Egypt give us much information about the daily running of a hospital, and what they do tell us is financial rather than personal or therapeutic. Nor does archaeology have much to add. Probably the biggest Byzantine hospital to have been excavated is that of St. Sampson in Constantinople. All that the portion dug reveals is a cluster of rooms around a courtyard – if the site has been correctly identi-fied. Separate wards and a substantial numbers of patients? Doubtless, but that is hardly new or surprising information. It has already come to us from the texts.[108]

VIII

Of such evidence, we want to ask the major question: what difference did hospitals make? By way of immediate answer, it is easy to advance some negative propositions and, in effect, cut hospitals down to size.

Did hospitals, for example, change the overall pattern of the transfer of alms between donors and recipients?[109] An earlier generation of hospital historians thought that hospitals and related types of institutionalized charity undermined the flow of spontaneous and ad hoc almsgiving from haves to have-nots. But support for both the poor and the clergy had, despite the contrary efforts of some aristocratic families, to a considerable extent been channelled through the bishop since the third century, if not the second. Church orders emphasize that the bishop is in a better position than the laity to identify recipients and organize connections and distributions. Not that begging on the streets or in church porticoes disappeared; far from it. The 'man of God' begged in church before sickness consigned him to the hospital. But whereas in the third century the bishops and deacons had to cajole to maintain collections of various forms, in the fourth century we find Chrysostom vehemently preaching that individual lay almsgiving has not been made redundant by such initiatives, and is still required. 'What I have to say about alms, I am not saying so that you bring them to me, but so that you yourself distribute with your own hands.'[110] The world of almsgiving remained a mixed economy, as it had been in pre-Constantinian times, a public-private partnership. The balance of ingredients varied in ways that will always elude us because of how little we know about the history of church finances. But it is at least reasonable to envisage hospitals as not, by themselves, having dramatically altered the overall blend.

On this somewhat negative side of the balance sheet, three further points of a comparative nature can tentatively be made.[111] First, there will have been many blanks on the map: areas where no hospitals or anything like them were to be found. Second, not only do the figures for size support the view that early medieval hospitals were small in comparison with, say, early modern ones; the figures for total numbers are small even by comparison with later periods within the Middle Ages. We know, for instance, of more than 300 hospitals for lepers alone founded in England between 1100 and 1250. That comfortably exceeds current estimates for the whole Byzantine empire, and over a much longer period.[112] Third, whether measured by average size or total numbers, the scale of hospital provision was easily dwarfed by other sources of social welfare. In late antiquity, the *annona* (dole) of grain and other foodstuffs in Rome, Constantinople, and even small towns such as Oxyrhynchus reached a far larger number of poorer people than any estimate we can hazard of the total hospital population. Hospital capacity was not only dwarfed by such state-run measures. It was also probably, in aggregate, surpassed even by the church's own 'outdoor' distributions to its local poor – those whose names were inscribed, sometimes in their thousands, on registers of the deserving (3,000 in Antioch, for instance).[113]

What can be said in a more positive vein? First, as argued before, we may entertain the possibility that, thanks to imperial patronage, the new establishments of the fourth century onward represented a massive increase in the scope of formal ecclesiastical charity by comparison with that of the pre-Constantinian centuries.

Second, hospitals could, as we have also seen, achieve in certain areas a considerable density. The patient turnover might also have been considerable. In Alexandria, John the Almsgiver established seven forty-bed hospitals for parturient women. The measure originated in a period of famine, but John's biographer writes as if the hospitals were intended to be permanent. So if the women each stayed for a week (as prescribed), the bishop could have facilitated more than 14,000 births a year.[114]

Third, we should envisage the economic and social difference that hospitals could make as not confined to the effects on inmates. Hospitals were sources of employment for priests, doctors (sometimes), nurses, attendants, gravediggers (if less often than has been imagined), builders, and maintenance staff of all kinds – many of whom will have been almost as poor as the designated inmates. A collectivity of quite small hospitals could, in aggregate, markedly have increased local opportunities in a world characterized by chronic underemployment.[115]

Fourth, hospitals reached beyond their walls in their services to the needy. Their functions sometimes (perhaps often) elided with those of 'outdoor' relief centres—soup kitchens, bathing facilities for the poor, charitable grain stores, and so forth. We should not think only in terms of inmates when assessing the impression they made.[116]

Fifth, we should register contemporary perceptions that hospitals had a significant effect on the poor. In the Christian kingdom of Armenia in the 350s, the decade in which the Christian hospital emerged in Byzantium, the patriarch Nerses, having very quickly appreciated the 'hospital idea', established a network of hospitals to help keep beggars off the streets. When the patriarch's enemy, King Pap, jealously destroyed these hospitals, the effect was, reportedly, to return the poor to beggary throughout the kingdom. The patriarch's hospitals are represented (admittedly more than a century after they were built) as having been all-embracing.[117]

What would have been the effect of a similar mass closure in Byzantium around 450 or 550? The answer must at least partly depend on our assessment of the effective demand for hospital places. This is not by any means necessarily coincident with the demand perceived by registrars of the poor, who tended to ignore or despise the 'labouring poor' (with large families) in favour of the biblically sanctioned categories of the needy, such as widows, orphans, and the sick. This effective demand must have varied markedly from area to area and, of course, cannot now be known with any precision.

Demand for hospital beds has often been measured by reference to estimates of the total population or of the likely number of poor and sick in the society in question—on which measure hospitals often fare poorly, because they could seldom have accommodated the 10 per cent or so in absolute penury, let alone the extra 20 to 30 per cent who might, at some point in the life cycle, need relief. But the massed ranks of the poor are, of course, only the potential demand. The effective demand – the actualization of that potential at any one time – will have been significantly less, because of self-help among the poor, on the one hand, and sources of charity other than hospitals, on the other.

These two sectors of help for the poor are easily mentioned and impossible to describe in detail.[118] Let us look first at what we can call the sources of 'vertical' relief – those from above, in social terms: from the state, the Church, individual benefactors. The respective proportions of these contributions can scarcely be estimated for any part of the period that concerns us. Moreover, it is not enough just to consider explicit sources of charity. The history of poor relief is much wider than the history of charity. We have to look for it in unlikely places and periods for instance, in the minimal care of sick slaves provided by owners (outside the few *valetudinaria*), in the whole grim history of debt bondage, in rural patronage, in distributions and benefactions that reached impoverished members of the citizen body and were provided by local pagan aristocrats who had no concept of charity, in distributions organized by temples. So in this context, to ask what difference hospitals made is hardly worthwhile. We cannot separate out the hospital contribution to the vertical component of poor relief. We cannot even say confidently that the establishment of Christianity and the proliferation of charitable institutions from the fourth century onward marked a decisive change in the relative strength of the vertical component, distinguishing later antiquity from classical antiquity, or the medieval from the ancient world. Charity may not have been a virtue in ancient pagan society, but poor relief could, whether directly or indirectly, have been practised – to an extent that is now wholly obscure.[119]

As for the 'horizontal' component in that relief – self-help and mutual aid among social equals – it has been argued on the basis of a wide comparative survey that we should not overestimate its strength or capacity. The large supportive households to which historians have unthinkingly attributed the overwhelming bulk of premodern support for the poor are hardly ever to be found. Pauper households were small and thus vulnerable. Networks of support operated between more than within them. And those networks were fragile and limited. They needed 'vertical' buttressing if their beneficiaries were to avoid sinking into criminality or terminal destitution.[120]

IX

The hospital is an idea, an invention, and not a reflex response to growing poverty in a Christianizing empire. That much is clear from the way the invention was diffused. It spread first, quite rapidly, around the Mediterranean from its Byzantine homeland in Asia Minor: westward to North Africa and Italy, and from Italy to Spain and parts of the Merovingian kingdoms.

And it spread eastward, more slowly, into the 'land of Islam' and, with Islam, across Asia. These hospitals are the distant but direct forebears of the modern biomedical hospital, the hospice, the night shelter, and a variety of other, related institutions. Their future does not belong here.[121] The history of hospitals has a beginning, which this chapter has attempted to trace, but, as yet, no end. Basil's ironic question, 'Are we harming anyone?' continues to resonate – as pertinent to the age of the so-called worried well as it was in the fourth century.

Notes

1 [Article reproduced by permission of Oxford University Press.] *Letter* 94, ed. Deferrari or Courtonne.
2 *Oration* 43, ed. Bernardi.
3 The literature on Basil's career and his philanthropy in this period, late 360s to early 370s, is copious, yet many aspects, not least chronology, remain controversial. The most helpful recent discussions are Finn 2006, 222–236; Holman 2001, 68–76; Brown 2002, 35–42. The best biography remains Rousseau 1994, but see also on philanthropy Giet 1941.
4 Garnsey 1988, 22–23; Stathakopoulos 2004, 200–202 (numbers 22, 23); Finn 2006, 222.
5 Homily VI.6, ed. Courtonne, with Holman 1999, 342.
6 Finn 2006, 224; Holman 2001, 4.
7 Mitchell 1993, 82; Holman 2001, 76.
8 Theodoret, *Historia Ecclesiastica* [hereafter *HE*] IV.16, ed. Parmentier and Hansen; Daley 1999, 440–441; for the imperial arms factory in Caesarea itself, see Mitchell 1993, 76.
9 Gregory Nazianzen, Letter 216, ed. Gallay.
10 *Oration* 43.63, ed. Bernardi; Sozomen, *HE* VI.34, ed. Bidez and Hansen.
11 Faroqhi 1987, 41; Daly 1999, 459; Finn 2006, 230–231.
12 Gregory Nazianzen, *Oration* 43.63.
13 Basil, *Letters* 94, 150, 176 (chapel), and cf. 143; Crislip 2005, 117; Holman 2001, 153–158. Orphans: Miller 2003, 115–116; Crislip 2005, 112–113.
14 Temkin 1991, 163, for Basil's own medical know-how.
15 Garnsey 1988, 23; Sen 1981.
16 *Chronicle of Pseudo-Joshua the Stylite*, 38, trans. Watt.
17 Faroqhi 1987, 43, 208.
18 Holman 2001, 70.
19 Neri 1998.
20 Brown 2002, 60, 65.
21 Patlagean 1977, chapter 1.
22 Finn, 2006, 69–70; Caner 2008, 228.
23 Holman 2001, 4–5.
24 Brown 2002, 61–2.
25 Holman 2001, 146–147; *Oration* 43.63.
26 *Letter* 43, ed. Calvet-Sebasti and Gabier.
27 Finn 2006, 3; *Sentences of Sextus* line 217, ed. Chadwick.
28 Henderson et al. 2007.
29 E.g. Miller 1997; van Minnen 1995.
30 Brown 2002, 26, 54–55. For the finances of the Cappadocian clergy, Hübner 2005.

31 Subtle discussion in Finn 2006, 224–226.
32 Zuiderhoek 2009, esp. 18, 156–159, 170.
33 Brown 2002; Rapp 2005, 219–228.
34 Basil, Letters 53, 142, 143; Hübner 2005, 62–63.
35 I shall not here look at early south Asian hospital history, on which see references in Henderson et al. 2007, 29–30; Horden 2005, 371.
36 Crislip 2005, 11, 20, with the Bohairic biography and the Greek *Vita prima* of Pachomius (sections 26, 28, respectively), trans. Veilleux. See also Chitty 1966, 22, with n. 22. On the Pachomian dossier, see Rousseau 1999, chapter 2. I am indebted also to forthcoming work by J. Grossmann.
37 Basil, Letter 223; Rousseau 1994, 54–55.
38 *Chronicon Paschale* s. a. 350, ed. Dindorf; trans. Whitby and Whitby.
39 Agreed by Brown 2002, 123, n. 121, *pace* Miller 1997, 21; note also p. 77 with 234, n. 62, for the possible mosaic evidence of another hospital 'of Leontius' in Daphne, a suburb of Antioch.
40 Elm 1994, 111; see also Dagron 1970, 238–239.
41 Sozomen, *HE* IV.20.2, ed. Bidez and Hansen.
42 Elm 1994, 112; Dagron 1970, 246–253.
43 Elm 1994, 106–110; Brown 2002, 36–39; Rousseau 1994, 233ff.
44 *HE* III.14.31.
45 Epiphanius, *Panarion* LXXV.3.7, ed. Holl and Dummer, with the skeptical comments on this evidence of Brown 2002, 37–38.
46 Miller 1997, 76, 93, attributes a 'network' of hospitals to the Arian George of Cappadocia after his consecration in 357 but is not supported by the passage from Epiphanius cited: LXXVI.1.6. This reads *ton xenon* (of strangers), not *ton xenonon* (of hospitals).
47 Trans. Garsoïan 1989, 115, 211, with Brown 2002, 42–44.
48 Garsoïan 1983, 166; Rousseau 1994, 64, 280; Brown 2002, 42–43. [The problems of chronology and the possible channels of reciprocal influence between Basil and Nerses are now discussed by Dumitraşcu 2018, 52–55.]
49 Miller 1997, 21, relies on an early-ninth-century, and on this topic unreliably late, text for hospitals supposedly founded or supported by Constantine: the *Chronicle* of Theophanes, sub A. M. 5824, ed. de Boor. Constantelos 1991, 89, uses a late biography of Constantine for that emperor's hospitals—again, I believe, unwisely. Constantelos also cites, p. 47, a canon (number 70) of the Council of Nicaea (325) that 'hospitals should be established in every city.' But this is a reference to the probably inauthentic Arabic text of over 80 canons, dependent on a Syriac original; hospitals do not appear in the original 20 canons. Compare Brown 2002, 123, n. 121.
50 The historiography is surveyed in Finn 2006, 26–31; Harnack 1908 remains classic. See also Grant 1977 chapter 6; Garnsey and Humfress 2001, 123–127.
51 Bowes 2008, 49–51; Doig 2008, 1–6.
52 Luijendijk 2008, 102–112.
53 *Apologeticum* XXXIX.5–6, ed. Dekkers.
54 *Letters* ed. Clarke, with Brown 2002, 24–25; Finn 2006, 258–259.
55 Eusebius, *HE* VI.43.11.
56 Finn 2006, 81.
57 van Minnen 1995; Luijendijk 2008; Serfass 2008.
58 1 Timothy 3:2; Titus 1:8.
59 *Similitude* IX.27.2, ed. Lake.
60 *Life of Johnson*, for 1784.
61 *HE* IV.23.10.

62 *Letter* 7.2, trans. Clarke, with Luijendijk 2008, 103–104.
63 Garsoïan 1981, 21–32.
64 Yarshater 1991, s.v. 'Charitable Foundations'. The first known Sasanian foundation of a hospital is that of the sixth century CE reported by (pseudo-)Zacharias Rhetor: *HE* XII.7, ed. Brooks.
65 *Letter* 22, ed. Wright; 84, ed. Bidez. For context, Kislinger 1984, and for a persuasive reassertion of this letter's authenticity in the face of some scholarly doubt, Bouffartigue 2005.
66 Gregory Nazianzen, *Oration* IV.111, ed. Bernardi, with Finn 2006, 87.
67 *HE* V.16.3; Luijendijk 2008, 111.
68 Hands 1968, 132.
69 For references to support what follows, see Horden 2005, 372–373.
70 Baker 2004.
71 Reinach 1920, 46–56; trans. from Fine 1996, 9.
72 Seccombe 1978, 140–143. For other synagogue hostels, see Kraeling 1979, 10ff.; Loewenberg 2001, 141ff., 153.
73 Safrai and Stern 1976, 943; Levine 2000, 381ff.
74 Reynolds and Tannenbaum 1987; Finn 2006, 267. On later Jewish hospitals, see Horden 2005, 374–375.
75 *On Matthew* VI.13; *PG* LIX.571.
76 *Letter* III.33; *PG* LXXIX.397; though see also Cameron 1976 on the textual problems presented by these letters.
77 *Lausiac History* 40, ed. Bartelink; Stathakopoulos 2004, 202–203 (number 23).
78 *Dialogue on the Life of St John Chrysostom* 5.128–139, ed. Malingrey and Leclercq.
79 Vööbus 1970, 129, 159; *Acts of the Council of Chalcedon*, canon 8, trans. Price and Gaddis.
80 *CIG* 9256 (Asia Minor).
81 Surveys and further references: Nutton 2004, 308; Constantelos 1991; Miller 1997.
82 *Life of the Man of God*, expanded Syriac version: Doran 2006, 38.
83 *Miracles of St Artemius* 21, trans. Crisafulli and Nesbit.
84 Horden 2005.
85 van Minnen 1995, 154; Temkin 1991, chapter 18.
86 Horden 2006, *contra* Miller 1997.
87 Du Cange 1680, 163–166; Janin 1969, 552–567.
88 Mentzou-Meimare 1982.
89 van Minnen 1995.
90 van Minnen 1995, 161, corrected from 8 to 7 by Serfass 2008, 101.
91 Brown 2002.
92 Horden 2007.
93 Brown 2003, 78; Augustine *Sermon* 356.10, *PL* XXXIX.1578.
94 *Life of the Man of God*, original Syriac version: Doran 2006, 20–23.
95 Lewit 2009; Laiou and Morrisson 2007, chapter 2; Decker 2009.
96 Gregory of Nazianzen, *Oration* 43.49.
97 Arterbury 2005; Hiltbrunner 2005, pt. 4; Dunning 2009; Constable 2003, 18–36.
98 Miller 1997, 76–85, largely and erroneously accepted in Horden 2004. See now Gwynn 2007.
99 For what follows, see Brown 1992, 94; 2002, 29–33; 2005.
100 Caner 2006; 2008.
101 Justinian, *Novel* 120; *Oxford Dictionary of Byzantium*, s.v. 'Euageis oikoi'.
102 *Life of the Man of God*, original Syriac version: Doran 2006, 24 (see also xv).

103 *The Heroic Deeds of Mar Rabbula*, Doran 2006, 100–101.
104 For context, see Janes 1998.
105 van Ommeslaeghe 1979, 151.
106 Rebillard 1999a; 1999b.
107 Hübner 2005, 32, 59.
108 Miller 1990; Lavan et al. 2007, 194–197.
109 For what follows, see Finn 2006, 27, 39, 40, 44, 107; Brown 1992, 95.
110 *Hom. on I Cor.* XXVI.6, *PG* LXI.179, with Finn 2006, 107.
111 For fuller references in support of what follows, see Horden 2004.
112 Rawcliffe 2006, 106–107.
113 Brown 2002, 27–28, 65; Herrin 1986, 153–154; Garnsey and Humfress 2001, 126–127; Finn 2006, 63.
114 *Life of John the Almsgiver* 7, ed. Festugière, trans. Dawes and Baynes.
115 Compare Patlagean 1977, 196–203.
116 For a hospital's distributions, see *P. Amh.* 154, *P. Bingen* 136, the latter discussed by Serfass 2008, 99–100.
117 Garsoïan 1989, 115, 211–212; Brown 2002, 42–43.
118 For what follows, see Horden 1998.
119 Brown 1992, 92–93; Atkins and Osborne 2006.
120 Horden 1998; Hübner 2012; see also for comparison Ben-Amos 2008.
121 But is sketched in Horden 2005; Henderson et al. 2007.

Bibliography

Arterbury, A. E. 2005. *Entertaining Angels: Early Christian Hospitality in its Mediterranean Setting.* Sheffield: Sheffield Phoenix.

Atkins, M., and R. Osborne, eds. 2006. *Poverty in the Roman World.* Cambridge: Cambridge University Press.

Baker, P. A. 2004. *Medical Care for the Roman Army on the Rhine, Danube, and British Frontiers.* Oxford: J. and E. Hedges.

Ben-Amos, I. K. 2008. *The Culture of Giving: Informal Support and Gift Exchange in Early Modern England.* Cambridge: Cambridge University Press.

Bouffartigue, J. 2005. 'L'authenticité de la Lettre 84 de l'empereur Julien', *Revue de philologie* 79: 231–242.

Bowes, K. 2008. *Private Worship, Public Values, and Religious Change in Late Antiquity.* Cambridge: Cambridge University Press.

Brown, P. R. L. 1992. *Power and Persuasion in Late Antiquity: Towards a Christian Empire.* Madison: University of Wisconsin Press.

Brown, P. R. L. 2002. *Poverty and Leadership in the Later Roman Empire.* Hanover, NH, and London: Brandeis University Press and Historical Society of Israel.

Brown, P. R. L. 2003. *The Rise of Western Christendom*, 2nd edn. Malden, MA: Blackwell.

Brown, P. R. L. 2005. 'Remembering the Poor and the Aesthetic of Society', *Journal of Interdisciplinary History* 35: 513–522.

Cameron, Alan. 1976. 'The Authenticity of the Letters of St Nilus of Ancyra', *Greek, Roman and Byzantine Studies* 17: 181–196.

Caner, D. 2006. 'Towards a Miraculous Economy: Christian Gifts and Material "Blessings" in Late Antiquity', *Journal of Early Christian Studies* 14: 329–377.

Caner, D. 2008. 'Wealth, Stewardship, and Charitable "Blessings" in Early Byzantine Monasticism', in *Wealth and Poverty in Early Church and Society*, ed. S. R. Holman, 221–242. Grand Rapids, MI: Baker Academic.

Chitty, D. 1966. *The Desert a City*. Crestwood, NY: St. Vladimir's Seminary Press.

Constable, O. R. 2003. *Housing the Stranger in the Mediterranean World*. Cambridge: Cambridge University Press.

Constantelos, D. J. 1991. *Byzantine Philanthropy and Social Welfare*, 2nd edn. New Rochelle, NY: Caratzas.

Crislip, A. 2005. *From Monastery to Hospital: Christian Monasticism and the Transformation of Health Care in Late Antiquity*. Ann Arbor: University of Michigan Press.

Dagron, G. 1970. 'Les moines et la ville: le monachisme à Constantinople jusqu'au concile de Chalcédoine (451)', *Travaux et mémoires* 4: 229–276.

Daley, B. E. 1999. 'Building a New City: The Cappadocian Fathers and the Rhetoric of Philanthropy', *Journal of Early Christian Studies* 7: 431–461.

Decker, M. 2009. *Tilling the Hateful Earth: Agricultural Production and Trade in the Late Antique East*. New York: Oxford University Press.

Doig, A. 2008. *Liturgy and Architecture: From the Early Church to the Middle Ages*. Aldershot: Ashgate.

Doran, R., trans. 2006. *Stewards of the Poor: The Man of God, Rabbula, and Hiba in Fifth-Century Edessa*. Kalamazoo, MI: Cistercian Publications.

Du Cange, C. Du F. 1680. *Historia Byzantina*, II: *Constantinopolis Christiana*. Paris: L. Billaine.

Dumitraşcu, N. 2018. *Basil the Great: Faith, Mission and Diplomacy in the Shaping of Christian Doctrine*. London: Routledge.

Dunning, B. H. 2009. *Aliens and Sojourners: Self as Other in Early Christianity*. Philadelphia: University of Pennsylvania Press.

Elm, S. 1994. *Virgins of God: The Making of Asceticism in Late Antiquity*. Oxford: Clarendon Press.

Faroqhi, S. 1987. *Men of the Modest Substance: House Owners and House Property in Seventeenth-Century Ankara and Kayseri*. Cambridge: Cambridge University Press.

Fine, S. ed. 1996. *Sacred Realm: The Emergence of the Synagogue in the Ancient World*. New York: Oxford University Press, Yeshiva University Museum.

Finn, R. 2006. *Almsgiving in the Later Roman Empire: Christian Promotion and Practice (313–450)*. Oxford: Oxford University Press.

Garnsey, P. 1988. *Famine and Food Supply in the Graeco-Roman World*. Cambridge: Cambridge University Press.

Garnsey, P., and C. Humfress. 2001. *The Evolution of the Late Antique World*. Cambridge: Orchard Academic.

Garsoïan, N. 1981. 'Sur le titre de *Protecteur des pauvres*', *Revue des études arméniennes*, n.s. 15: 21–31.

Garsoïan, N. 1983. 'Nersês le Grand, Basile de Césarée et Eustathe de Sébaste', *Revue des études arméniennes*, n.s. 17: 145–169.

Garsoïan, N., trans. 1989. *The Epic Histories Attributed to P'awstos Buzand*. Cambridge, MA: Harvard University Press.

Giet, S. 1941. *Les idées et l'action sociale de Saint Basile*. Paris: J. Gabalda.

Grant, R. M. 1977. *Early Christianity and Society*. New York: Harper and Row.

Gwynn, D. 2007. *The Eusebians*. Oxford: Oxford University Press.

Hands, A. R. 1968. *Charities and Social Aids in Greece and Rome*. London: Thames and Hudson.

Harnack, A. 1908. *Mission and Expansion of Christianity in the First Three Centuries*, 2nd edn. London: Williams and Norgate.

Henderson, J., P. Horden, and A. Pastore, eds. 2007. *The Impact of Hospitals 300–2000*. Oxford: Peter Lang.

Herrin, J. 1986. 'Ideals of Charity: Realities of Welfare', in *Church and People in Byzantium*, ed. R. Morris, 151–164. Birmingham: Centre for Byzantine, Ottoman and Modern Greek Studies.

Hiltbrunner, O. 2005. *Gastfreundschaft in der Antike und im frühen Christentum*. Darmstadt: Wissenschaftliche Buchgesellschaft.

Holman, S. R. 1999. 'The Hungry Body: Famine, Poverty, and Identity in Basil's *Hom.* 8', *Journal of Early Christian Studies* 7: 337–363.

Holman, S. R. 2001. *The Hungry Are Dying: Beggars and Bishops in Roman Cappadocia*. New York: Oxford University Press.

Horden, P. 1998. 'Household Care and Informal Networks: Comparisons and Continuities from Antiquity to the Present', in *The Locus of Care*, ed. P. Horden and R. M. Smith, 21–67. London: Routledge.

Horden, P. 2004. 'The Christian Hospital in Late Antiquity: Break or Bridge?' In *Gesundheit-Krankheit: Kulturtransfer medizinischen Wissens von der Spätantike bis in die Frühe Neuzeit*, ed. F. Steger and K. P. Jankrift, 76–99. Cologne: Böhlau.

Horden, P. 2005. 'The Earliest Hospitals in Byzantium, Western Europe, and Islam', *Journal of Interdisciplinary History* 35: 361–389.

Horden, P. 2006. 'How Medicalised were Byzantine Hospitals?' *Medicina e storia* 10: 45–74.

Horden, P. 2007. 'Alms and the Man: Hospital Founders in Byzantium', in *The Impact of Hospitals 300–2000*, ed. J. Henderson, P. Horden, and A. Pastore, 59–76. Oxford: Peter Lang.

Hübner, S. R. 2005. *Der Klerus in der Gesellschaft des spätantiken Kleinasiens*. Stuttgart: Steiner.

Hübner, S. R. 2012. *The Family in Roman Egypt: A Comparative Approach to Solidarity and Conflict*. Cambridge: Cambridge University Press.

Janes, D. 1998. *God and Gold in Late Antiquity*. Cambridge: Cambridge University Press.

Janin, R. 1969. *La géographie ecclésiastique de l'empire byzantin, première partie*, III: *Les églises et les monastères*, 2nd edn. Paris: Institut français d'études byzantines.

Kislinger, E. 1984. 'Kaiser Julian und die (Christlichen) Xenodocheia', in *BYZANTIOΣ: Festschrift für Herbert Hunger*, ed. W. Hörandner et al., 171–184. Vienna: Ernst Becvar.

Kraeling, C. H. 1979. *The Synagogue. The Excavations at Dura-Europos*, Final Report VIII, Part I, Aug. edn. New Haven, CT: Yale University Press.

Laiou, A., and C. Morrisson. 2007. *The Byzantine Economy*. Cambridge: Cambridge University Press.

Lavan, L., E. Swift, and T. Putzeys, eds. 2007. *Objects in Context, Objects in Use: Material Spatiality in Late Antiquity*. Leiden: Brill.

Levine, L. I., ed. 2000. *The Jewish Synagogue: The First Thousand Years*. New Haven, CT: Yale University Press.

Lewit, T. 2009. 'Pigs, Presses and Pastoralism: Farming in the Fifth to Sixth Centuries AD', *Early Medieval Europe* 17: 77–91.

Loewenberg, F. M. 2001. *From Charity to Social Justice: The Emergence of Communal Institutions for the Support of the Poor in Ancient Judaism*. New Brunswick, NJ: Transaction.

Luijendijk, A. 2008. *Greetings in the Lord: Early Christians and the Oxyrhynchus Papyri*. Cambridge, MA: Harvard University Divinity School.

Mentzou-Meimare, K. 1982. 'Eparchiaka evage idrymata mechri tou telous tes eikomomachias', *Byzantina* 11: 243–308.

Miller, T. S. 1990. 'The Sampson Hospital of Constantinople,' *Byzantinische Forschungen* 15: 101–135.

Miller, T. S. 1997. *The Birth of the Hospital in the Byzantine Empire*, 2nd edn. Baltimore: Johns Hopkins University Press.

Miller, T. S. 2003. *The Orphans of Byzantium: Child Welfare in the Christian Empire*. Washington, DC: Catholic University of America Press.

Mitchell, S. 1993. *Anatolia: Land, Men, and Gods in Asia Minor*, vol. 2. Oxford: Oxford University Press.

Neri, V. 1998. *I marginali nell'occidente tardoantico*. Bari: Edipuglia.

Nutton, V. 2004. *Ancient Medicine*. Abingdon: Routledge.

Patlagean, E. 1977. *Pauvreté économique et pauvreté sociale à Byzance 4e–7e siècle*. Paris: Mouton.

Rapp, C. 2005. *Holy Bishops in Late Antiquity*. Berkeley: University of California Press.

Rawcliffe, C. 2006. *Leprosy in Medieval England*. Woodbridge: Boydell.

Rebillard, E. 1999a. 'Église et sépulture dans l'antiquité tardive (occident latin, 3e–6e siècles)', *Annales* (Sept.–Oct.): 1027–1046.

Rebillard, E. 1999b. 'Les formes de l'assistance funéraire dans l'empire romain et leur évolution dans l'antiquité tardive', *Antiquité tardive* 7: 269–282.

Reinach, T. 1920. 'L'inscription de Théodotos', *Revue des études juives* 71: 46–56.

Reynolds, J., and R. Tannenbaum. 1987. *Jews and God-Fearers at Aphrodisias*. Cambridge: Cambridge Philological Society.

Rousseau, P. 1994. *Basil of Caesarea*. Berkeley: University of California Press.

Rousseau, P. 1999. *Pachomius*, rev. edn. Berkeley: University of California Press.

Safrai, S., and M. Stern, eds. 1976. *The Jewish People in the First Century*, vol. 2. Assen: Van Gorcum.

Seccombe, D. 1978. 'Was There Organized Charity in Jerusalem Before the Christians?' *Journal of Theological Studies*, n.s. 29: 140–143.

Sen, A. 1981. *Poverty and Famines*. Oxford: Oxford University Press.

Serfass, A. 2008. 'Wine for Widows: Papyrological Evidence for Christian Charity in Late Antique Egypt', in *Wealth and Poverty in Early Church and Society*, ed. S. R. Holman, 88–102. Grand Rapids, MI: Baker Academic.

Stathakopoulos, D. C. 2004. *Famine and Pestilence in the Late Roman and Early Byzantine Empire*. Aldershot: Ashgate.

Temkin, O. 1991. *Hippocrates in a World of Pagans and Christians*. Baltimore: Johns Hopkins University Press.

Van Minnen, P. 1995. 'Medical Care in Late Antiquity', in *Ancient Medicine in its Socio-Cultural Context*, ed. P. van der Eijk, H. F. J. Horstmanshoff, and P. H. Schrijvers, vol. 1: 153–169. Amsterdam: Rodopi.

van Ommeslaeghe, F. 1979. 'Jean Chrysostome en conflit avec l'impératrice Eudoxie', *Analecta Bollandiana* 97: 131–159.

Vööbus, A. 1970. *Syrische Kanonessammlungen*, vol. 1. Louvain: Secrétariat du CSCO.

Yarshater, E. ed. 1991. *Encyclopaedia Iranica*, vol. 5. London: Routledge and Kegan Paul.

Zuiderhoek, A. 2009. *The Politics of Munificence in the Roman Empire*. Cambridge: Cambridge University Press.

3

THE EARLIEST HOSPITALS IN BYZANTIUM, WESTERN EUROPE, AND ISLAM

I

What difference did hospitals make? A question of that form has a distinguished pedigree in late antique studies. E. A. Judge reported in 1980: 'when I once told A. H. M. Jones that I wanted to find out what difference it made to Rome to have been converted [to Christianity], he said he already knew the answer: None.' In 1986 Ramsey MacMullen published a more open-minded enquiry into the possible impact of the newly established religion on fourth-century changes in secular life. He took as his title 'What Difference Did Christianity Make?' My appropriation of MacMullen's phrasing pays oblique homage – not only to him, but to Peter Brown, who has taught us that it may not be the appropriate question to ask of the period. The implied imagery of Christianity as a single powerful tide progressively sweeping away the vestiges of paganism, and thus effecting a distinct and measurable difference, owes too much to the primary-colored triumphalist narrative of Christianization bequeathed to us by fifth-century historians. It does not reflect the complex grisaille of the actual religious history of the fourth and fifth centuries.[1]

Does the history of hospitals belong under the aegis of MacMullen or under that of Brown? Can we assess the impact of these institutions for the overnight accommodation and relief of the poor and sick from the mid-fourth century onwards? Or is the 'problem of hospitals' as labyrinthine as 'the problem of Christianization'? In this paper I try to address the question I have set myself while all the time keeping a skeptical eye in its validity. The inspiration for it has come from studies of hospitals of the later Middle Ages and Renaissance, as well as of the nineteenth century – studies that bring hospitals from the margins to the very centre of the concerns of social and religious historians, while remaining chary of according such establishments any clear primacy in the explanation of major change. My approach is deliberately broad and comparative, encompassing the beginnings of traditions of hospital foundations in early Byzantium (late antiquity), in early medieval western Europe, and (to a lesser extent) in the early Islamic caliphate, as well as in Jewish communities.[2]

II

To ask what difference hospitals made is immediately to prompt other questions: difference of what kind? And to whom? Brown's work has offered an answer in terms of 'crowds and power' in the urban churches of the post-Constantinian world. What seemed to us like an almost natural *evolution* from a pagan to a Christian 'folk sociology' is presented instead as a *revolution*. In this revolution the bishops are the leaders. And one of the means by which they assert their leadership, from the mid-fourth century onwards, is the founding and patronage of hospitals. The self-image of the inhabitants of the ancient city had space for local notables sharing a common rhetorical culture with provincial governors and imperial courtiers. In both centre and periphery the 'big men' spoke the same language. At a local level, this marked the big men off from those who entrusted themselves to their care. The local 'big man' was a 'nourisher' of his citizen body, the *demos*. In this collective representation of urban society the poor had no conceptual place. Those who could expect 'nourishment' did so as citizens, not as paupers: that is, on legal grounds, not economic ones. With the establishment of the Christian Church by Constantine, the way was to some extent prepared for Christian bishops to usurp the already weakened power of local lay notables. They achieved this through a 'Christian populism': the deliberate replacement of a civic model of society with a universal citizenship (a prelude to that of heaven) in which the poor emerged from the conceptual shadows and symbolized the Church's embrace of the whole of society, to its very margins. The bishop as 'lover of the poor' supplanted the nourisher of the citizenry. This was a stronger image in both its emotional charge and its social ramifications. It shattered the ancient civic model.[3]

Hospitals for the poor figure in this revolution in urban leadership because, under Constantine and Constantius II, churches and clerics benefited from enormously valuable tax immunities. They needed a highly visible symbol of their deployment of the wealth generated not only by these immunities but also through the patronage of emperors and from the much smaller donations of ordinary citizens. The hospital highlighted the poor as the defining group in the new Christian representation of society. It legitimated the Church's wealth by showing that it was being channelled into purposes few could reasonably question. Other scholars have noticed and indeed carefully described the changes in the late antique city that accompanied Christianization. Brown is distinctive in interpreting these changes, less as epiphenomenal to a growth in numbers of the urban poor and as the obvious culmination of pre-existing Christian charity, and much more as ingredients in a quite deliberate episcopal arrogation of power, both material and symbolic.[4]

So Brown's answer to the question 'What difference did hospitals make?' is presumably a very large one. Hospitals stood for, and contributed to, a quiet social revolution in the ancient city.

It is important to stress two features of this answer. One is that it is not specific to hospitals. The other is that it does not necessarily implicate the poor directly. If the poor felt pleasure at their novel symbolic standing, they were not inevitably less hungry or more powerful. In the Christian crowds over whom and through whom the bishop exercised power, the heavyweight supporters who could intimidate the opposition were not the hospital patients. They were, in Alexandria at least and perhaps elsewhere too, the corps of hospital stretcher-bearers. It was through them rather than through the sick that the hospital had achieved genuine 'clout'.[5]

Brown's view is, then, a view of poverty and charity through the prism of a broad ideology. While he by no means sets aside painful social and economic realities, he is concerned with the conceptual space occupied by poverty in 'self-image of the age'. 'In a sense,' he ventures, 'it was the Christian bishops who invented the poor.' My concerns in what follows are related but slightly different. I want to ask what practical difference hospitals might have been perceived to make – perceived, first, by their founders, then by the recipients of poor relief and charity. To approach these topics, however, some further consideration is needed of what a hospital is.[6]

III

One definition, which has the merit of forming a transition from Brown's conceptual account to my own, can be couched in terms of the 'production of space'. The space is physical, not conceptual. A hospital is a pauper enclosure: it gathers in and, for a time (perhaps only overnight), removes the poor from exposure to the elements and the view of society. It does not do this in the Foucauldian manner of a great *renfermement* of beggars behind hospital walls. (Such containment was seldom attempted on any scale in the fourth or fifth centuries any more than, *pace* Foucault, it was in the seventeenth.) Rather, the hospital defines a new space as being for the poor or it sets barriers round a space already loosely demarcated by custom as the resort of the sick or needy. In major cases, such as St Basil's cluster of philanthropic foundations outside Caesarea in the early 370s, hospitals can even provide new focuses for urban or sub-urban space. When the *Basileias* was lauded as a 'new city', this was not only because, in Brownian terms, it exemplified the novel conceptual weight attached to episcopal 'love of the poor', but also because, like some extramural shrine or new church building, the hospital complex really was a topographical challenge to the established centre of Caesarea.[7]

The hospital as a means of reconfiguring urban space cannot, however, be viewed in isolation. It should be set in the context of parallel transformations that are all part of 'the problem of Christianization'. Since the fourth century, hospitals have been imaged, not altogether fairly, as stairways to heaven, and the obvious context within which to view the hospital as space is death. Eric Rebillard has painstakingly examined the limited evidence for the development of ecclesiastical cemeteries for the poor and strangers. What deserves emphasis here is that the chronology of this development matches very closely what has been called, in an influential monograph, 'The Birth of the Hospital in the Byzantine Empire'. It seems clear that Constantine had, in the early fourth century, instituted a system for the provision of free burial to the inhabitants of Constantinople. Yet not until the latter part of that century is there any sign of burial grounds set aside for indigents and strangers. That is very much the story of early hospitals too.[8]

IV

Their chronology should, therefore, next be explored in a little more detail. In doing so, I shall start in the early Byzantine empire and then push the boundaries of the enquiry beyond late antiquity to look at hospital history right across the early Middle Ages, geographically as well as chronologically. My purpose here is not to repeat a well-established narrative; it is to bring out some of the geographical and chronological gaps that must be included, yet are seldom stressed in modern accounts. I am exploring hospital history from the presumed viewpoint of founders, looking for the circumstances in which the establishment of a hospital came to seem desirable. Brown has given us an explanation of the first Christian hospitals in terms of their furtherance of an urban revolution; it remains to be seen how far such an approach can be applied to later hospitals. This is an oblique approach to the question of what difference hospitals made – by way of an enquiry into their perceived importance to founders. We are not, therefore, in the world of hospital patients. Although we shall come a little closer to the patients later on, it is essential not to conflate their likely perceptions with those of their benefactors. We have learned from studies of later periods how different the two sets of perceptions could be.[9]

It is fruitless to search for one specific foundation with which the Christian charitable tradition of hospital foundations can be said to begin. So far as we can tell, no one claimed absolute priority. Perhaps the infirmary of what is usually taken as the first monastery, that of Pachomius at Tabennesi (north of Thebes in Egypt), should count as the first Christian hospital. If so, the institution may date from around 325. But the evidence of that infirmary, like much else in the Pachomian dossier, is ambiguous and, worse, may actually speak to us of developments after his death. In any case, this not a 'public' hospital for the poor. Probably the first such hospital that we happen to know about was that erected by Bishop Leontius of Antioch (in modern south-eastern Turkey). Leontius was bishop from 344 to 358, so let us accept 350 as the round date for the emergence (at least into the light of the evidence) of *xenodocheia* or *xenones*, hospitals for strangers or migrants. At about the same time a deacon called Marathonius, protégé of the newly elected bishop

Macedonius, was put in charge of the hospitals and monasteries of an extreme wing of urban asceticism in Constantinople. A little later, in the late 350s or 360s, Eustathius of Sebaste (Sivas in northern Turkey) built a *ptochotropheion*, literally a place in which beggars are nourished. Shortly after, St Basil established his charitable 'multiplex' for the sick, lepers, the paralysed, and strangers, as a 'new city', in extramural Caesarea. The evidence for Leontius, Marathonius, and Eustathius is brief, partial, and vulnerable to scepticism. We know little beyond the basic information just given, and perhaps not even that much. We do not know the ideas and decisions that preceded the foundations. Some historians have seen the origins of the idea of the hospital, as a sign of commitment to charity, in urban monasticism. Others have related it to the rival claims to popular support of orthodox and Arian 'heretics' in the fourth-century Church. Brown has nudged the pendulum in the direction of imperial patronage as the context for, above all, Basil's foundations. The dispute cannot be properly conveyed, let alone settled, other than through rehearsal of textual minutiae, so I shall leave it to one side. What matters for present purposes is that, on any plausible account, hospitals – whether for poor or sick – seem to develop quite suddenly, and in specific areas. If the poor of this period are an invention of bishops, so too, with all deference to Pachomius, is the hospital.

It is worth pausing to digest the significance of this round date of 350. We are in the reign of Constantius II, not that of Constantine. Despite the enormous patronage that the latter expended on the newly established Christian Church, hospitals did not flourish in his time. Nor had they developed in the early (pre-Constantinian) Church, although this was clearly capable of elaborate charitable distributions. Nor, seemingly, were they a prominent feature of Jewish communities in rabbinic times (a point to which I shall return).[10]

We might next ask why the invention occurs exactly where it does. If the hospital was a visual justification of imperial largesse to the Church, a symbol of its embrace of the whole of society and not just of the citizen body, then we might have expected its very first appearance in Constantinople, and in a more emphatic manner. Perhaps the pressure to justify and symbolize was greater in smaller centres, where the transfers of resources required were relatively greater. We shall never know. All we do know is that this invention seems to have been diffused rapidly. Indeed, as we shall see later, it may have arrived in the Christian kingdom of Armenia at about the same time as it arrived in the capital.[11]

The next discernible phase in early hospital history takes us outside the eastern empire. There is no need for detail: I want merely to draw attention to one major aspect. That is, the hospital is received as an invention, as a novelty the adoption of which was presumably thought to make some important difference, whether to inmates or to founders. We can see this invention being quite rapidly diffused around the Mediterranean, at the end of the fourth and the beginning of the fifth century. It is diffused to areas in contact with Byzantium – to Italy (Ostia and Rome) and to North Africa (Augustine's Hippo). Whereas the earliest hospitals are lost in obscurity and, so far as we can tell, no one claimed priority, it now becomes worth asserting, as Jerome did of the great Roman lady Fabiola, that 'primo omnium *nosokomion* instituit'. That is, observers want to say that this person was 'the first of all to found a hospital'. Jerome's accuracy in the particular case of Fabiola does not matter. What is significant is that he thought the 'primo omnium' deserving of emphasis.[12]

At that point, geographically the northern and westward lines of transmission peter out. It is as if this new 'hospital idea' has become less attractive. The hospital in Hippo inaugurated no vigorous North African tradition of foundation. Outside Rome there are few Italian hospitals until the Lombard period. In Visigothic Spain, the only prominently attested hospital is the remarkable establishment of Bishop Masona of Mérida, who died in 605. In Gaul, no hospital, either monastic or episcopal, is well evidenced before 500 – that is, almost a century after the idea started its westward spread. The earliest recorded foundation, that of Caesarius of Arles, can be seen as the beginning of a more resilient hospital tradition in the Merovingian realms than is detectable elsewhere in the post-Roman West; but this tradition embraces only some 34 documented establishments.[13]

Of course, it may reasonably be objected that these are only the visible summits of a mountain range whose lower slopes and valleys are covered by the mists of time. It is highly likely that, in any given period or place within late antiquity or the early Middle Ages, there were many more hospitals than those we know about. Counting establishments, even for the much better documented later Middle Ages, is fraught with difficulty, because the foundations are still very often obscure and ephemeral. Yet the early hospital trail is so quickly and comprehensively lost as we follow it across the Mediterranean from east to west and south to north that it is hard not to see the transmission of the idea as having faltered. [14]

I shall come back to these gaps both geographical and evidential. Before I do so, however, let us look eastwards. Hospital historians, like other early medievalists, are familiar with the adage that the evidence improves as one moves eastwards, in cultural terms if not always strictly in geographical ones. If we want some idea – however heightened from life – of the interior of a small hospital of the early Byzantine period, we must look not to Greek evidence, but to that written in Syriac. The *Life* of Rabbula of Edessa (modern Urfa), for example, records the clean bedding and clothes available to the inmates of Rabbula's two hospitals, one for men, one for women, and the attentive and kindly regime of the deacons and deaconesses employed in them. Such establishments and their later imitations in Byzantine Syria and Egypt, as well as in Sassanid Iran, form the link between the hospital history of Byzantium and that of Islam.[15]

I turn briefly to Islam after looking at the West because it is in the land of Islam that the idea of the hospital can next be seen to arrive in a relatively clear-cut manner. The hospital is presumably thought to make a difference if it is seen as distinctive enough for self-conscious adoption. It is received in this spirit in Italy and Gaul. But the story of the Islamic hospital is slightly different. Here, there is indeed a direct and relatively speedy transmission – but in what proves to be only legend. That is, a retrospective account was elaborated during the Middle Ages according to which the idea of the hospital was conveyed by Greek physicians to the Persian court at Jundeshapur in Khuzistan. There, during the second and third centuries, two shahs both contributed to the development of a hospital and medical school. The school's pre-eminence was supposedly reinforced during the sixth century by the arrival of Nestorian Christians; and, after the Arab conquests, the associated hospital was the chief model for the yet more elaborate foundations of Islamic caliphs. The durability of this myth of origins shows how readily the hospital could be conceived as an invention passed from one specific location to another. The narrative has been so seductive in its simplicity that only recently has a more messy and realistic analysis been substituted. The details do not matter. What here deserves emphasis is the multiplicity of Christian charitable foundations active within the land of Islam after the conquests, and the plurality of medical centres that could have served as inspiration for them. Still, the fact that the Arabic word for a hospital, *bimaristan*, means 'house [or place] of the sick' in New Persian points to a connection between the Christian hospitals of Iran/Iraq and the first Islamic foundations. There were indeed several different kinds of Zoroastrian charitable foundation characteristic of pre-Islamic Iran. But the hospital does not seem to have been among them. A sixth-century Syriac chronicle (that probably reached its surviving form in Amida) announces that the Shah Chosroes Anushirvan 'on the advice of the Christian doctors who are close to him, has now, departing from custom, made a hospital [*xenodocheion*]'. One hundred and fifty camels are to transport its supplies and it is to be staffed by twelve doctors. The implication of the passage is that, in founding this hospital, the king was departing not only from his own custom, but from Sassanian royal custom generally. So the hospital idea as it were leaps from the eastern Christian to the Zoroastrian world, although not quite at the time or in the place that the myth of origins asserted.[16]

It did not take root. Indeed, there is instead another long gap in hospital history. Christian hospitals form a background continuum. But there seem to have been no hospitals founded by either later Sassanian or early Islamic rulers (or other benefactors) between the mid-sixth and the late eighth or early ninth century. In other words, there were no Umayyad hospitals, and no early Abbasid ones either, until the Barmakid hospital in ninth-century Baghdad – the first Islamic hospital. Why the hospital was not a more immediately attractive expression of the piety of Islamic ruling elites is a matter for conjecture. The explanation may lie with medical history because (unlike many of these of Byzantium and the West) the typical Islamic hospital in the great cities such as Baghdad and Cairo came to be staffed by Galenic physicians. And that was only possible after the absorption of Greek medical learning, which in turn could not have occurred before the court-inspired translation movement of the later eighth century CE.[17]

V

I do not want to pursue the early medieval history of hospitals around the Mediterranean or in the Middle East any further at this point. My argument has been that the hospital was, at least, special enough to make a difference to the modes of thought of potential founders: special in the sense that it was a distinct idea, a type of project that inspired imitation and recreation; an idea that was transmitted across space in a way that could incite contemporaries to record: 'X was the first to build a hospital here.' The hospital was indeed an invention of fourth-century bishops to the same extent that 'the poor' were an invention of the same.

To what extent, though? Let us briefly try to put the hospital in a global context. By the term 'hospital', to confirm, I mean simply a more or less distinct and permanent structure for the overnight accommodation and relief of the poor and/or sick. A hospital is not, in pre-modern times, an obvious or natural thing to build. It requires a certain type of economy, with stable, usually urban, centres; a certain concentration of resources, human and material – most obviously space, conceptual, and topographical – for the building and its purposes; a perception of the inadequacy or inappropriateness of dispersed forms of support ('outdoor' relief in the terminology of the English poor law; 'care in the community' in modern discourse), linked to a belief that economies of scale are possible through the concentration of support within a building; a perception of the value of the project and its beneficiaries, whether spiritual value (e.g. the poor as intercessors for the rich) or economic value (the maintenance of a labour force).

All these perceptions and calculations have been rare in ancient and medieval times. In the New World, in pre-Columbian central Mexico, some bathhouses may have doubled as reception centres for the sick. In the Old World, the idea of the hospital did not (so far as I can tell) occur to the Babylonians or any other pre-classical Near Eastern civilization, to the Egyptians, or to the ancient Greeks. Further east, hospitals are principally found as expressions of the charity of Buddhist rulers, for example in India, Sri Lanka, and Cambodia. Where hospitals appear in Hindu or neo-Confucian milieux, this is likely to reflect Buddhist influence. So, although hospitals can be found within the cultural realms of all the world religions, the global map of their foundations has huge blanks on it until the formation of European overseas empires.[18]

There is one main exception outside the realms of world religions. It may hint at why, on a global scale, hospitals have been so rare. They appear in only highly restricted circumstances. In the majority of cases these circumstances derive from a particular inflexion of an ideology of charity. The ancient case is different, but the circumstances are no less specific and unusual. For a relatively brief period, the Romans occasionally built hospitals (*valetudinaria*) for slaves and soldiers: buildings within which the two categories of labourers who mattered most to the functioning of the empire might be repaired when broken down and then sent back to work. Slave hospitals were favoured by some of the richest owners from the first century BC to the end of the first CE. That is, they came to be built when the supply of slaves through conquest had diminished, prices had risen, and it was worth maintaining those who could work and breed. When the empire's crucial labour force became the *coloni*, tied to the land and living in quasi-peasant households, slave hospitals were no longer economical or indeed necessary. The rise and fall of military hospitals comes a little later, but can be explained in similar structural-cum-economic terms. These date from the time of Augustus until around the middle of the third century CE. They correspond to the period in which the army was often operating well beyond the empire's northern frontiers in areas largely bereft of friendly settlements where sick and wounded soldiers could be usefully accommodated. When, in the third century, the army was reorganized and a local militia, supported where needed by a mobile field army, defended the frontier, the construction of fortress hospitals ceased. Sick soldiers were thereafter cared for by their families or in their own tents – just as sick *coloni* were tended by their wives or relatives. The age of Roman hospitals was over. Even at its height, moreover, neither kind of hospital was at all widespread. The anonymous (?) second-century Roman writer now known as pseudo-Hyginus included a hospital in his description of the standard Roman tented camp. Yet it is far from clear that such hospitals under canvas were any more common than the permanent fortress type. Further literary evidence for them is lacking; and the archaeological evidence for military hospitals of any kind is slight – slighter than used to be thought because the identification of a number of proposed sites of *valetudinaria* is now being questioned. About the number and distribution of slave hospitals even less is known. These hospitals – to repeat – belong to a highly specific 'niche' in Roman history. They reflect a calculation of the economies of scale to be made by the centralized reconstituting of the work force. Such a calculation will not be made again until the later Middle Ages in Italy, when hospitals once again attempted a rapid patient turnover.[19]

No one in the mid-fourth century is likely to have seen the buildings that were formerly *valetudinaria* (if the structures survived at all). Hardly anyone is likely to have read or heard anything about them. The Christian hospital of the fourth century is essentially a new creation in European, Mediterranean, or Middle Eastern history.

VI

Perhaps there is another way of looking at this phenomenon: a way that might account for the gaps in the line of transmission of the hospital idea, and for the apparent lack of a 'pre-history' of this sudden invention? To show what this other way might look like, I turn to Jewish hospitals. I have asserted that, Roman *valetudinaria* apart, there were no hospitals in the ancient world before the Christian foundations of the reign of Constantius II. That is a slight exaggeration:

> Theodotos, son of Vettenos the priest and synagogue leader [*archisynagogos*] . . . built the synagogue . . . and as a hostel with chambers and water installations for the accommodation of those who, coming from abroad, have need of it.

So runs a well-known inscription from first-century Jerusalem. Some have wanted to claim it as the first Jewish medical hospital. But there is no reason to think that doctors attended those staying in it.

Several paradoxical aspects of the establishment should, rather, be stressed. First, as a 'hostel with chambers' it resembles the accommodation for visitors that could be found beside any major shrine in the ancient world, such as that of Epidaurus. The Temple in Jerusalem was perhaps the largest temple of its time, and virtually the sole focus of Jewish pilgrimage. It doubtless attracted far more visitors than did most pagan shrines, which would come fully to life only once or twice a year for a great festival. Its facilities were presumably offered in a more charitable spirit than were the pagan ones. Still, it is no surprise that the Jerusalem synagogue of the first century CE, whether before or after the destruction of the Second Temple in the year 70, should cater for needy visitors. More surprisingly, secondly, there seems to have been no wider system of organized charity in Jerusalem at the time; individual initiatives such as that of Theodotos were crucial. Thirdly, there is little or no specific evidence of other such hospices attached to synagogues in the first five or six centuries CE – despite a number of rabbinic texts which show that travellers might be lodged within a synagogue precinct. Clear archaeological, epigraphic and 'documentary' evidence is simply lacking. The first well-attested Jewish hospitals come from a letter of 598 of Pope Gregory the Great, in which he investigates Christian appropriation of synagogues and their guesthouses in Palermo. In the mid-fourth century the pagan emperor Julian had, famously, paid Jewish and Christian philanthropy the compliment of imitation. He had ordered the establishment of hospitals because 'it is disgraceful that, when no Jew ever has to beg, and the impious Galileans [i.e. Christians] support not only their own poor but ours as well, all men see that our people lack aid from us.' We should not read too much into the distinction he draws between Jews and Christians there. Yet it is still perhaps notable that he associates with the Christians the generalized support for the poor that would be manifested, *inter alia*, in hospitals, and with the Jews the relief of potential beggars. For the latter is a form of relief at least consistent with an absence of indoor, hospital care, and with an emphasis on outdoor distribution (for example, the characteristic *quppah*, the weekly dole to resident poor, or the soup kitchen perhaps found in the synagogue at Aphrodisias). In other words, the paradox of the Jerusalem hostel is that it blends far better into a pagan than a Jewish context. And it looks forward to Christian hospitals of almost three centuries later rather than standing in a demonstrable tradition of its own.[20]

This paradox is, at first sight, only compounded by bringing in evidence from subsequent periods. In the later Middle Ages, Jewish hospitals were quite widespread – following Christian example, I suspect – in those parts of Europe where Jews were tolerated. These hospitals were often referred to as *heqdeshim*; but the *heqdesh*, 'the holy', was more broadly the property and assets of the community. There was no more specific designation for Jewish hospitals. Earlier, in the tenth to thirteenth centuries, the gaonic period illuminated for us so wonderfully – and uniquely – by the archive of the Geniza of old Cairo, similar ambiguities prevail. There was apparently only one major hospital in the city, a hospital with doctors attached. It was a Muslim foundation, and the city's Jewish population had nothing like it – at least, there is no mention of such a hospital in the Geniza. Nor is there any reference to Jews as patients in the Muslim hospital, even though some of its physicians would have been Jewish. Whether Jews ever in fact placed themselves in the hands of the Muslim foundation, overcoming the dietary problem by having their own food brought in by friends or relatives, is a matter for conjecture. If an impoverished Jew needed sustained nursing or medical attention, he or she was much more likely to have received it in the home or in the doctor's surgery. As for transients, they might be put up in a *funduq*. *Funduq* is an Arabic word meaning caravanserai, but derived from the Greek *pandocheion* or inn (close to the Christian term for a hospital, *xenodocheion*). Equally, needy guests might be accommodated in vacant rooms within houses that were part of the synagogue's endowment, or in rooms set aside ad hoc within the synagogue.[21]

The contrast between this type of establishment and the Christian *xenodocheion* is a marked, and diagnostic, one. To oversimplify, doubtless: the Christian *xenodocheion* packed an ideological punch out of all proportion to its size and distribution. Even if we qualify Brown's account of its symbolic weight, it is still a deliberate reminder of the established Christian Church's affront to ancient civic values. The Jewish hostel within or adjacent to the medieval synagogue complex seems to have been the converse of this. Here is a hospital whose history is very difficult to write precisely because substance outweighs symbolism. It has no specific name, unlike the Christian *xenodocheion* or *nosokomeion*. It is not a means to social revolution, but a quick and unobtrusive adjunct to the range of social services by which Jewish communities tried to protect their more valuable new arrivals from the shame of poverty.

The Geniza evidence also suggests that the synagogue *heqdesh* cannot (when it is detailed at all) be viewed in isolation from other hospitals or quasi-hospitals scattered across the Jewish households of the city. The hospice, the converted room in the synagogue complex, the room used ad hoc for a transient in a building otherwise rented out commercially, the room in a private household for which the synagogue pays rent – all these seem to lie on a smooth spectrum, rather than to represent divergent and unequal possibilities. Nor was the synagogue the only provider of such varieties of indoor support. A twelfth-century Jewish judge in old Cairo, for instance, kept a private hospice for the sick and elderly within his home.[22]

These examples suggest a point that is a wider application. We should not only envisage the best-documented hospitals as ideological inventions which, in any given culture or century, either exist or do not exist. We should also try to peer 'behind' the ideology and search out traces of the less formal, or less permanent, establishments; for these make up the hinterland of hospitals and help explain their appearance. Hospital historians have characteristically expended energy on trying to determine when, and in what circumstances, hospices for the poor became 'true' hospitals for the sick – truth being defined (quite inappropriately, as I argue below) by the documented attendance of doctors. I think we should look for the emergence of hospitals in a different direction, less at personnel than at structure, or perhaps morphology. I propose that we think of the hospital as a solidification – architectural, ideological, or both together – of part of the spectrum of what I shall now call 'sub-hospitals' – hospitals in all but name, perhaps not quite independent structures but fulfilling many or all of the functions of pre-modern hospitals. These could be domestic hospitals, arising from the conversion of one part of a house or villa, as with Fabiola in late fourth-century Rome or that judge in twelfth-century Cairo. They could involve the covering over of a portico or the atrium of a church, or the erection of temporary shelters in time of famine. They could even be initiated by a group of paupers in taking over some derelict building – foundation from below, as it were. They could include some of those locations in which ancient historians have searched diligently for pagan hospitals in order to show that neither Jews nor Christians 'got there first': the area around healing shrines in which the sick 'incubators' might by day need some basic care from attendants (even if by night they lodged elsewhere, in the sort of hostel mentioned earlier); or the small *iatreion* in which the doctor lodged some patients overnight. Our analysis can embrace such locations because our 'rules of engagement' do not oblige us to decide whether each was or was not a true hospital. We are simply placing them on a spectrum of more or less hospital-like facilities, and seeing the *xenodocheion* and its successors as a highly self-conscious privileging of one particular part of that spectrum.[23]

Hospital history of this more inclusive kind complements the ideological history of invention and diffusion. It helps explain some of the gaps in that history. We have seen that with respect to hospitality in the synagogue. The bishop's house (to revert to Christianity) is likely to have been the matrix of mid-fourth-century hospitals in Byzantium, or fifth- to sixth-century hospitals in Gaul. The change of style in poor relief from rooms in the bishop's house or its surrounding outbuildings to conceptually or architecturally freestanding hospitals could have been a very slight change indeed. Augustine's complex at Hippo in the early fifth century had, for instance, 120 rooms: surely plenty of scope for a *xenodochium* even though the energy of a priest whom Augustine had consecrated, not directly that of the great man himself, was required to bring into being his city's first Christian hospital. When they emerged, synagogue hospices probably related to their surroundings in a similar way. In the world of Islamic elites the change was one of initiative – from letting Christians do the founding to founding a hospital oneself; perhaps it was additionally an implementation of the newly received Galenic medical programme.[24]

VII

Conjecturally filling in some of the gaps in this way raises in a slightly altered form the question of what difference hospitals made. So far I have rehearsed two kinds of answer. The first is ideological. Hospitals were seen to have symbolic potency in eastern Mediterranean cities of the mid-300s. Partly for that reason, they can, now, be interpreted as an invention that was, with interruptions, transmitted both eastwards and westwards over subsequent centuries. The attractiveness of the invention at least tells us that its adoption was thought to make a difference of some kind. The second answer to our question is more materialist. Hospitals were simply an intensification or solidification of one part of a blurred spectrum of hospital-like provisions. Seen in this way, presumably, the hospital makes a less significant difference because of its context of 'sub-hospitals'. The transition from the background noise of the latter to the clearer signal of named hospitals could have entailed no more than a modest increase in visibility. The visibility might attract greater charity, and hence lead to an increase in size. Such a change was not, however, necessarily inherent in the emergence of the *xenodocheion* into the light of the surviving evidence.

The skeptic might assert at this point that the hospital made no difference at all. But that would be solely on the basis of a supply-side history that has focused on founders, their attitudes, and the 'raw materials' (the sub-hospitals) with which they sometimes operated. What is needed to round out the picture is a demand-side account, which looks at the impact of hospitals on the poor.

From the viewpoint of the poor or sick – those who, in these early centuries of hospital history, can be presumed as the great majority of inmates – the prospect might seem unpromising. If one wants to cut hospitals down to size, so that they can have made little difference to the ranks of the impoverished, it is easy to do so.

First, many, and perhaps most, late antique and early medieval hospitals were very small. An apostolic dozen beds is quite commonly attested. Hospitals with 200 are very much the exception and are confined to Constantinople, or to such major pilgrimage centres as Jerusalem, and the sphere of influence of such major founders as the emperor Justinian. Overall, even in large foundations, beds are usually to be numbered in tens, not hundreds, and doubling the numbers of beds to arrive at a number of inmates (who often slept two to a bed) still does not produce very impressive totals.[25]

Secondly, early hospitals were apparently not numerous. Counting them began in 1680 when Du Cange published his *Constantinopolis Christiana*, listing some 35 charitable institutions. Janin's more recent tabulation for the capital – not wholly reliable – finds 31 *xenones* and hospitals, and 27 old people's homes. The most recent survey for the provinces of the Byzantine empire, up to the mid-ninth century, gives a total of over 160 charitable facilities of various kinds, of which the most numerous are *xenodocheia* and *xenones* (71), *nosokomeia* (44), and *ptocheia* (poor-houses; 21). There are no modern and comprehensive surveys covering Italy or Spain (with respect to the latter, as we have seen, only one institution is ever discussed, though some others are attested). From the textual and archaeological deposit of Merovingian Gaul, there are, as noted above, signs of only 34 hospitals, the majority in the north-east of the country. Jewish hospitals of the early Middle Ages are too elusive for the statistician. As for Islam: we are assured that 'a hospital was an essential feature of any large Islamic town'. Yet that generalization can be applied only to the twelfth century and after. We have no genuinely comprehensive survey of the evidence, but it is salutary to note that only ten or eleven hospital foundations are attested before the year 1000 CE. Seven of them were in Baghdad, three in Iran, one (perhaps) in old Cairo. Only from the eleventh century onward did the Islamic 'hospital idea' spread to Mesopotamia and Syria, and westwards around the southern Mediterranean.[26]

These figures are potentially misleading in contradictory ways. On one hand, there are likely to have been more small establishments than we know of. In particular, we should add a quantity of 'sub-hospitals' on the brink of distinctive and independent existence. On the other hand, hospitals could be ephemeral. We usually do not know how many establishments were functional at any one time. Their number is likely always to have been smaller than the number of earlier foundations, since some of these will already have gone out of business.

Two further points of a comparative nature can tentatively be made. First, not only do the figures for size support that the view that early medieval hospitals were small in comparison with say, early modern ones; the figures for total numbers are small even by comparison with later periods within the Middle Ages. We know, for example, of almost 300 hospitals for lepers alone founded in England between 1100 and 1250. That comfortably exceeds current estimates for the whole Byzantine empire, and over a much longer period. Secondly, whether measured by average size or total numbers, the scale of hospital provision was easily dwarfed by other sources of social welfare. In late antiquity, the *annona* (dole) of grain and other foodstuffs in Rome, Constantinople, and even small towns such as Oxyrhynchus reached a far larger number of poorer people than any estimate we can hazard of the total hospital population. Hospital capacity was not only dwarfed by such state-run measures. It was probably, in aggregate, surpassed even by the Church's own 'outdoor' distributions to its local poor – those whose names were inscribed, sometimes in their thousands, on registers of the deserving.[27]

To strengthen this 'minimalist' interpretation, we might draw attention to the large blanks that remain on the map. Our field for comparison is northern Europe, the Mediterranean, and the Middle East. So we ought to survey the whole map. There are no clearly attested hospitals in Celtic Ireland or Anglo-Saxon Britain before their respective Norman conquests, other than monastic infirmaries (run by monks for sick brethren). I believe that much the same can be said of the Scandinavian world during the early Middle Ages (despite an anecdote to be presented below). The East Frankish lands and eastern Europe generally present another great void, although there are some notable exceptions such as Erembert's hospital at Bremen. With the exception of West Frankish lands, only as we move south and eastwards around the Mediterranean does the map become relatively crowded.[28]

Even some of the explanations for the fourth-century proliferation of hospitals that modern historians have devised turn out to have the effect of playing down the difference they can have made. Some have, for example, posited a population boom in fourth-century eastern empire that generated substantial migration to the cities. Now, if this happened and the hospital-building in Caesarea and elsewhere can be seen as part of the response, then it must have been an inadequate response. If it did *not* happen at quite such a pace, as seems increasingly likely from new interpretations of the archaeology and the texts, then the new hospitals are left without a particular *raison d'être* – at least, one that we can state in simple economic and demographic terms.[29]

In general, it seems, periods of more intense hospital foundation correlate poorly with big trends in population or the economy. The foundations of the fourth to fifth century around the Mediterranean mesh quite well not with Malthusian crisis in the countryside, but rather with sustained growth and prosperity – which should, if anything, have reduced the numbers of unemployed migrants while increasing the numbers and wherewithal of potential founders. The economic expansion of twelfth-century Europe would see another phase of hospital construction, perhaps the most intense until the Renaissance. Otherwise, it cannot be said that the establishments of Italy, Gaul, or Spain in the first half of the Middle Ages clearly reflect changes of economic gear, whether towards growth or contraction. And the hospitals of early Abbasid Islam mirror more closely the intellectual and religious environment than the character of the caliphate's economy, which had already prospered for some time.[30]

Were hospitals, then, an irrelevance in the centuries of which we have been taking an aerial view? Did they make no difference to the poor because, overall, the history of poor relief (hospitals included) must be understood above all in terms of the ideology of the founders rather than of the actual history of poverty? Perhaps we cannot invoke general economic history to explain changes in hospital history. But that is not to say that economics made no difference to founders' attitudes. In some areas, obviously, the poor may have been relatively few – too few to prompt that peculiar concentration of services we call a hospital. This seems to have been increasingly the case the further north and west we move across the early medieval map. It may account for some of the blanks already mentioned. In many more areas, the 'perceived need' – the result of filtering out the undeserving, disreputable poor – may have been small. It is a strangely persistent historiographical myth that charity was undiscriminating before the twelfth century or, in some accounts, the Reformation. The widespread keeping of lists (*matriculae*) of local poor supported by the Church is sufficient testimony to discrimination; genuinely open-handed, unquestioning distributions were the exception. A story in Rimbert's *Life* of Anskar, the ninth-century 'apostle of the north', may illustrate both the absence of poverty and the blinkered perception of need. A wealthy, pious, and elderly lady of Birka on Lake Mäleren, Sweden, instructed her daughter to distribute all her mother's possessions to the poor after her death. Since there were very few poor in the immediate area, she, the daughter, should go to the much larger emporium at Dorestad where there was a multitude of clergy and paupers. When the time came, the daughter did as she was bidden – in the company of some devout women of Dorestad who took her around the local churches and pointed out those to whom she should give alms. They are, we might guess, meant to be taken as not just identifying paupers for her but selecting them: as telling her who was on the *matricula* and who was not. Although Rimbert was writing only shortly after his subject's death, his background details are fanciful: the archaeology of Dorestad reveals wharves and warehouses, not churches. Clearly, though, he reckoned that a geography of poverty in which areas of 'scarcity' coexisted with areas of 'abundance' (the latter associated with churches) would be entirely plausible to his audience. The important point for us is this. The selectivity in almsgiving that he implicitly portrays has the effect of scaling down the acknowledged demand for all forms of ecclesiastical charity – the sub-hospital of the bishop's house, the *matricula*, as well, of course, as the hospital.[31]

VIII

On that point, the argument may be allowed to change tack. Having now defended the proposition that hospitals made little detectable difference socially or economically to the poor, I want to see what can be said in a more positive spirit. This defence of hospitals has to be limited in scope, limited to the geographical areas where some hospitals are attested.

First, it might be noted that even in the historiography of the infinitely better-documented nineteenth century, the general impact of institutional charity remains hard to assess. Was charity ever a regular source of income for the poor, or was formal relief totally inadequate? Did charity exercise a negative or a positive influence on the wider economy? The debate contin-ues. We should not be too disappointed by the ambiguity of much earlier and more obscure periods. That is, we should not assume from the lack of evidence to settle the question that hospitals had no impact apart from improving the otherworld prospects of founders.[32]

Second, we may entertain the possibility that, thanks to imperial patron-age, the new establishments of the fourth century onwards represented a massive increase in the scope of formal ecclesiastical charity by comparison with that of the pre-Constantinian centuries. In the period before *c.*300 we hear of some spectacular feats of routine organization (as in third-century Rome), and some very impressive episcopal initiatives in times of crisis (es-pecially famine). Yet these are likely to have been the remarkable instances that stood in high relief against a duller background of small-scale and somewhat introverted philanthropy. The local distributions, sick visiting, and (often strictly limited) hospitality to transients of the Pauline commu-nities and their successors over the next century did not, perhaps, amount to much in aggregate. In his fundamental *Mission and Expansion of Chris-tianity in the First Three Centuries*, Harnack emphasized the attractions of an open-handed charity as a primary factor in Christian success. More recently, Rodney Stark and others have offered similar analyses. Yet it is not clear that the size of the Christian population on the eve of Constantine's conversion was so great that it requires a special explanation of this kind, or that charity was so much more potent a factor in conversion and diffusion than, say, charismatic healing.[33]

Third, hospitals could, despite the modest aggregates cited above, achieve in certain areas a considerable density. Medievalists studying later centuries often find existing estimates of the number of hospitals to be, on closer archival inspection, much too low. One study of later medieval to post-Reformation East Anglia in England has, for instance, doubled the number of known philanthropic foundations. In similar fashion, traces of more and more local hospitals turn up in the papyri recovered from the rubbish tips of late antique Egypt. As in Gaul and elsewhere, they are clustered – in this case in Middle Egypt. In Hermopolis, for instance, there seem to have been at least eight *nosokomeia* (specifically for the sick) and some other *xenodocheia*: a generous provision in a conurbation of at most 40,000. Moreover, hospitals of varying sorts could also be found in relatively small villages. The patient turnover might be considerable. In Alexandria, John the Almsgiver established seven forty-bed hospitals for post-parturition women. The measure originated in a period of famine; but John's biographer writes as if the hospitals were intended to be permanent. So if the women each stayed for a week (as prescribed) the bishop could have facilitated over 14,000 births a year. Gregory Nazianzen called the hospital a stairway to heaven, implying these early hospitals aimed only to facilitate a good death rather than a rapid recovery, and that they admitted chiefly the chronically or terminally ill. But comparative evidence suggests that hospitals were not always 'the end of the road'. And some anecdotes imply that, for example, Byzantine hospitals aimed at cure of acute cases.[34]

Fourth, we should envisage the economic and social 'difference' that hospitals could make as not confined to the effects upon inmates. Hospitals were sources of employment for priests, doctors (sometimes), nurses, attendants, gravediggers (if less often than has been imagined), builders and maintenance staff of all kinds – many of whom will have been as poor as the designated inmates. A collectivity of quite small hospitals could, in aggregate, markedly have increased local opportunities in a world characterized by chronic underemployment.[35]

Fifth, hospitals reached beyond their walls in their services to the needy. Their functions sometimes (perhaps often) elided with those of 'outdoor' relief centers – soup kitchens, bathing facilities for the poor, charitable grain stores, and so forth. We should not think only in terms of inmates when assessing the impression they made.[36]

Finally, we should register contemporary perceptions that hospitals had a significant effect on the poor. The emperor Julian thought that 'pagan' hospitals were well worth establishing. In the 350s, the decade in which the Christian hospital emerged in Byzantium, in the Christian kingdom of Armenia, the patriarch Nerses, having very quickly appreciated the 'hospital idea', had established a network of hospitals to keep beggars off the streets. When the patriarch's enemy, King Pap, jealously destroyed these, the effect was, reportedly, to return the poor to beggary throughout the kingdom. The patriarch's hospitals are represented (admittedly over a century after they were built) as having been all-embracing.[37]

IX

What would have been the effect of a similar mass closure in Byzantium of around 450, or of Frankish ones in 650, or of Islamic hospitals around 1200 CE? The answer must at least partly depend on our assessment of the effective demand for hospital places. This is not by any means necessarily coincident with the demand perceived by registrars of the poor, who tended to ignore or despise the 'labouring poor' with large families in favour of the biblically sanctioned categories of the needy such as widows, orphans and the sick. This effective demand must have varied markedly from area to area, perhaps (as already indicated) diminishing as we move from the Middle East to north-western Europe. But it is of course unknowable with any precision.[38]

Demand for hospital beds has often been measured by reference to estimates of the total population or of the likely number of poor and sick in the society in question – on which measure hospitals often fare poorly, because they could seldom have accommodated the 10% or so in absolute penury, let alone the extra 20–30% who might, at some point in the life cycle, need relief. But the massed ranks of the poor are, of course, only the potential demand. The effective demand – the actualization of that potential at any one time – will have been significantly less, because of self-help among the poor on one hand and other sources of charity than hospitals on the other.

These two 'sectors' of help for the poor are easily mentioned, impossible to describe in detail. To look first at what we can call the sources of 'vertical' relief – those from above, in social terms: from the state, the Church, individual benefactors. The respective proportions of these contributions are impossible even to estimate for any part of the period that concerns us. Moreover, it is not enough just to consider explicit sources of charity. The history of poor relief is much wider than the history of charity. We have to look for it in unlikely places and periods – for instance in the minimal care of sick slaves provided by owners (outside the few *valetudinaria*), in the whole grim history of debt bondage, in rural patronage, in distributions and benefactions that reached impoverished members of the citizen body and were provided by local pagan aristocrats who had no concept of charity, in distributions organized by temples. So in this context, to ask what difference hospitals made is scarcely worthwhile. We cannot separate out the hospital contribution to the vertical component of poor relief. We cannot even say confidently that the establishment of Christianity and the proliferation of charitable institutions from the fourth century onwards marked a decisive change in the relative strength of the vertical component, separating classical from late antiquity, or the ancient from the medieval world. Charity may not have been a virtue in ancient pagan society; but poor relief could, whether directly or indirectly, have been practised – to an extent that is now wholly obscure to us.[39]

As for the 'horizontal' component in that relief – self-help and mutual aid among social equals – I have argued elsewhere, on the basis of a wide comparative survey, that we should not overestimate its strength or capacity. The large supportive households to which historians have unthinkingly attributed the overwhelming bulk of pre-modern support for the poor are hardly ever to be found. Pauper households were small: they were vulnerable to 'nuclear hardship'. Networks of support operated between more than within them. And those networks were fragile and limited. They needed 'vertical' buttressing if their beneficiaries were to avoid sinking into criminality or terminal destitution.[40]

The best evidence of this weakness is 'high' medieval: the Cairo Geniza, or the Miracles of Saint Louis as brilliantly analysed by Sharon Farmer. Specifically late antique or early medieval evidence on this score is hard to find. We have general exhortations to neighbourliness but very few representations of the poor in groups, other than as faceless beggars or criminal gangs. Early medieval western hagiography is perhaps the least unhelpful type of source. There are isolated vignettes showing the scope and the limits of neighbourly and familial assistance in some Dark Age texts not hitherto exploited in this context, such as the aforementioned Anskar's *Miracles* of St Willehad. But, for the most ample illustration, we should look to the corpus of hagiographies written by Gregory, bishop of Tours, in the later sixth century. In Gregory's miracle narratives, pauper households appear predictably small, and mostly conjugal. Neither the immediate family nor the wider kin group is ever depicted as supportive. Instead, there is seemingly a ready resort to institutional or informal charity. For example: 'a woman named Foedamia was restricted by swelling due to paralysis and felt pain whenever she moved any part of her body. Her relatives brought her and put her on display at the blessed church [of St Julian in Brioude], so that she might earn her keep from almsgivers.' The martyr Julian appeared to her and she was cured. Gregory fails to tell us how old she was, but he does say that she had been paralysed for eighteen years. So we should not accuse her relatives of too hastily ridding themselves of the burden of an unproductive member, in need, presumably, of continual nursing. But it is very striking how entirely matter of fact and non-judgemental Gregory is in his report of their decision to put the woman out to beg.[41]

In another story, from the *Miracles* of St Martin of Tours, Gregory does offer an excuse for a similar familial response to incapacity. A blind child was 'given to beggars, so that he might wander about with them and receive some alms; for his parents were very poor'. Elsewhere in Gregory's writings, neighbourly support is represented as somewhat out of the ordinary. A slave named Veranus, stricken with gout, lost the use of his feet. 'After Veranus was afflicted for an entire year with such pains that even his neighbors located nearby carried him [*ut etiam vicina in proximo posita commoveret*], suddenly his nerves stiffened and he was completely crippled.' That is why his master, 'grieved at the loss of a faithful slave' (or rather, one surmises, at the loss of his labour), had him brought to the shrine of St Martin.[42]

These stories focus on healing shrines, not on an institution of poor relief in the usual sense. And they are, like so much of the evidence of informal, 'horizontal' poor relief, skewed toward failure: they show us networks of support only at the moment of breakdown. Yet Gregory's narratives do have the merit of telling us how an early medieval hagiographer recorded or imagined the prior biographies of those who benefited at his favoured shrines. There was, in that process, no reason why he should have filtered larger support groups out of his narrative if he actually encountered them – no pastoral or theological need to represent only the nuclear family.

If 'horizontal' poor relief was *relatively* weak in the early Middle Ages (as it seems to have been in later and better-evidenced periods), then our estimate of the aggregate need for the vertical should be correspondingly increased. That new estimate gives greater emphasis to the role of hospitals in helping to meet the need. But that is as far as the argument can be pressed.

X

I have left until last the subject that many hospital historians would have put first: medicine. Van Minnen has wondered why such a 'major revolution . . . in medical care' as the hospital should have had no discernible impact on the medical writing of late antiquity. Miller has made spectacular claims for the Byzantine hospital from the reign of Justinian onwards. For him, Byzantine hospitals, like later Islamic ones but unlike their contemporary western European foundations, were centres of medical excellence, staffed by the leading physicians of the time; centres of medical education; even centres of medical learning with libraries and scriptoria. These claims, I have urged in another paper, are largely unfounded. The response to both Van Minnen and Miller is that Byzantine hospitals were indeed a new source of medical care in the fourth century. *Valetudinaria* could not have matched them in this respect. But the medicine of these hospitals is 'low-level' medicine to judge by the surviving manuscripts associated with them: simple, atheoretical, little concerned with etiology or prognosis. There is nothing distinctive about it. It blends into the wider landscape of late antique medicine and thus excited no comment from medical writers. Even the much-vaunted medicine of the Islamic *bimaristan* may not have been so superior as was once thought, to judge by the case books of a ninth-century hospital physician, the great Razi. As we have seen, several of the earliest hospitals often had physicians to attend to their inmates. But such healers had no professional qualifications – there were none to be had – so were not necessarily much different in competence from nurses and other attendants.[43]

XI

At the outset, I asked whether the subject of early hospital history belongs under the aegis of MacMullen or Brown. A clear decision is hardly possible. With MacMullen, it would be easy to conclude that, overall, hospitals seem to have made more difference in Christian milieux than in Jewish or Islamic ones (early Jewish hospitals are too obscure, Islamic ones too few); or that eastern Mediterranean hospitals were more significant than north-western European ones. I also hope to have shown that, although hospital history must always be understood in terms of founders' interests and motivations, hospitals were no irrelevance to the life of the poor, not least because of the limitations of their self-help mechanisms. Charitable hospitals reached out into their local populations in a variety of ways – a variety that has often been ignored because of historians' emphasis on medical functions. Such conclusions must always, however, be tempered by a Brownian awareness of the labyrinthine nature of the subject. The hospital, a simple structure to house a few people with basic needs, is a surprisingly complex phenomenon: at once an invention and an evolution, patchy in its geography yet far-reaching in the types of history that it implicates.

Notes

1 [©2005 by the Massachusetts Institute of Technology and the editors of the *Journal of Interdisciplinary History*.] E. A. Judge, *The Conversion of Rome: Ancient Sources of Modern Social Tensions* (North Ryde, Sydney, 1980), 10, quoted by Ramsay MacMullen, *Christianizing the Roman Empire (AD 100–400)* (New Haven, CT, 1984), 154, n. 25; MacMullen, 'What Difference Did Christianity Make?', *Historia* 35 (1986), 322–343, repr. in idem, *Changes in the Roman Empire* (Princeton, NJ, 1990), 142–155; Peter Brown, *Authority and the Sacred: Aspects of the Christianisation of the Roman World* (Cambridge, 1995), esp. x, 6–7, 47.

2 Brown, *Authority*, 3. Carole Rawcliffe, *Medicine for the Soul: The Life, Death and Resurrection of an English Medieval Hospital. St Giles's, Norwich, c. 1249–1550* (Thrupp, 1999); John Henderson, *The Renaissance Hospital* (New Haven, CT, 2006); Marco H. D. van Leeuwen, *The Logic of Charity: Amsterdam, 1800–1850* (Basingstoke, 2000). What follows touches on too many areas and periods to be fully documented in the available space. Footnotes are therefore largely confined to recent work that opens up, to the non-specialist, both the primary evidence and a wider secondary literature.

3 Peter Brown, *Poverty and Leadership in the Later Roman Empire* (Hanover, NH, 2002), partly anticipated in idem, *Power and Persuasion in Late Antiquity: Towards a Christian Empire* (Madison, WI, 1992), 75–103.

4 Contrast e.g. Evelyne Patlagean, 'The Poor', in Guglielmo Cavallo (ed.), *The Byzantines* (Chicago, 1997), 18; eadem, *Pauvreté économique et pauvreté sociale à Byzance 4e–7e siècle* (Paris, 1977), 185–188, 231–235. For some critical reflections on Brown's views, which may be thought to present a too reductive analysis of power and its uses in the late antique city, see Eric Rebillard, 'La "conversion" de l'empire romain selon Peter Brown', *Annales* (July–Aug. 1999), 813–823. See also, anticipating Brown, Brian E. Daley, 'Building a New City: The Cappadocian

Fathers and the Rhetoric of Philanthropy', *Journal of Early Christian Studies* 7 (1999), 431–461, at 432–433.

5 Christopher Haas, *Alexandria in Late Antiquity: Topography and Social Conflict* (Baltimore, MD, 1997), 235–238, 314.

6 Brown, *Poverty*, 8.

7 Henri Lefebvre, *The Production of Space* (Oxford, 1991). On Foucault, see, among numerous discussions by the late Roy Porter, his *Mind Forg'd Manacles: A History of Madness in England from the Restoration to the Regency* (London, 1987). Basil's philanthropic foundations are discussed in Brown, *Poverty*, 38–42; Susan R. Holman, *The Hungry Are Dying: Beggars and Bishops in Roman Cappadocia* (Oxford, 2001), 74–75; Timothy S. Miller, *The Birth of the Hospital in the Byzantine Empire*, 2nd edn (Baltimore, MD, 1997), 85–88. See also, among more recent works, Raymond Van Dam, *Kingdom of Snow: Roman Rule and Greek Culture in Cappadocia* (Philadelphia, 2002), ch. 2.

8 Éric Rebillard, 'Église et sépulture dans l'antiquité tardive (occident latin, 3e–6e siècles)', *Annales* (Sept.–Oct. 1999), 1027–1046 at 1037–1038; idem, 'Les formes de l'assistance funéraire dans l'empire romain et leur évolution dans l'antiquité tardive', *Antiquité tardive* 7 (1999), 269–282 at 274–278. Hospital as path up to heaven: Gregory Nazianzen, *Oratio* 43.63 (*Funeral Oration for Basil the Great*), in Jean Bernardi (ed. and trans.), *Grégoire de Nazianze, Discours 42–43* (Paris, 1992), 262.

9 Sandra Cavallo, *Charity and Power in Early Modern Italy: Benefactors and their Motives in Turin, 1547–1789* (Cambridge, 1995).

10 Brown, *Poverty*, 2, 25, 34, with Eusebius, *Ecclesiastical History*, VI.43.11, for the often-remarked sizeable distributions of the church in third-century Rome. Armenia: see below at n. 37.

11 For a fuller discussion of the evidence see Peregrine Horden, 'The Christian Hospital in Late Antiquity: Break or Bridge?' in Florian Steger and Kay Peter Jankrift (eds), *Gesundheit–Krankheit: Kulturtransfer medizinischen Wissens Von der Spätantike bis indie Frühe Neuzeit* (Cologne, 2004), 77–99. For Pachomius see Andrew T. Crislip, 'The Monastic Health Care System and the Development of the Hospital in Late Antiquity', PhD dissertation (Yale University, 2002), esp. 20 (now published as *From Monastery to Hospital: Christian Monasticism and the Transformation of Health Care in Late Antiquity* (Ann Arbor, 2005)), with the 'first' Greek and Bohairic *Lives* of Pachomius (sections 28, 26), trans. Armand Veilleux, *Pachomian Koinonia*, I (Kalamazoo, 1980), 315, 48. See also Demetrios J. Constantelos, *Byzantine Philanthropy and Social Welfare*, 2nd revised edn (New Rochelle, NY, 1991), pt 3; Miller, *Birth*, 21–22, ch. 5 (favouring as explanation the competition for pauper support of orthodox and Arians); Brown, *Poverty*, 36–38. The explanation in terms of asceticism was propounded by Gilbert Dagron, 'Les moines et la ville: le monachisme à Constantinople jusqu'au concile de Chalcédoine (451)', *Travaux et mémoires* 4 (1970), 229–276, repr. in Dagron, *La romanité chrétienne en Orient: héritages et mutations* (London, 1984), ch. 8, and criticized in Brown, *Poverty*, 38 with n. 138. See now also Daniel Caner, *Wandering, Begging Monks: Spiritual Authority and the Promotion of Monasticism in Late Antiquity* (Berkeley, CA, 2002), 96–101, 175–176.

12 Vivian Nutton, 'From Galen to Alexander: Aspects of Medicine and Medical Practice in Late Antiquity', *Dumbarton Oaks Papers* 38 (1984), 9; Brown, *Poverty*, 65, for Hippo; Jerome, *Letter* 77.6, in *Sancti Eusebii Hieronymi epistulae*, ed. Isidore Hilberg, *Corpus Scriptorum Ecclesiasticorum Latinorum* LV, 2nd edn (Vienna, 1996), 43.

13 Thomas Sternberg, *Orientalium More Secutus: Räume und Institutionen der Caritas des 5. bis 7. Jahrhunderts in Gallien, Jahrbuch für Antike und Christentum Ergänzungsband* 16 (Münster, 1991), of much wider geographical reference than its title suggests. For the 'oriental custom' in hospital endowment in Francia, see 277–279. For Caesarius, 196–199. On Spain, see now Peter Heather (ed.), *The Visigoths from the Migration Period to the Seventh Century: An Ethnographic Perspective* (Woodbridge, 1999), 196, 272, with *Vitas Sanctum Patrum Emeretensium*, V.3, 4–6, ed. A. Maya Sánchez, *Corpus Christianorum* CXVI (Turnhout, 1992); trans. A. T. Fear, *Lives of the Visigothic Fathers* (Liverpool, 1997).

14 On the counting of late medieval hospitals, I am above all indebted to the work both published and unpublished of Marjorie McIntosh.

15 Susan Ashbrook Harvey, 'The Holy and the Poor: Models from Early Syriac Christianity', in Emily Albu Hanawalt and Carter Lindberg (eds), *Through the Eye of a Needle: Judeo-Christian Roots of Social Welfare* (Kirksville, MO, 1994), 49–51.

16 Michael W. Dols, 'The Origins of the Islamic Hospital: Myth and Reality', *Bulletin of the History of Medicine* 61 (1987), 367–390; Peregrine Horden, 'Nestorians, Gondeshapur, and Islamic Medicine: A Sceptical Comment' (unpublished). I am also much indebted to an unpublished paper by Lawrence I. Conrad, 'The Institution of the Hospital in Medieval Islam: Ideals and Realities'. On Zoroastrian charity see Ehsan Yarshater (ed.), *Encyclopaedia Iranica* V (Costa Mesa, CA, 1991), s.v. 'Charitable Foundations'. The quotation is from (pseudo-) Zacharias Rhetor, *Ecclesiastical History* 12.7, ed. E. W. Brooks, *Corpus Scriptorum Christianorum Orientalium* II (1921), 217–218. I am most grateful to Andrew Palmer for help with the translation.

17 The supposed evidence for an *early* eighth-century Islamic hospital is neatly demolished by Lawrence I. Conrad in 'Did al-Walīd found the First Islamic Hospital?' *Aram* 6 (1994), 225–44. For the Barmakid hospital see Dols, 'Origins', 382–383. On the translation movement a convenient and authoritative summary is Conrad, 'The Arab-Islamic Medical Traditon', in Conrad et al., *The Western Medical Tradition 800 BC to AD 1800* (Cambridge, 1995), 103–110.

18 Thelma D. Sullivan, 'Tlazolteotl-Ixcuina: The Great Spinner and Weaver', in Elizabeth Hill Boone (ed.), *The Art and Iconography of Late Post-Classic Central Mexico* (Washington, DC, 1982), 19–22. Pre-classical Mediterranean and Middle East: I shall not use a footnote to try to prove a negative. There has been no proper comparative discussion of this subject since Hendrik Bolkestein, *Wohltätigkeit und Armenpflege im vorchristlichen Altertum: ein Beitrag zum Problem 'Moral und Gesellschaft'* (Utrecht, 1939). Nor to my knowledge is there any reliable modern global survey. The literature is variable in quality and mostly rather elderly. See e.g. Karl Sudhoff, 'Aus der Geschichte des Krankenhauswesens im früheren Mittelalter in Morgenland und Abendland', *Sudhoffs Archiv* 21 (1929), 164–203; Renihold F. G. Müller, 'Über Krankenhäuser aus Indiens älteren Zeiten', *Sudhoffs Archiv* 22 (1930), 135–151; K. E. Rehm, *Die Rolle des Buddhismus in der Indischen Medizin und das Spitalproblem* (Zurich, 1969); G. Cœdès, 'Les hôpitaux de Jayavarman VII', *Bulletin de l'École française d'extrême orient* 50 (1940, published 1941), 344–349.

19 Georg Harig 'Zum Problem der "Krankenhaus" in der Antike', *Klio* 53 (1971), 179–195 at 188–193; Vivian Nutton, 'Healers in the Medical Market Place: Towards a Social History of Graeco-Roman Medicine', in Andrew Wear (ed.), *Medicine in Society: Historical Essays* (Cambridge, 1992), 50–52. I am also indebted to an unpublished paper by Nutton, 'Hospitals in Antiquity', of which the author kindly sent me a typescript, as well as to Patricia Anne Baker, 'The Roman

Military *Valetudinaria*: Fact or Fiction?' in Robert Arnott (ed.), *The Archae-ology of Medicine* (Oxford, 2002), 69–80. For context: Leonhard Schumacher, *Sklaverei in der Antike: Alltag und Schicksal der Unfreien* (Munich, 2001); Jon-athan P. Roth, *The Logistics of the Roman Army at War (264 B.C.–A.D. 235)* (Leiden, 1999), 86. Hyginus, *Liber de Munitionibus Castrorum*, IV, in *Polybius and Pseudo-Hyginus: The Fortification of the Roman Camp*, ed. and trans. M. C. M. Miller and J. G. DeVoto (Chicago, 1994), 68–69. For the later Middle Ages see again Henderson, *The Renaissance Hospital*.

20 The Theodotos inscription was first published by T. Reinach in *Revue des études juives* 71 (1920), 46–56; translation quoted here is from Steven Fine (ed.), *Sacred Realm: The Emergence of the Synagogue in the Ancient World* (New York, 1996), 9. Context is discussed by Nutton, 'Hospitals in Antiquity', and idem, 'From Galen to Alexander', 9. Unlike some others, I remain persuaded by the nega-tive answer defended by David Seccombe in 'Was There Organized Charity in Jerusalem Before the Christians?', *Journal of Theological Studies*, n.s. 29 (1978), 140–143. On the minimal and ambiguous evidence of other synagogue hostels, see Carl H. Kraeling, *The Synagogue: The Excavations at Dura-Europos Final report VIII, Part I*, augmented edn (New Haven, CT, 1979), 10–11. The only re-cent discussion known to me is Frank M. Loewenberg, *From Charity to Social Justice: The Emergence of Communal Institutions for the Support of the Poor in Ancient Judaism* (New Brunswick NJ, 2001), 141–142, 153. On synagogue hospitality see also S. Safrai and M. Stern (eds.), *The Jewish People in the First Century: Historical Geography, Political History, Social, Cultural and Religious Life and Institutions*, II (Amsterdam, 1976), 943; Lee I. Levine, *The Ancient Syn-agogue: The First Thousand Years* (New Haven, CT, 2000), 381–382. Hospitals in Gregory the Great: *Register*, 9.38, in *Gregorii I Papae registrum epistolarum*, ed. M. Hartmann, II (Berlin, 1899), 67. Julian's *Letter* 22 to the high priest of the province of Galatia (ed. and trans. Wilmer Cave Wright, *The Works of the Emperor Julian*, III (London, 1953), 70–71) is here cited in the translation by Menahem Stern, *Greek and Latin Authors on Jews and Judaism*, II (Jerusalem, 1980), no. 482. On the controversial 'soup kitchen' see Joyce Reynolds and Robert Tannenbaum, *Jews and Godfearers at Aphrodisias* (Cambridge, 1987), 28–29, 41.

21 I do not know of a satisfactory modern study of Jewish hospitals in the later Middle Ages. Mark Cohen generously shared with me in advance of publication his section on medical care for the needy in his *Poverty and Charity in the Jewish Community of Medieval Egypt* (Princeton, NJ, 2005). On that community the fundamental study remains S. D. Goitein, *A Mediterranean Society: The Jew-ish Communities of the Arab World as Portrayed in the Documents of the Cairo Geniza*, 5 vols (Berkeley, CA, 1977–88), II, 99, 113–14, 135–6, 153–4, 251. For the *funduq*, see Olivia Remie Constable, *Housing the Stranger in the Mediterranean World: Lodging, Trade, and Travel in Late Antiquity and the Middle Ages* (Cam-bridge, 2003), 85–88.

22 Goitein, *Mediterranean Society*, II, 251–2.

23 True hospitals as medicalized: Miller, *Birth*. Hospital in Spanish villa: Brown, *Poverty*, 130, n. 22. Paulinus of Nola and portico hospital in early fifth century: Paulinus, *Poem* 21, ll. 384–386, in *The Poems of St. Paulinus of Nola*, trans. P. G. Walsh (New York, 1975), 185. Foundation from below: I infer the general possi-bility from its discovery in twelfth-century England by Max Satchell, 'The Emer-gence of Leper Houses in Medieval England, 1100–1250', unpublished DPhil thesis (University of Oxford, 1998). Temporary hospitals and famine relief: Pal-ladius, *Historia Lausiaca* 40, in *The Lausiac History of Palladius*, ed. Cuthbert

Butler, II (Cambridge, 1904), 126–7. For pagan quasi-hospitals: Nutton, 'Hospitals in Antiquity.'

24 Bishop's house, Sternberg, *Orientalium More Secutus*, ch. 2. Augustine, *Sermon* 356.10, in *Patrologia Latina*, ed. J.-P. Migne, XXXIX, col. 1578, with Brown, *The Birth of Western Christendom*, 2nd edn (Oxford, 2003), 78; idem, *Poverty*, 65.

25 Roland de Vauz, 'Les hôpitaux de Justinien à Jérusalem d'après les dernières fouilles', *Comptes rendus de l'Académie des Inscriptions et Belles-Lettres* (1964), 202–207; Constantelos, *Byzantine Philanthropy*, 122. For a multi-storied hospital see Timothy S. Miller, 'The Sampson Hospital of Constantinople', *Byzantinische Forschungen* 15 (1990), 101–135 at 113. I am also indebted to the brief discussion of the matter in Vivian Nutton, *Ancient Medicine* (London 2004), ch. 19, of which the author kindly showed me the typescript.

26 Charles Du Fresne Du Cange, *Historia Byzantina*, II, *Constantinopolis Christiana* (Paris, 1680), bk. 4, no. 9; Robert Janin, *La géographie ecclésiastique de l'empire byzantin, première partie*, III, *Les églises et les monastères*, 2nd edn (Paris, 1969), 552–567; Konstantina Mentzou-Meimare, 'Eparchiaka evage idrymata mechri tou telous tes eikonomachias', *Byzantina* 11 (1982), 243–308; Sternberg, *Orientalium More Secutus*, 291 (map); Walther Schönfeld, 'Die Xenodochien in Italien und Frankreich im frühen Mittelalter', *Zeitschrift der Savigny-Stiftung für Rechtsgeschichte, Kanonistische Abteilung* 12 (1922), 1–54; Lawrence I. Conrad, 'Arab-Islamic Medicine', in W. F. Bynum and Roy Porter (eds), *Companion Encyclopaedia of the History of Medicine*, II (London, 1993), 716; idem, 'Institution of the Hospital'.

27 Satchell, 'The Emergence of Leper Houses'; Brown, *Poverty*, 27–8, 65; Judith Herrin, 'Ideals of Charity, Realities of Welfare: The Philanthropic Activity of the Byzantine Church', in Rosemary Morris (ed.), *Church and People in Byzantium* (Birmingham, 1991), 153–154; Peter Garnsey and Caroline Humfress, *The Evolution of the Late Antique World* (Cambridge, 2001), 126–127.

28 Wendy Davies, 'The Place of Healing in Early Irish Society', in Donnchadh Ó Corráin, Liam Breatnach, and Kim McCone (eds), *Sages, Saints and Storytellers: Celtic Studies in Honour of Professor James Carney* (Maynooth, 1989), 43, notes the absence of 'any strong tradition of sick care in early Irish monastic rules'. On Anglo-Saxon hospitals see esp. Audrey Meaney, 'The Practice of Medicine in England about the Year 1000', *Social History of Medicine* 13 (2000), 224–227. For the Bremen hospital Rimbert, *Vita S. Anskarii*, 35, ed. W. Trillmich, *Quellen des 9. und 11. Jahrhunderts zur Geschichte der Hamburgische Kirche und des Reiches* (Darmstadt, 1978).

29 Patlagean as in n. 4 above. Brown, *Poverty*, 128, n. 13, gives some more recent bibliography on the prosperity of the later Roman empire in the east, to which add Jairus Banaji, *Agrarian Change in Late Antiquity: Gold, Labour, and Aristocratic Dominance* (Oxford, 2001), 214–215. I am also indebted to Peter Sarris for sight in advance of publication of his 'Rehabilitating the Great Estate: Aristocratic Property and Economic Growth in the Late Antique Eastern Empire', in L. Lavan and W. Bowden (eds), *Recent Research in the Late Antique Countryside* (Leiden, 2004), 55–71.

30 I shall not try to buttress that brief overview. Some of the issues raised are touched on in Peregrine Horden and Nicholas Purcell, *The Corrupting Sea: A Study of Mediterranean History* (Oxford, 2000), ch. 5. See now also Michael McCormick, *Origins of the European Economy: Communications and Commerce AD 300–900* (Cambridge, 2001).

31 Rimbert, *Vita S. Anskarii*, 20, in Trillmich (ed.), *Quellen*, 64–66, with Ian Wood, *The Missionary Life: Saints and the Evangelisation of Europe 400–1050* (Harlow,

2001), 123–132. The lesser scale of poverty in western Europe as compared with Byzantium is touched on by Peter Brown, *The Cult of the Saints: Its Rise and Function in Latin Christianity* (London, 1981), 40, although Brown, *Poverty*, now takes a different view of the scale of poverty in the east and would presumably downplay his earlier stark contrast. For context see Valerio Neri, *I marginali nell'occidente tardoantico: poveri, 'infames' e criminali nella nascente società cristiana* (Bari, 1998), esp. 97–102 for the *matricula pauperum* in Gaul, a topic of which much heavy weather has previously been made.

32 van Leeuwen, *The Logic of Charity*, 20, 26.

33 Garnsey and Humfress, *Evolution*, 123–7; Brown, *Poverty*, 17, 27. With Adolf von Harnack, *Mission und Ausbreitung des Christentums* (Leipzig, 1924), 1st edn trans. J. Moffat (London, 1904–5); compare now Rodney Stark, *The Rise of Christianity: A Sociologist Reconsiders History* (Princeton, NJ, 1996), and the papers by him discussed in William R. Garrett, 'Sociology and New Testament Studies: A Critical Evaluation of Rodney Stark's Contribution', *Journal for the Scientific Study of Religion* 29 (1990), 377–384; also Gary B. Ferngren, 'Early Christianity as a Religion of Healing', *Bulletin of the History of Medicine* 61 (1992), 1–15; MacMullen, *Christianizing*, ch. 4; R. M. Grant, *Early Christianity and Society* (London, 1977), ch. 6.

34 Elaine Phillips, 'Charitable Institutions in Norfolk and Suffolk', PhD thesis (University of East Anglia, 2001); Peter van Minnen, 'Medical Care in Late Antiquity', in Philip J. van der Eijk, H. F. J. Horstmanshoff, and P. H. Schrijvers (eds), *Ancient Medicine in Its Socio-Cultural Context*, I (Amsterdam, 1995), 153–169. I am also greatly indebted to an unpublished paper by Richard Alston on charity in late antiquity. John the Almsgiver: Leontius of Neapolis, *Life*, 7, trans. Elizabeth Dawes and Norman Baynes, *Three Byzantine Saints* (London, 1948). Gregory Nazianzen, n. 8 above. In the (?) tenth-century *Life* of Luke the Stylite a patient with severe head injuries is discharged as incurable from one major Constantinople *xenon* to end his days in some other unnamed institution: H. Delehaye (ed.), *Les saints stylites*, Subsidia hagiographica XIV (Paris, 1923), 218.

35 Compare Patlagean, *Pauvreté*, 196–203. Rawcliffe, *Medicine for the Soul* is again here exemplary for the early medievalist.

36 For a hospital's distributions, see Bernard P. Grenfell and Arthur S. Hunt (eds), *The Amherst Papyri*, II (London, 1901), 188–189, no. 154, with Alston, unpublished paper; compare Nicholas Orme and Margaret Webster, *The English Hospital 1070–1570* (New Haven, CT, 1995), ch. 3.

37 Julian: see note 20 above. Armenia: Nina G. Garsoïan (trans.), *The Epic Histories Attributed to P'awstos Buzand* (Cambridge, MA, 1989), 115, 211–212; Brown, *Poverty*, 42–3. [See now also Nicu Dumitraşcu, *Basil the Great: Faith, Mission and Diplomacy in the Shaping of Christian Doctrine* (London, 2018), 52–55.]

38 Fuller documentation of what follows can be found in Peregrine Horden, 'A Discipline of Relevance: The Historiography of the Later Medieval Hospital', *Social History of Medicine* 1 (1988), 359–74; idem, 'Household Care and Informal Networks: Comparisons and Continuities from Antiquity to the Present', in Peregrine Horden and Richard Smith (eds), *The Locus of Care: Families, Communities, Institutions and the Provision of Welfare since Antiquity* (London, 1998), 21–67.

39 Brown, *Persuasion*, 92–3. Nutton, 'From Galen to Alexander', 10, hypothesizes a crisis of patronage in the third to fourth centuries that could help explain the rise of the hospital in the later Roman empire. I do not know how such a crisis could readily be detectable.

40 To the bibliography given in my 'Household Care' add Adriann Verhulst, *The Carolingian Economy* (Cambridge, 2002), ch. 2, on the early medieval western peasant family, and Neri, *Marginali*.

41 Geniza: for a sample of the material see Goitein, *A Mediterranean Society*, II, 460; V, 74, 110, 117, 122 etc. I should stress that I take a different view of this evidence from that of Mark Cohen, to whom I am indebted for discussion and references. See again his *Poverty and Charity in the Jewish Community of Medieval Egypt*. Louis: Sharon Farmer, *Surviving Poverty in Medieval Paris: Gender, Ideology and the Daily Lives of the Poor* (Ithaca, NY, 2002). Note also William Chester Jordan, *Women and Credit in Pre-industrial and Developing Societies* (Philadelphia, 1993), too little known in this context. *Miracula S. Willehadi auctore S. Anskari episcopo Bremensi* IX, XII, *Acta Sanctorum* (Nov.), III, 349. Wood, *Missionary Life*. Gregory, *De virtutibus Juliani* IX, trans. Raymond Van Dam, *Saints and their Miracles in Late Antique Gaul* (Princeton, NJ, 1993), 170.

42 *De virtutibus Martini*, III.16, II.4; trans. Van Dam, 266–267, 231.

43 Van Minnen, 'Medical Care', 153; Miller, *Birth*. I summarize here my paper, 'How Medicalized Were Byzantine Hospitals?', in Neithard Bulst (ed.), *Sozialgeschichte mittelalterliche Hospitäler, Vorträge und Forschungen*, LIII (Stuttgart), 213–236. Also P. Horden, 'The Millennium Bug: Health and Medicine around the Year 1000', *Social History of Medicine* 13 (2000), 201–219 at 214–215; Peter E. Pormann, 'Theory and Practice in the Early Hospitals in Baghdad: Al-Kaškari on Rabies and Melancholy', *Zeitschrift für Geschichte der Arabisch-Islamischen Wissenschaften* 15 (2002/2003), 198–199.

4

SICKNESS AND HEALING [IN THE CHRISTIAN WORLD, *c*.600–*c*.1100]

1. Saints and others

In early medieval Basra (Iraq), a story circulated about a handsome deacon with a speech impediment.[1] Sorcerers were blamed for his eight years' suffering.

> His mother took him round to a monastery to be healed, but he received no healing, either from the monastery, or from anyone else. So she went off to the doctors, followers of Plato, but she received no help from Plato or his followers. So she set off on a journey . . . to some sorcerers, she [got] nothing either from them or from the wicked whom the demons had deceived.

Finally, she heard about a visiting holy man, John of Dailam. The outcome can be guessed. Merely laying his cross on the deacon's tongue, the saint triumphed where others – monks, doctors, 'witch doctors' – had failed. (The doctors, as purveyors of philosophical medicine, were supposedly followers of Plato; more realistically they were disciples of Galen.) The following Sunday, to universal astonishment, the deacon read the Epistles in church.

Such was the miracle story included in a panegyric of John. Composed well after his death in the early eighth century, it apparently incorporates material from his own time. In England, much later on, a similar tale was told: of a girl who suffered for two years from an ulcer on each foot.[2] 'She endured such great pain and swelling that . . . she could not touch the ground with either foot.' Her father carried her about among 'doctors and holy places' – living physicians and dead saints. Eventually she found miraculous relief at the shrine of Gilbert of Sempringham (*c*.1083–1189, canonized 1202).

Hagiographical narratives like these open windows onto the therapeutic landscape of the early Middle Ages. True, they offer only a partial view of illness and handicap. They were recorded by those hoping to promote a saint's cult by extolling his or her miracles; almost every story thus has the same happy ending. Normally, too, the background detail of the pilgrim sufferer's previous, unsuccessful, attempts at cure is set out in a predictable sequence that echoes the Gospel prototype of Christ's healing of the woman with an issue of blood.[3] The pilgrim has tried doctors, who are expensive and useless, then turns to saintly medicine, which is free and immediately effective.

Still, the incidental details of the run-up to the cure must have been plausible. That was essential for the miracle narrative to persuade its audience of the attractiveness of the shrine. The various healers to whom the pilgrims had reportedly first turned may have been caricatured, but they could not have been totally misrepresented. Their costly failures would not have been worth cataloguing so heavy-handedly if they did not offer a credible, popular alternative to a miracle at a shrine. The hagiographers are the first to admit that the sick tried secular therapy first and its heavenly counterpart second.

The two stories retold above, however, differ slightly in structure from the standard type of miracle narrative. The deacon of Basra is led to monks, then to physicians, then to sorcerers. The hagiographer does not rearrange his mother's preferences into a neat progression, from superstition (sorcery) to earthly medicine (doctors) to religious healing (first monks, then saint). The English girl with the painful feet is taken indiscriminately to both doctors and saints. Such departures from the biblical prototype may increase our confidence in the accounts' broad veracity.

The saint does not even have to be the end of the story. In Anatolia, Theodore of Sykeon (d. 613), a living holy man, sometimes avoided miracle-working by referring his patients to others:[4]

> If any required medical treatment for certain illnesses or surgery or a purging draught or hot-springs, this God-inspired man would prescribe the best thing for each, for even in technical matters he had become an experienced doctor. He might recommend one to have recourse to surgery and he would always state clearly which doctor they should employ.

Similarly, in the early eighth century, John, bishop of Hexham (northern England), did not hesitate to call upon physicians and surgeons as supplements to his own miraculous cures.[5] And throughout our period, dead saints, appearing to pilgrims in dreams and visions, would continue to instruct sufferers to embrace the techniques of secular medicine.

Since the 1980s medical historians have used the metaphor of the marketplace to characterize this therapeutic pluralism. For some tastes, that is too redolent of modern economics: it implies that patients could exercise more freedom of choice than will often have been possible. One advantage of the metaphor is, however, that it brings out the simultaneous availability of many different types of healer and the competition between them. This competition is well attested from the ancient and late antique worlds, and we sense it, from the early Middle Ages, in snippets of hagiography. A further advantage is that the metaphor accentuates the role of the patient – or the immediate carer – in deciding his or her own 'hierarchy of resort':[6] a hierarchy in which the positions of saints, doctors, and sorcerers are not predetermined.

Granted, then, that there was a marketplace for healing in the early medieval world, obvious questions suggest themselves. Who was selling what to whom? What were the relative proportions of the different 'sectors', and how did these vary over time and space? How important were gender differences among healers? Above all, what was the role of Christianity?

None of these questions is readily answered. Hagiography provides our best evidence for the 'everyday life' of the period, and thus for healing, but does not take us far enough. For medicine in the various learned traditions, we have a substantial number of texts, but in most cases we do not know how they were used or by whom. The daily practice of the average healer – who learned his craft orally, through apprenticeship – is even more obscure. We do not have the inscriptions and papyri that elucidate the lower reaches of the medical 'profession' in the classical world, or the archives that reveal their later medieval successors. Sorcerers and other magical healers, of the kind whom the deacon of Basra visited, are yet more obscure.

Overall, the relative scale that we can attribute to each type or source of healing is in inverse proportion to the volume of evidence for it that survives. Saints, so well documented, were demanding in their prerequisites (the pilgrim must have demonstrated full repentance of sin to merit cure). They can have catered for only a minority of the sick. At the other end of the spectrum, the 'informal' sector of self-help or reliance on family and neighbours for basic nursing was presumably the largest, even if, among the poorer members of society, such support networks were fragile. Yet this sector is seldom documented. A few texts survive that are explicitly for the self-medication of those without access to doctors. The possibly magical impedimenta – pieces of cloth, herbs, animal substances, rings – found in women's graves, in boxes that hung from the waist, across barely Christianized northern Europe at the start of our period have been interpreted as signs of female domestic therapy.[7] But if aristocratic ladies dispensed remedies to their household in the seventh century, as we know that they would in the seventeenth,[8] there is no direct trace of such activity. Hagiography once again offers suggestive glimpses of domestic support, in its narration of who helped whom on pilgrimage. For example in Anskar's *Miracles* of St Willehad, the first bishop of Bremen (north-western Germany), written in the 860s, one poor woman is shown helping her neighbour, blind for seven years, to travel to the saint's shrine because she had no one else.[9] It is not much to go on, and for detailed and evocative material we have to wait for the thirteenth century and the *Miracles of St Louis*.[10] Even then, the material is necessarily skewed towards showing informal support only at its moments of failure. And what it tells us is hardly more than could have been intuited – that co-resident household members and neighbours were more help in sickness than distant kin.

This bias of the evidence is not the only challenge. Unavoidably, the medical historian is embroiled in debates about the relationship between magic, science, and religion that have been running inconclusively since the nineteenth century. To give just one illustration: in a ninth-century Carolingian manuscript from a French monastery, seventeen remedies derived from the body of a freshly killed vulture are inserted on a blank page in the middle of a Latin version of the *Materia Medica* of the great first-century pharmacologist Dioscorides. Before decapitating the vulture to make e.g. a remedy for migraine one should say 'Angel, Adonai, Abraham'.[11] Such a ritual utterance, with its implied coercion of hidden powers, its air of mechanical efficacy, bears all the hallmarks of the magical. How then do we conceptualize this short text's relationship to the surrounding medicine of Dioscorides? And how do we interpret its Biblical elements? Is this Christianized magic or 'magic-ized' Christianity, some unorthodox outgrowth of proper observance? Or does more depend on the way the text would have been used rather than on the words on the page? The triple invocation can be enunciated in a prayerful way, as ideally was the liturgy, rather than in a mechanical way that paid no attention to the words. The only path through these difficulties is found in respecting local definitions and conceptions, so far as we can establish them. For early medieval sufferers, the real contrast was less between incompatible systems of ideas – theology, medicine, magic – than between different authorities. Few disputed that ritual words and gestures had power over invisible forces – but whose words, and which forces?[12]

In what follows, then, headings are given – medicine, magic, religion – but they should be taken only as indicating movement along a continuum, not clear transitions from one category to another.

2. Medicine

In the history of medical learning, our period falls between two peaks of impressive activity, each of which marks a major transformation in the way medicine was conceived. At the start, more or less complete by 600, had come the subjugation of medical learning, at least in the Byzantine world, by Galenism. The achievement of Galen of Pergamum (129–216/17) was so comprehensive, his solutions to almost all the big medical questions seemingly so complete, that most subsequent medical scholarship in the Greek East was devoted to distilling his vast output and harmonizing its contradictions – rendering it 'user-friendly'.

At the end of our period, in the second half of the eleventh century in southern Italy, the first steps were taken in the great translation movement that made Greek medicine and philosophy, preserved in Arabic, fully accessible to western scholars in Latin. That translation movement, initially associated with the name of Constantine the African (d. before 1099), laid the basis for a philosophically robust medicine capable of being taught in schools such as the famous one at Salerno (southern Italy) and later in universities. It ensured that Galenic medicine would dominate European medical learning for another 800 years.

In between these two developments, what was medicine like? The first general observation to make is that, early on in our period, learned medicine was not only shorn of its earlier pagan associations, it was domesticated by Christianity. Hippocrates had said that the doctor's fate was to harvest sorrow of his own from others' miseries.[13] In some respects obviously applicable to Jesus, the complaint subtly changed, and by around AD 400 had become a description of the ideal physician. So broadly compatible were the ethics of ancient medicine with those of Christianity that an eleventh-century Greek manuscript (now, appropriately, in the Vatican) includes a text of the Hippocratic Oath in the shape of a cross.[14]

The second, related, observation to make is that this medicine was very often practised by priests and monks. It is a cliché that the medicine of the early Middle Ages was *exclusively* monastic; this may underplay the role of secular priests, especially at the end of our period, and it certainly underplays the role of lay healers. It is also a cliché that there was, on the other hand, some deep antithesis between the religious life and medical practice. Yet in Christianized Russia of the eleventh century (according to some later redactions of the 'Law of Vladimir', d. 1015) healers were among those over whom the Church was given exclusive jurisdiction.[15] As we shall see, the largest and medically most impressive hospital of its age, the hospital of the Pantocrator, was based within a monastery; and the whole medical history of the period would look very different were it not for the texts copied and preserved in monastic scriptoria and libraries. Moreover, when canon law on the matter began to solidify, just after the end of our period, it placed relatively few restrictions on the practice of medicine by monks and clerics.

The third generalization that can be hazarded about the medical literature of the period is that the theory has largely been drained out of it. Overall, not counting Galen and a handful of others, theorists and practitioners had slowly been parting company for some centuries in classical Mediterranean medicine. The medical literature of the early Middle Ages takes this to an extreme. In the East the characteristic major product, in vogue at the start of our period and again, to a lesser extent, in the tenth and eleventh centuries, is the encyclopaedic collection – artfully arranged excerpts from Galen and from the other authors needed to fill in the gaps that he left. On a lesser level, perhaps closer to everyday practice, is the treatment list. From both, all genuine discussion of medical ideas has been eliminated, as, mostly, has consideration of symptoms. 'Against headache and migraine', read one much copied Greek remedy, 'crush cress in vinegar with oil of roses; make an ointment of it. Rub it thoroughly into the head.'[16] Plain and simple, and no vultures required.

The literate medicine of early medieval western Europe is harder to sum up. In formal terms the written medicine is more various than that of Byzantine medicine – from a few extended translations of ancient treatises to very short miscellanies. The latter texts are highly unstable: hardly any two surviving manuscripts resemble one another closely. And their stated authorship – Galen or Hippocrates in many cases – is frequently questionable. Some collections, such as the late eighth-century *Book of Medicine* (essentially a substantial recipe book) copied in the great Carolingian abbey of Lorsch (south-western Germany), with its defence of medicine and brief introductory sections on medical ethics, the humours, etc., were intended to have an air of comprehensiveness and order.[17] Other, lesser, texts often degenerate into unintelligibility through repeated copying. They survive in, to us, unlikely ways – as did gynaecological treatises in monastic libraries. And many texts were quite unsuited to medical training. Consider *The Book of Medicine from Urines*, a short treatise by 'Hermogenes', an author probably of the ninth century dignified with a classical name. It is preserved uniquely in a late tenth-century manuscript at the Italian abbey of Monte Cassino.

> For there are many signs and kinds of illness associated with white urine. And white urine denotes dissolution of vigour . . . And there is another white urine which denotes a weakness lasting many days, and the blockage of the body's veins; and this illness often happens because of excessive drinking of wine. Where you see urine which is thick and white, you should know that one of the four humours is being liquefied . . . And if you see urine with a strong yellow colour it proclaims the body is sick because of red melancholy . . .[18]

There are traces there of the ancient theory according to which ill health reflected an imbalance of humours. Yet the text is vague about what diseases result from the imbalances mentioned, and silent on what should be done about them. It is hard to imagine at whom the treatise was aimed or how it could, without a great deal of supplementary instruction, be turned to practical advantage.

We know more about the medicine of the period, for all its obscurities, than we do about doctors. We know, of course, the names (and sometimes the writings) of a modest number of physicians at court or in the great monasteries: for instance Theophanes Chrysobalantes, who addressed a medical handbook to a Byzantine emperor, probably Constantine Porphyrogenitus (905–959).[19] We also know about those whom we might call gentlemen amateurs, beginning with the emperor Charlemagne himself, knowledgeable about medicine as a part of a wider liberal education and occasional dispensers of advice to friends, yet hardly doctors. But nothing survives that would enable us to address the big sociological questions that bear on the full spectrum of practice.

The fundamental problem is one of definition: what was it to be a doctor? The attempted legal definitions of antiquity scarcely apply in our centuries. There were some medical guilds in the Greek East, especially in Constantinople.[20] Yet no evidence suggests that they were able to enforce professional standards at all widely. Elsewhere, the designation 'doctor' had simply to be claimed, and then retained through successful practice. Often it will have been a part-time activity; and so a great number of practitioners will escape our notice because they are never labelled as such.

One consequence of that is our inability to say much about women's practice. In this period as later, women were far more likely to be part-time carers, nurses, or healers. Like most other female workers, they had 'weak occupational identity' as well as inferior status. Hence on the rare occasions when they surface in the documentation they are unlikely to be identified as medical practitioners. It is impossible even to sketch the history of midwifery, a category of much broader scope in the early Middle Ages than it would later become. The one exception to all this obscurity is the nascent medical school of eleventh- to twelfth-century Salerno, with its handful of known women healers, especially Trota (the famous 'Trotula' is not her name but the collective title of the texts attributed to her).

We should not imagine that the majority of male practitioners are any better placed. To look only at western Europe: Ireland in this period comes across as a land almost without medicine. Of course, practitioners of various kinds, some of them female, are attested (bone-setters, blood-letters etc.). But of literate medical practice, or even of basic herbalism, there is little trace.

Anglo-Saxon medicine was much inspired by Latin medical wisdom and some one thousand manuscript pages of it survive; yet in pre-Conquest England, too, the prosopography of doctors is slender. Only for France is the record more full: some 45 named medical men for the period 600–1000; 87 for the eleventh century (showing how far the picture can be distorted by the increasing survival rate of documents and widening literacy). But the careers of individuals in question are for the moment mostly unknowable. Perhaps charter evidence will shed more light on the French, German, and Spanish 'medical' scene, as it has already begun to do for southern Italy.

On these fragile foundations it would be rash to erect any grand conclusions. Healers in the West were probably overall fewer in number and lower in status than those of the more urbanized East, with its concentrations of wealthier sick people. It was demonstrably like this in antiquity. It probably remained so in the early Middle Ages.

What was the reach, socially and economically, of the medicine dispensed? Archival work done on later medieval societies suggests that there could be a surprisingly intense and widespread appetite for medical learning. It could be imitated by illiterate 'empirics' – or even by parish priests. A manual produced by the abbey of Lorsch c.900, perhaps for parish priests being sent out onto some of its estates, includes the 'Egyptian days', on which one should not be bled or given any medicine. It also lists preventative regimes for each month of the year.[21]

3. Magic

Beyond the frontier of this parish medicine should we place sorcery – a distinct alternative to Galenism or its western equivalents, as in the Syriac tale of a search for cure with which we began? It would be convenient to hold up the sorcerer as the poor person's physician: easier of access because there were more sorcerers than physicians and they were cheaper. Or again it would be convenient to accept that sufferers tried sorcerers or magicians when naturalistic medicine had failed and something more powerful was needed. Much of the hagiography (though not my two opening examples) suggests as much. But hagiography, as we saw, has a particular slant on the topic and cannot be taken at face value. Anyone can in principle pronounce a spell or charm or construct an amulet; but that does not make magic simply the pauper's medicine. Sorcerers demand fees, too; and magic is not disdained by the educated. Like the manuscript referred to earlier, in which incantatory vulture medicine is found in the middle of an ancient treatise on drugs, many of the most learned and expensive texts copied in our period include remedies that we might classify as magical.

We know little, however, about the circumstances in which the sick resorted to magical remedies. Byzantium provides tantalising vignettes. The first comes from the threshold of our period. The learned sixth-century physician Alexander of Tralles happily condoned the use of charms and amulets. He included in his medical encyclopaedia a traditional remedy for epilepsy that required the blood of a dead gladiator. This had been rejected by Galen. Yet for Alexander, writing centuries after the death of the last gladiator, it remained an 'excellent and well-tried remedy'.[22] As for colic:

> since many patients, and especially the wealthy ones, object . . . to treating their bowels with enemas, they force us to cure the pain with the help of magical amulets. That is why I have thought it worthwhile to give you an account of these also, both the ones which I know from my own experience and those whose effectiveness is vouched for by trusted friends.[23]

Thus magic was not restricted to cases where Galenic methods had failed, but could be used when patients found conventional methods unpleasant. The good doctor, Alexander says, should omit nothing from his arsenal that might contribute to healing. For him, magic is characterized by its material vectors and its aura of secrecy. But he crosses the boundary between it and medicine without fear of censure from any medical or ecclesiastical authority. We have heard much about 'the rise of magic' in the early Middle Ages. But magic did not rise as if engulfing the supposed rationalism of ancient medicine. It had always been there. Only Galen and a few like-minded souls rejected all but naturalistic explanations of phenomena. Alexander was enough of a Galenist to pigeonhole his magical remedies – not enough of one to eliminate them altogether.

Moving forward to just after the end of our period, we can, highly unusually, hear from a magician in his own words. Michael Italikos, a teacher of many subjects including medicine before he became a high-ranking churchman around 1145, writes to one Tziknoglos.[24] This man's sister has developed some chronic condition (perhaps a tumour) that conventional medicine cannot cure. She and her brother have heard about a magician who offers to help, and they consult Italikos about the wisdom of accepting the offer. Italikos counsels against resort to magic, which is contrary to Christian law. Even so, he clearly knows a great deal about it, and has read many books on it:

> I have also extended my eagerness for such knowledge to the daft babbling of the old women at the crossroads, and anything else going round the common people. I am in possession of charms, binding-magic, and a good many useful symbols which contain unspoken commands, and cures for stinking viscera, and relief for swellings.

Then he starts to protest too much: 'but I have never acquired any of these for my own benefit, nor have I ever had any faith in them.' Anxious to avoid direct involvement in the cure of Tziknoglos's sister, he has asked another magician to do him 'a favour'. He now has in his possession some ancient remedy which he will describe when he and Tziknoglos next meet because it would, he says, take too much space to write down.

Between Alexander and Michael, magic has been more broadly defined and vigorously prohibited than it was around 600. Hence Italikos's prudent reluctance to put his spell in writing. In the West, also, magical healing of this kind had been outlawed. A substantial body of hagiography, secular as well as canon law, penitentials, sermons, and polemic repeats, stereotypically, a catalogue of prohibited practices – sooth-saying, divining, lot-casting, enchanting, witchcraft. Sometimes it provides memorable examples in specifying punishment. 'If a woman places her daughter on the roof or in an oven as a cure for fever, let her do penance for seven years.'[25] Yet how widespread were such practices? Evidence suggesting their ubiquity is of two kinds. First, there is the frequency and stridency with which the practices were condemned throughout our period. Second, there is the extent to which the Church increasingly accommodated some of their more beneficent forms, notably astrology. In the West much of the reality of everyday magic is obscure to us because we see it only through inflamed clerical eyes. Yet the sheer pressure that it apparently exerted on the Church can at least be taken as testimony to its prevalence.

That prevalence may, however, have been a 'regional' phenomenon. The argument does not apply so readily to the Byzantine world. There, the prohibitions were perhaps more all-embracing and more effective, as we can infer from Italikos's anxiety. Quasi-pagan charms and amulets largely disappeared after the ninth or tenth century in Byzantium, to be replaced by small portable crosses and other such orthodox items. There was not quite the same accommodation that has been detected in the West, even though magical beliefs were obviously by no means extirpated. Perhaps in the West, as has been suggested, sorcerers really were more numerous then priests at the start of the period, especially in the frontier zones of Christianity.[26] Dare we then conclude that there was more magical healing in the West than in the East? We have no means of measuring.

4. Religion

After science (medicine), and after magic, where can the chapter turn next but to religion? How did religion and healing interrelate in our period? Christianity began, in the gospels, as a religion of healing. And although historians dispute the relative importance of healing miracles in Christianity's early propagation, there is no doubting the subsequent centrality of the wonder working of holy persons and their relics to both the expansion of Christendom and its internal dynamics.

The miracles with which the chapter opened were, however, only one element in the array of therapies developed by the early medieval Church – therapies directed primarily at the immortal soul, rather than the body, and dependent on prayer and the sacraments rather than drugs and ointments. Between medicine and theology there was thus enormous potential for tension. At the start of our period the 'profession' of medicine was too imbued with paganism to be acceptable to many church rigorists. Later on its implicit naturalism may, it has been argued, have rendered medical theory suspect in a different way. Our period ends before, in the West, the recovery of Aristotle established philosophical common ground for theology and university medicine.

Was resort to medicine therefore really permissible? For Pope Gregory the Great, composing c.590 his enormously influential manual for bishops, the sick among Christian congregations should be told that they must endure suffering on this earth if they were ever to reach heaven. 'The health of the heart' (or soul) is bodily affliction, a great gift in that it 'cleanses sins'. Illness should be endured as Christ endured the Cross. It is a way of disciplining or educating the soul. It removes the sins that, by implication, might have caused it and hinders the committing of further sins.[27] This seems to leave no room for secular medicine.

And yet Gregory himself, martyr to chronic pain, ascribed one of his own illnesses to melancholy, not to moral failing, and had a physician from the great medical school of Alexandria in permanent attendance. Nor did he hesitate to recommend physicians and their remedies to friends or colleagues.[28] The connection between sin and disease was far less often to the fore in early medieval accounts of sickness than has usually been imagined. Since the Fall, the general 'background' sinfulness of humanity had brought disease into creation, but by no means all illnesses were to be related to specific sins. In a seventh-century Greek collection of 'questions and answers' attributed to Anastasius of Sinai, it is asked why there are more maimed, arthritic, gouty, and leprous people among Christians than among infidels.[29] The answer is equivocal. Some say that God has sent these afflictions to test his devotees' faith and love. Others, though, argue that it is a question of climate, habitat, and diet. No one mentions sin.

The tensions between religion and medicine should thus not be overstressed. When few forms of secular healing could accomplish much, illness almost always had to be endured to some extent, thus leaving considerable scope for meditation on its spiritual significance. Of the various types of therapy that we have been reviewing, there was none, from learned medicine to simple herbalism or the use of Christian charms, that was widely seen as *in principle* incompatible with the Christian life. (Even the forms of 'magic' that the Church tried to prohibit fell within the framework of theological explanation, because they were, by definition, demonic.) There was only one axiom: sufferers and healers alike should always recall that true healing ultimately comes from God. The message that earthly medicine would fail if the soul had not previously been tended did not have to wait to be proclaimed by the fathers assembled at the Fourth Lateran Council (1215).[30] It had been enunciated some 1,400 years earlier in the Book of Ecclesiasticus (38.1–15). 'Honour the physician,' we are told in a proof text for the Christian reception of medicine. God created medicines from the earth and the prudent man will not disdain them. But then: 'in sickness . . . pray to the Lord, and he will cure you. Turn away from sin . . . and then give place to the physician.' The physician will succeed when he too prays. Even so, he is best avoided, by following the path of goodness: 'he that sins before his maker, let him fall into the hands of the physician!'

The most forceful demonstration of this qualified compatibility between medicine and religion lies in the frequency with which theologians used the physician as a 'role model'. Christ is not described as a physician in the gospels. But within only decades of his death he had become one. From the early first century to – decisively for the West – Augustine (354–430), a sequence of Church Fathers elaborated the idea of *Christus medicus* or *iatros*, originally perhaps as a riposte to the cult of the pagan healing god Asclepius. Our period is replete with literary imagery reflecting the assumption that the careful physician is an effective and powerful figure. This respect is a more positive counterpart to the obloquy heaped on doctors (as effective rivals) by custodians of shrines. Both derive from the perception that the physician's therapy must be taken seriously. It was not only Christ and his saints who were associated with physicians in this way. The priest as confessor was also thought to benefit by association with the healer who carefully weighed symptoms and circumstances so as to arrive at a medicine wholly suited to the individual patient. In the early 1000s, Burchard of Worms tellingly gave the penitential included as book 19 in his collection of canon law the heading *Corrector et medicus*. It listed 'corrections' for bodies and 'medicines' for souls, the converse of what we might have expected.[31]

This medicine for souls was no less medicine than it was soteriology. Any given individual in the period under discussion may have held one or more 'lay' notions of what constituted health – a balance of humours, freedom from demons or (in the Anglo-Saxon case) the attacks of elves, ability to work or procreate sufficiently, mere longevity, etc. But any properly catechized Christian will also have added 'freedom from un-atoned sin'. The health of the soul was no mere metaphor. Attention to it was a form of preventative medicine. In the East, where the Galenic tradition of 'hygiene' or diet in the broadest sense remained unbroken, one could commission from a doctor a regimen, showing what to do and eat month by month. In the West, with its lack of such a central tradition and its emphasis on simple remedies, there are few signs of any comparable approach. But, in West as well as East, protective amulets could be worn, and loricas (protective verbal shields) could be chanted. The Old English text known as the *Lorica of Gildas* calls for example on heaven's army for defence against a wide range of dangers, enumerating all body parts internal and external.[32]

Nor is this just a matter for individuals. The early medieval chapter in the history of public health belongs under the heading of religion rather than medicine. The period is mostly lacking in the usual ingredients of public health history. It falls between the famous markers of Roman public-health concerns – aqueducts, baths, sewers – and the legislation of the Italian cities of the high Middle Ages for the regulation of noxious (and thus pestilential) smells. In the gap between the Romans and the 'Italians' we see occasional signs of a materialist approach. In the early seventh century, for instance, a Frankish bishop, Desiderius of Cahors, anticipated later medieval Italian measures. He set up checkpoints to stop pestiferous merchants from importing the plague. He also wrote to another bishop asking for the loan of specialist craftsmen who would make the wooden tubing needed for planned refurbishment of his city's water supply.[33] More often, though, we encounter what remained a principal ingredient in the public health of the later Middle Ages too: the collective response to impending or actual epidemic manifested in processions and litanies and led by the bishop. Once more it is a question of seeing religion not as a substitute for 'the real thing' (according to our modern definition) but as the real thing itself.

Far more common than the processions, and the miracles some saints wrought to ward off disease, was the administration of the sacraments. Indeed, the Church's one great, truly essential, means of promoting good health was baptism. Baptism was the equivalent of early inoculation: the means to forgiveness of original sin and an exorcism, a rebirth into health. It was not the only sacrament relevant here. We have already sampled the therapy of penance. In both eastern and western rites, the potentially therapeutic effects of the eucharist were also recognised. From the earlier Fathers on, the eucharistic liturgy was a *pharmakon* (drug or medicine), and the prayers for the healing of the sick incorporated into its text were unambiguous.

5. Hospitals

In no therapeutic setting was the interpenetration of medicine of the soul and that of the body so clear as in the hospital. Today's hospital is characterized above all by technological intensity, and concentration of medical expertise on the seriously ill. Such a definition would have embraced only some of the institutions that were called hospitals in the Christian world before around 1800. Still less can it apply before 1100. The medievalist must conceive the hospital more broadly, as an establishment for the overnight accommodation of the poor and/or sick – hospice as much as hospital, charitable first and therapeutic only second.

The hospital in that sense – the hospital before the great 'medicalization' of the modern age – was by origin a Christian invention, and in our period its history is overwhelmingly a Christian history. It was therapeutic by medieval medical standards as a beneficial regulator of the environment in which the needy poor lived and slept. But still more was it therapeutic by medieval theological standards in that it looked after the health of the soul: the founder's soul through the prayers of patients; the patients' souls through the spiritual and physical healing of the liturgy and the sacraments.

The majority of early medieval hospitals would not have passed the test of medicalization imposed by the historiography of their nineteenth- and twentieth-century successors. But the presence of physicians is, however, recorded in a long sequence of them, from that of St Basil of Caesarea established in Anatolia around 370 to the great projected hospital of the Pantocrator monastery founded in Constantinople by John II and his wife, Irene, in the 1120s. In the latter, if the imperial couple's plans were fully realized, a huge staff of some 50 eminent physicians and supporting personnel cared for no more than 50 patients in astonishingly modern-seeming specialized wards.[34]

This 'medicalization' – the intended presence, in some hospitals, of figures labelled doctors – is above all a phenomenon of the East in our period. It is a phenomenon of Byzantium primarily, and then of the cultures to which the model of the Byzantine hospital was exported, especially Sassanian and then Islamic Iran and Iraq. In the West, the explicit involvement of doctors with hospitals is rarer and comes mostly from the earlier part of our period. We must look to Visigothic Spain for an example recorded in any detail. Bishop Masona (d. 605) of Mérida

> built a *xenodocium* ['house for strangers', hospital], enriching it with a large patrimony and appointing ministers and doctors to serve travellers and the sick, giving them this command: that the doctors should go through the entire city without ceasing and whosoever they found that was sick . . . they were to carry in their arms to the *xenodocium*, and having prepared there a well-made bed set the sick man on it and give him light and pleasant food until, with God's help, they returned the patient to his former health.[35]

Although its doctors were thought to offer nothing but rest and diet, this hospital at least was somewhat removed from the stereotype of the pre-modern hospital as no more than a gateway to death.

We should not overestimate the impact of such institutions on the aggregates of sickness and deprivation among the poor. Hospitals were few in number, generally small, and restricted in geography (mostly to the larger cities of Byzantium, and to parts of Italy and Francia). Our period falls between the first wave of hospital foundations of the eastern Mediterranean in the fourth to fifth centuries on the one hand and, on the other, the great vogue for hospital-building evident in twelfth-century Europe.

Despite these caveats, great claims for the precocious modernity of early medieval hospitals have been made. On one influential recent account,[36] the hospital was 'born' in the Byzantine empire – not just as a charitable institution, not just as a place where doctors functioned, but (by the late sixth century) as a centre of medical excellence, medical scholarship, and medical education. The tiny portion of surviving Byzantine medical manuscripts that can in any way be associated with hospitals tell a different story. Hospital medicine in Byzantium was not evidently superior to non-hospital medicine; indeed, the two were very similar, and mostly rather basic.

6. Conclusion

Around the year 1000 one of the most famous physicians in Europe was a monk of St Gall (Switzerland) called Notker. The duke of Bavaria knew of his reputation for accurate prognosis and decided to consult him. First, though, he tested the monk's expertise. He sent him a urine sample – not his own, but that of a servant girl. Having examined it carefully, Notker fell to his knees proclaiming a miracle: in 30 days the duke would give birth to a son. The duke's emissaries returned to court where they found that the servant had in fact been delivered of a boy. They later came back to St Gall with the duke's own urine.[37]

The monastery of St Gall lay about 150 miles from the Bavarian court. This story can thus be taken to suggest the extreme scarcity of good doctors. Yet then as now, the elite will travel, or send a specimen, any distance to secure the very best in treatment. All the signs are that the therapeutic landscape of Notker's age was in fact rather crowded. Notker was a monk-physician of a religious house the library of which contained several medical volumes, including a small portable manual that still survives. His house was the home of the St Gall plan, a famous ninth-century blueprint for the ideal monastery, including a sizeable infirmary. It was also the home of what specialists now reckon an important manuscript of the sixth-century monastic Rule of St Benedict, in which the abbot's pastoral role is likened to that of 'a wise physician'.[38] Notker's skill at prognostication, akin to prophecy, was one that, in less respectable hands, might have seemed more magical than medical. He and his monastery are emblematic of the complex interplay of medicine and religion, the orthodox and the deviant in therapy, the individual and the institutional, the literate and the oral (for his was more than bookish skill), all of which makes sickness and healing in the early Middle Ages such a rich if recalcitrant topic.

Notes

1 [© Cambridge University Press. Reproduced with permission.] Brock, 'A Syriac Life of John of Dailam', 127, 166–167, 187–188. I am much indebted to Klaus-Dietrich Fischer for comments on a draft of this chapter.
2 *The Book of St Gilbert* 19, ed. Foreville and Keir, pp. 324–325.
3 *Mark* 8.25–28; *Luke* 8.43–44.
4 *Vie de Théodore* (Life of Theodore) 145, ed. Festugière, p. 114; tr. Dawes and Baynes, p. 182.
5 Bede, *Ecclesiastical history*, V.2, 6, ed. Colgrave and Mynors, pp. 458–459, 468–469.
6 Horden, 'Saints', 12–13.
7 Meaney, 'Women', pp. 9–12, 29–30.
8 Pollock, *With Faith*.
9 *Miracula* 9, *AASS* 8 Nov., III, p. 849.
10 Guillaume de Saint-Pathus, *Miracles de Saint Louis*; Farmer, *Surviving Poverty*.
11 MacKinney, 'An unpublished treatise', 495; Möhler, *'Epistula de vulture'*.
12 Jolly, 'Medieval magic', p. 16.
13 Hippocratic *On Breaths* 1, ed. Heiberg, p. 91; Temkin, *Hippocrates*, p. 247.
14 Leven, 'Attitudes', p. 76.
15 *The Laws of Rus'*, ed. Kaiser, ch. 16, p. 44; Franklin and Shepard, *Emergence*, p. 234.
16 Jeanselme, 'Sur un aide-mémoire', p. 148; Bennett, 'Xenonica', p. 409, no. 2.
17 *Das Lorscher Arzneibuch*, ed. Stoll.

18 Wallis, 'Signs and senses', 273.
19 Theophanes Chrysobalantes, *Epitome*, ed. St Bernard.
20 Constantine Porphyrogenitus, *Book of Ceremonies*, ed. Vogt, I, p. 10.
21 Paxton, *Bonus liber*.
22 *Alexander von Tralles*, ed. Puschmann, I, p. 565.
23 *Alexander*, ed. Puschmann, II, p. 375, tr. Duffy, 'Byzantine medicine', p. 26.
24 *Michel Italikos*, ed. Gautier, *Letter* 31, pp. 201–203; *The Occult*, tr. Maxwell-Stuart, pp. 148–149.
25 *Penitential of Theodore*, I.15.2, in *Councils and Ecclesiastical Documents*, ed. Haddan and Stubbs, *Councils*, III, p. 190, tr. McNeill and Gamer, *Medieval Handbooks*, p. 198, modified.
26 Flint, *Rise of Magic*, p. 79.
27 Gregory the Great, *Regula pastoralis*, III.12, ed. Judic et al., II, pp. 326–332.
28 Richards, *Consul of God*, pp. 46–47.
29 Anastasius, *Questions and answers* 94, *PG* LXXXIX.732–733.
30 Canon 22, *Decrees of the Ecumenical Councils*, ed. Tanner, I, pp. 245–246.
31 Burchard, *Corrector, PL*, CXL.949, tr. McNeill and Gamer, *Medieval Handbooks*, p. 323.
32 *Anglo-Saxon Remedies*, ed. Pettit, I, pp. 40–56.
33 Horden, 'Ritual', p. 31.
34 'Le typikon', ed. Gautier, 82–112; *Byzantine Monastic Foundation Documents*, tr. Thomas and Hero, no. 28, vol. II, pp. 757–766.
35 *Vitas Patrum Emeretensium*, V.3, ed. Maya Sánchez, pp. 50–51; tr. Fear, *Lives*, pp. 74–75.
36 Miller, *Birth*.
37 Ekkehard, *Casus*, ed. Haefele, p. 240.
38 *Regula Benedicti*, ed. Probst, pp. 79–81 (chs 27, 28).

Bibliography

Abbreviations

AASS = *Acta Sanctorum*
CC = *Corpus Christianorum*
DOP = *Dumbarton Oaks Papers*
PL = *Patrologia Latina*
PG = *Patrologia Graeca*
SC = *Sources chrétiennes*

Primary evidence cited

Alexander von Tralles, Original-text und Übersetzung, edited by Theodor Puschmann, 2 vols (repr. Amsterdam: M. Hakkert, 1963).
Anastasius, *Questions and Answers*, *PG* LXXXIX.311–823.
Anglo-Saxon Remedies, Charms, and Prayers from British Library MS Harley 585: The Lacnunga, edited by Edward Pettit, 2 vols, Mellen Critical Editions and Translations 6a (Lewiston, VA: Edwin Mellen Press, 2001).
Anskar, *Miracula Sancti Willehadi*, in *AASS dies octavus Novembris*, vol. III, pp. 847–851.

Bede, *Ecclesiastical History of the English People*, edited and translated by Bertram Colgrave and Roger A. B. Mynors (Oxford: Clarendon Press, 1969).

The Book of St Gilbert, edited by Raymonde Foreville and Gillian Keir (Oxford: Oxford University Press, 1987).

Brock, Sebastian P., 'A Syriac Life of John of Dailam', *Parole de l'Orient* 10 (1981–2), 123–189.

Burchard of Worms, *Corrector et Medicus* (*Decretum* book 19), *PL* CXL.943–1018.

Byzantine Monastic Foundation Documents: A Complete Translation of the Surviving Founders' Typika and Testaments, edited by John Thomas and Angela Constantinides Hero with the assistance of Giles Constable, 5 vols (Washington DC: Dumbarton Oaks, 2000), and at <www.doaks.org/etexts>.

Constantine Porphyrogenitus, *Book of Ceremonies* (*Constantin VII Porhyrogénète, Le livre des cérémonies*), edited by Albert Vogt, 4 vols (Paris: Les Belles Lettres, 1935–40).

Councils and Ecclesiastical Documents Relating to Great Britain and Ireland, edited by A. W. Haddon and William Stubbs, 3 vols (Oxford: Clarendon Press, 1869–78).

Das 'Lorscher Arzneibuch': ein medizinisches Kompendium des 8. Jahrhunderts (Codex Bambergensis medicinalis 1). Text, Übersetzung und Fachglossar, edited by Ulrich Stoll, Sudhoffs Archiv Beiheft 28 (Stuttgart: Franz Steiner, 1992).

Decrees of the Ecumenical Councils, edited by Norman Tanner, 2 vols (Washington DC: Georgetown University Press, 1990).

Ekkehard IV, *Casus sancti Galli*, edited and translated by Hans F. Haefele, Ausgewählte Quellen zur deutschen Geschichte des Mittelalters 10 (Darmstadt: Wissenschaftliche Buchgesellschaft, 1980).

Gregory the Great, *Regula pastoralis* (*Grégoire le Grand, Règle pastorale*), edited and translated by Bruno Judic, Floribert Rommel, and Charles Morel, 2 vols, *SC* 381, 382 (Paris: Éditions du Cerf, 1992).

Guillaume de Saint-Pathus, *Les miracles de Saint Louis*, edited by Percival B. Fay (Paris: J. Champion, 1931).

Hippocratic author, *On Breaths*, ed. I. L. Heiberg, Corpus Medicorum Graecorum I.1 (Leipzig: Teubner, 1927).

Jeanselme, Edouard, 'Sur un aide-mémoire de thérapeutique byzantin contenu dans un manuscrit de la Bibliothèque Nationale de Paris (Supplément grec 764): traduction, notes et commentaires', in *Mélanges Charles Diehl*, 2 vols (Paris: E. Leroux, 1930), vol. I, pp. 147–170.

The Laws of Rus', Tenth to Fifteenth Centuries, edited and translated by Daniel H. Kaiser (Salt Lake City: Charles Schlacks, Jr., 1992).

MacKinney, Loren C., 'An Unpublished Treatise from the Age of Charlemagne', *Speculum* 18 (1943), 494–496.

McNeill, John T., and Helena M. Gamer, tr., *Medieval Handbooks of Penance* (New York: Columbia University Press, 1938, repr. New York: Octagon Books, 1979).

Michel Italikos, Lettres et discours, edited by Paul Gautier (Paris: Institut français d'études byzantines, 1972).

The Occult in Mediaeval Europe, edited and translated by P. G. Maxwell-Stuart (Basingstoke: Palgrave Macmillan, 2005).

Regula Benedicti, de codice 914 in bibliotheca monasterii S. Galli servato, edited by Benedikt Probst (St Ottilien: EOS, 1983).

107

Theophanes Chrysobalantes, *Theophanis Nonni epitome de curatione morborum Graece ac Latine*, edited by J. St Bernard, 2 vols. (Amsterdam: Gotha, 1794–5).

'Le typikon du Christ Sauveur Pantokrator', edited by Paul Gautier, *Revue des études byzantines* 32 (1974), 1–145.

Vie de Théodore de Sykéôn, edited by André-Jean Festugière, 2 vols, Subsidia hagiographica 48 (Brussels: Société des Bollandistes, 1970), translated by Elizabeth Dawes and Norman Baynes, *Three Byzantine Saints* (Oxford: Mowbray, 1977), pp. 87–192.

Vitas sanctorum patrum Emeretensium, ed. A. Maya Sánchez, *CC* CXVI (Turnhout: Brepols, 1992); translated by A. T. Fear, *Lives of the Visigothic Fathers* (Liverpool: Liverpool University Press, 1997).

Secondary sources cited and further reading

Agrimi, Jole, and Chiara Crisciani, 'Medicina del corpo e medicina dell'anima: note sul sapere del medico fino all'inizio del sec. XIII', *Episteme* 10 (1976), 5–102.

Amundsen, Darrel. W., *Medicine, Society, and Faith in the Ancient and Early Medieval Worlds* (Baltimore, MD: Johns Hopkins University Press, 1996).

Arbesmann, Rudolph, 'The concept of *Christus medicus* in St Augustine', *Traditio* 10 (1954), 1–28.

Bennett, David, 'Medical practice and manuscripts in Byzantium', *Social History of Medicine* 13 (2000), part 2, special issue, *The Year 1000*, edited by Peregrine Horden and Emilie Savage-Smith, 279–291.

Bennett, David, 'Xenonika: medical texts associated with *xenones* in the late Byzantine period', PhD thesis, University of London (2003) [revised version published as *Medicine and Pharmacy in Byzantine Hospitals: A Study of the Extant Formularies* (Abingdon: Routledge, 2017)]

Biller, Peter, and Joseph Ziegler (eds), *Religion and Medicine in the Middle Ages* (Woodbridge: Boydell Press, 2001).

Constantelos, Demetrios J., *Byzantine Philanthropy and Social Welfare*, 2nd edn (New Rochelle, NY: Aristide D. Caratzas, 1991).

Constantine the African and 'Alī ibn al-'Abbās al-Maǧūsī: The Pantegni and Related Texts, edited by Charles Burnett and Danielle Jacquart (Leiden: Brill, 1994).

Cunningham, Graham, *Religion and Magic: Approaches and Theories* (Edinburgh: Edinburgh University Press, 1999).

Davies, Wendy, 'The place of healing in early Irish society', in *Sages, Saints and Storytellers: Celtic Studies in honour of Professor James Carney*, edited by Donnchadh Ó Corráin, Liam Breatnach, and Kim McCone (Maynooth: An Sagart, 1989), pp. 43–55.

Dawtry, Anne F., 'The *modus medendi* and the Benedictine order in Anglo-Norman England', *Studies in Church History* 19 (1982), 25–38.

Déroche, Vincent, 'Pourquoi écrivait-on des recueils de miracles? L'exemple des miracles de Saint Artémios', in *Les saints et leurs sanctuaires à Byzance: textes, images, et monuments*, edited by Catherine Jolivet-Lévy, Michel Kaplan, and Jean-Pierre Sodini, Byzantina Sorbonensia XI (Paris: Sorbonne, 1993), pp. 95–116.

Dickinson, Tania M., 'An Anglo-Saxon "cunning woman" from Bidford-on-Avon', in *In Search of Cult: Archaeological Investigations in honour of Philip Rahtz*, edited by Martin Carver (Woodbridge: Boydell Press, 1993), pp. 45–54.

Campbell, Sheila, Bert Hall, and David Klausner, *Health, Disease and Healing in Medieval Culture* (Basingstoke: Macmillan, 1992), pp. 12–33.

Duffy, John, 'Byzantine medicine in the sixth and seventh centuries: aspects of teaching and practice', *DOP* 38 (1984), 21–27.

Duffy, John, 'Reactions of two Byzantine intellectuals to the theory and practice of magic', in *Byzantine Magic*, edited by Henry Maguire (Washington DC: Dumbarton Oaks, 1995), pp. 83–97.

Farmer, Sharon, *Surviving Poverty in Medieval Paris: Gender, Ideology and the Daily Lives of the Poor* (Ithaca, NY: Cornell University Press, 2002).

Ferngren, Gary B., 'Early Christianity as a religion of healing', *Bulletin of the History of Medicine* 66 (1992), 1–15.

Finucane, Ronald C., *Miracles and Pilgrims: Popular Beliefs in Medieval England* (London: J. M. Dent, 1977).

Flint, Valerie I. J., 'The early medieval *medicus*, the saint – and the enchanter', *Social History of Medicine* 2 (1989), 127–145.

Flint, Valerie I. J., *The Rise of Magic in Early Medieval Europe* (Oxford: Oxford University Press, 1991).

Franklin, Simon, and Jonathan Shepard, *The Emergence of Rus 750–1200* (Harlow: Longman, 1996).

Gil-Sotres, Pedro, 'The regimens of health', in *Western Medical Thought from Antiquity to the Middle Ages*, edited by Mirko D. Grmek (Cambridge, MA: Harvard University Press, 1998), pp. 291–318.

Glaze, Florence Eliza, 'The perforated wall: the ownership and circulation of medical books in medieval Europe, ca. 800–1200' (unpublished PhD thesis, Duke University, 1999).

Green, Monica H., *Women's Healthcare in the Medieval West: Texts and Contexts* (Aldershot: Ashgate, 2000).

Grmek, Mirko D. (ed.), *Western Medical Thought from Antiquity to the Middle Ages* (Cambridge, MA.: Harvard University Press, 1998).

Grumel, Venance, 'La profession médicale à Byzance à l'époque des Comnènes', *Revue des études byzantines* 7 (1949), 42–46.

Haldon, John, 'The works of Anastasius of Sinai: a key source for the history of seventh-century east Mediterranean society and belief', in *The Byzantine and Early Islamic Near East*, I: *Problems in the literary source material*, edited by Averil Cameron and Lawrence I. Conrad (Princeton, NJ: Darwin Press, 1992), pp. 107–147.

Horden, Peregrine, 'Saints and doctors in the early Byzantine empire: the case of Theodore of Sykeon', *Studies in Church History* 19 (1982), 1–13.

Horden, Peregrine, 'Household care and informal networks: comparisons and continuities from antiquity to the present', in *The Locus of Care: Families, Communities, Institutions and the Provision of Welfare since Antiquity*, edited by Peregrine Horden and Richard Smith (Abingdon: Routledge, 1998), pp. 21–67.

Horden, Peregrine, 'Ritual and public health in the early medieval city', in *Body and City: Histories of Urban Public Health*, edited by Sally Sheard and Helen Power (Aldershot: Ashgate, 2000), pp. 17–40.

Horden, Peregrine, 'Family history and hospital history in the Middle Ages', in *Living in the City*, edited by Eugenio Sonnino (Rome: Università La Sapienza, 2004), pp. 255–282.

Horden, Peregrine, 'The Christian hospital in late antiquity – break or bridge?' in *Gesundheit–Krankheit: Kulturtransfer medizinischen Wissens von der Spätantike bis in die frühe Neuzeit*, edited by Florian Steger and Kay Peter Jankrift, Beiheft zum Archiv für Kulturgeschichte 55 (Cologne: Böhlau, 2004), pp. 77–99.

Horden, Peregrine, 'The earliest hospitals in Byzantium, western Europe, and Islam', *Journal of Interdisciplinary History* 35 (2005), 361–389 [reprinted in the present volume].

Horn, Walter, and Ernest Born, *The Plan of St. Gall: A Study of the Architecture and Economy of and Life in a Paradigmatic Carolingian Monastery*, 3 vols (Berkeley: University of California Press, 1979).

Jacquart, Danielle, *Le milieu médical en France du XII au XVe siècle, en annexe 2e supplément au 'Dictionnaire' d'Ernest Wickersheimer* (Geneva and Paris: Droz and Champion, 1981).

Jolly, Karen [Louise], 'Medieval magic: definitions, beliefs, practices', in *The Athlone History of Witchcraft and Magic in Europe*, vol. III: *The Middle Ages*, edited by Karen Jolly, Catharina Raudvere, and Edward Peters (London: Athlone Press, 2002), pp. 1–71.

Jolly, Karen Louise, *Popular Religion in Late Saxon England: Elf Charms in Context* (Chapel Hill: University of North Carolina Press, 1996).

Knipp, David, 'The chapel of physicians at Santa Maria Antiqua' [eighth-century Rome], *DOP* 56 (2002), 1–23.

Kroll, Jerome, and Bernard Bachrach, 'Sin and the etiology of disease in pre-crusade Europe', *Journal of the History of Medicine and Allied Sciences* 41 (1986), 395–414.

Leven, Karl-Heinz, 'Attitudes towards physical health in late antiquity', in *Coping with Sickness: Perspectives on Health Care, Past and Present*, edited by John Woodward and Robert Jütte (Sheffield: European Association for the History of Medicine and Health, 1996), pp. 73–89.

MacKinney, Loren C., *Early Medieval Medicine with special reference to France and Chartres* (Baltimore, MD: Johns Hopkins Press, 1937).

MacMullen, Ramsay, *Christianity and Paganism in the Fourth to Eighth Centuries* (New Haven, CT: Yale University Press, 1997).

Magoulias, H. J., 'The lives of the saints as sources of data for the history of Byzantine medicine in the sixth and seventh centuries', *Byzantinische Zeitschrift* 57 (1964), 127–150.

Maguire, Henry, 'Introduction', in *Byzantine Magic*, edited by Henry Maguire (Washington, DC: Dumbarton Oaks, 1995), pp. 1–7.

McVaugh, Michael R., 'Bedside manners in the Middle Ages', *Bulletin of the History of Medicine* 71 (1997), 201–223.

McVaugh, Michael R., *Medicine Before the Plague: Practitioners and their Patients in the Crown of Aragon, 1285–1345* (Cambridge: Cambridge University Press, 1994).

Meaney, Audrey L., *Anglo-Saxon Amulets and Curing Stones*, British Archaeological Reports British series 96 (Oxford: British Archaeological Reports, 1981).

Meaney, Audrey L., 'Women, witchcraft and magic in Anglo-Saxon England', in *Superstition and Popular Medicine in Anglo-Saxon England*, edited by D. G. Scragg (Manchester: University of Manchester Centre for Anglo-Saxon Studies, 1989), pp. 9–40.

Meaney, Audrey L., 'The Anglo-Saxon view of the causes of illness', in *Health, Disease and Healing in Medieval Culture*, edited by Sheila Campbell, Bert Hall, and David Klausner (Houndmills: Macmillan, 1992), pp. 12–33.

Meaney, Audrey, 'The practice of medicine in England about the year 1000', *Social History of Medicine* 13 (2000), part 2, special issue, *The Year 1000*, edited by Peregrine Horden and Emilie Savage-Smith, 224–227.

Meens, Rob, 'Magic and the early medieval world view', in *The Community, the Family and the Saint: Patterns of Power in Early Medieval Europe*, edited by Joyce Hill and Mary Swan (Turnhout: Brepols, 1998), pp. 285–295.

Miller, Timothy S., *The Birth of the Hospital in the Byzantine Empire*, 2nd edn (Baltimore, MD: Johns Hopkins University Press, 1997).

Möhler, Rainer, *'Epistula de vulture': Untersuchungen zu einer organotherapeutischen Drogenmonographie des Frühmittelalters* (Pattensen: Horst Wellm, 1990).

Murray, Alexander, 'Missionaries and magic in Dark-Age Europe', *Past and Present* 136 (1992), 186–205.

Nutton, Vivian, 'Archiatri and the medical profession in antiquity', *Papers of the British School at Rome* 45 (1977), 191–226; repr. in Nutton, *From Democedes to Harvey: Studies in the Social History of Medicine* (London: Variorum, 1988).

Nutton, Vivian, 'From Galen to Alexander: aspects of medicine and medical practice in late antiquity', *DOP* 38 (1984), 1–14.

Nutton, Vivian, 'Healers in the medical market place: towards a social history of Graeco-Roman medicine', in *Medicine in Society*, edited by Andrew Wear (Cambridge: Cambridge University Press, 1992), pp. 15–58.

Nutton, Vivian, *Ancient Medicine* (London: Routledge, 2004; 2nd edn, 2013).

Park, Katherine, 'Medicine and society in medieval Europe 500–1500', in *Medicine in Society*, edited by Andrew Wear (Cambridge: Cambridge University Press, 1992), pp. 59–90.

Paxton, Frederick S., *'Bonus liber*: a late Carolingian clerical manual from Lorsch (Bibliotheca Vaticana MS Pal. lat. 485)', in *The Two Laws: Studies in Medieval Legal History Dedicated to Stephan Kuttner*, edited by Laurent Mayali and Stephanie A. J. Tibbetts (Washington, DC: Catholic University of America Press, 1990), pp. 1–30.

Paxton, Frederick S., 'Anointing the sick and the dying in Christian antiquity and the early medieval west', in *Health, Disease and Healing in Medieval Culture*, edited by Sheila Campbell, Bert Hall, and David Klausner (Houndmills: Macmillan, 1992), pp. 93–102.

Paxton, Frederick S., 'Liturgy and healing in an early medieval saint's cult: the Mass *in honore sancti Sigismundi* for the cure of fevers', *Traditio* 49 (1994), 23–43.

Paxton, Frederick S., 'Curing bodies – curing souls: Hrabanus Maurus, medical education, and the clergy in ninth-century Francia', *Journal of the History of Medicine* 50 (1995), 230–252.

Pollock, Linda, *With Faith and Physic: The Life of a Tudor Gentlewoman, Lady Grace Mildmay 1552–1620* (London: Collins and Brown, 1993).

Richards, Jeffrey, *Consul of God: The Life and Times of Gregory the Great* (London: Routledge and Kegan Paul, 1980).

Riché, Pierre, *Education et culture dans l'occident barbare, 6e–8e siècle* (Paris: Seuil, 1962), translated as *Education and Culture in the Barbarian West, Sixth through Eighth Centuries* (Columbia: University of South Carolina Press, 1976).

Riddle, John M., 'Theory and practice in early medieval medicine', *Viator* 5 (1974), 158–184.

Sigal, Pierre-André, *L'homme et le miracle dans la France médiévale XIe–XIIe siècle* (Paris: Éditions du Cerf, 1985).

Siraisi, Nancy G., *Medieval and Early Renaissance Medicine: An Introduction to Knowledge and Practice* (Chicago: University of Chicago Press, 1990).

Skinner, Patricia, *Health and Medicine in Early Medieval Southern Italy* (Leiden: Brill, 1997).

Skinner, Patricia, *Women in Medieval Italian Society 500–1200* (Harlow: Longman 2001).

Sonderkamp, Joseph A., 'Theophanes Nonnus: medicine in the circle of Constantine Porphyrogenitus', *DOP* 38 (1984), 29–41.

Sternberg, Thomas, *Orientalium more secutus: Räume und Institutionen der Caritas des 5. bis 7. Jahrhunderts in Gallien* (Münster: Aschendorff, 1991).

Stolte, Bernard H., 'Magic and Byzantine law in the seventh century', in *The Metamorphosis of Magic from Late Antiquity to the Early Modern Period*, edited by Jan N. Bremmer and Jan R. Veenstra (Louvain: Peeters, 2002), pp. 105–115.

Sumption, Jonathan, *Pilgrimage: An Image of Mediaeval Religion* (London: Faber and Faber, 1975).

Talbot, Alice-Mary, 'Pilgrimage to healing shrines: the evidence of miracle accounts' [Byzantine], *DOP* 56 (2002), 153–173.

Temkin, Owsei, *Hippocrates in a World of Pagans and Christians* (Baltimore, MD: Johns Hopkins University Press, 1991).

The Trotula: A Medieval Compendium of Women's Medicine, edited and translated by Monica H. Green (Philadelphia: University of Pennsylvania Press, 2001).

Vikan, Gary, 'Art, medicine and magic in early Byzantium', *DOP* 38 (1984), 65–86.

Voigts, Linda, 'Anglo-Saxon plant remedies and the Anglo-Saxons', *Isis* 70 (1979), 250–268.

Wallis, Faith, 'The experience of the book: manuscripts, texts, and the role of epistemology in early medieval medicine', in *Knowledge and the Scholarly Medical Traditions*, edited by Don Bates (Cambridge: Cambridge University Press, 1995), pp. 101–126.

Wallis, Faith, 'Signs and senses: diagnosis and prognosis in early medieval pulse and urine texts', *Social History of Medicine* 13 (2000), part 2, special issue, *The Year 1000*, edited by Peregrine Horden and Emilie Savage-Smith, 265–278.

Ziegler, Joseph, *Medicine and Religion, c.1300: The Case of Arnau de Vilanova* (Oxford: Clarendon Press, 1998).

5

THE LATE ANTIQUE ORIGINS
OF THE LUNATIC ASYLUM?

I

> Now, if an English clergyman with such a reputation for miraculous powers were placed for some days in a London hospital, and in that time succeeded in quieting only one lunatic, his pretensions, to say the least, would be somewhat discredited.[1]

Such was the caustic response of the Reverend Frederick Holmes Dudden, BD, to an episode recorded in the 590s in Rome by Pope Gregory the Great in the *Dialogues*.[2] Dudden's magisterial and still unreplaced book on Gregory – in his own words 'not merely . . . a biography . . . but also', thanks to the amplitude of its source quotation, 'in some degree . . . a work of reference' – generally evinces admiration for 'the most remarkable man of a remarkable age'.[3] Still, for Dudden, in this episode of a healer in a hospital Gregory showed a lamentable incapacity for weighing evidence given by others and for drawing valid inferences from personal observation.[4] Dudden was an Oxford scholar of wide sympathies who deserves the attention of historiographers.[5] His monographs ranged in subject from Gregory (1905) and Ambrose (1935) to an equally substantial biography of Henry Fielding (1952) as well as an address on 'The Influence of Women in the Home and Society' (1913) and wartime sermons on 'the future life' (1915) and 'the heroic dead' (1917). Yet, faced with Gregory's degree of credulity, his standards held firm. He would, one guesses, have shared the renewed wariness of 'holy men' that Hensley Henson voiced in 1925: 'a strong tide is running in the religious world; "faith healing" is now patronised by Society [and] approved by bishops.'[6] A sixth-century bishop of Rome, himself sick from birth with, in Dudden's resonant diagnosis, 'the malady of the Middle Ages', was thus never to attain 'a perfect sanity of view'. He could not correctly appraise a report of a charismatic cure.[7]

By what cure was Dudden so unimpressed? At this point in the *Dialogues*, Gregory has been telling his interlocutor, the deacon Peter, about his friend and fellow monk Eleutherius, a man of great simplicity and compunction.[8] This man's prayers had reportedly raised someone from the dead; and he personally told Gregory of his success in eventually ridding a little boy in a convent of the 'malign spirit' that tormented him every night, but that remained quiet while the healer slept next to him.[9] Moreover, Gregory himself had been a beneficiary of Eleutherius's therapeutic prayer. While still a mere monk he suffered from stabbing pains in his guts – 'for which doctors use the Greek word *syncope*'[10] – pains so sharp that he feared death. More seriously yet, as Easter approached, Gregory was anxious that he would be unable to fast on Holy Saturday. He went into the monastery chapel with Eleutherius, who prayed with him. He thereby recovered the strength to fast.

After an excursus on compunction, we come to the story at issue.[11] Gregory is asked whether there are other saints of the same calibre still around. Again he recalls personal experience. The story repeats several motifs from its predecessors while introducing some significant changes. First, Gregory invokes Floridus, bishop of Tifernum Tiberinum (Città di Castello):

> He told me that he had with him a priest called Amantius, a man of extraordinary simplicity, who seemed to have such power that, in the manner of the apostles, he would lay his hands on the sick and restore them to health.

Floridus added that the man also possessed apostolic authority over even the most dangerous serpents, which he could kill with the sign of the Cross. It was natural that Gregory should want to see such a powerful healer for himself.

> I had him brought to me to stay for a few days in the house of the sick [*in infirmorum domo*], where, if he had a gift [*gratia*] for healing, it could quickly be verified. For among the other sick people there lay a madman [*mente captus*], the sort whom medicine calls by the Greek word *freneticus*. One night the insane man [*insanus*] let out great cries and disturbed the other sick people with his immense clamour, so that none could get any sleep there. What a wretched business; because one person was very ill everyone grew worse.

Now Bishop Floridus was also staying in this house of the sick, presumably having accompanied his prize exhibit Amantius to Rome in response to Gregory's invitation. From Floridus, and also from the lad (*puer*) who was looking after the sick that night, Gregory received an exact report of what happened next:

> That venerable priest got up from his own bed, went silently to that of the frenetic man and, with his hands placed upon him, prayed.

Soon the man got better. Amantius took him with him into the oratory in the upper part of the house. There the priest more freely gave himself up to prayer for him and then at once took him back, cured, to his own bed. He did not make any more noise and disturb the other sick people. Nor did he who had completely recovered his own senses exacerbate the sickness of another.

'From this one act of his' – Gregory concludes, now in Dudden's disapproving rendition – 'I learned to believe all the stories I had heard of him.'[12]

In a volume dedicated to Peter Brown, there is no need to reopen the question of Gregory's presumed credulity, the place of miracles in his thought, the authenticity of the *Dialogues*, or the relation between them and his exegetical labours.[13] In this vignette of Amantius, as with almost all the miracles recounted in the *Dialogues*, witnesses are invoked and Gregory insists on their credibility, placing himself, he avers, at no greater distance from his subject than the evangelists Mark and Luke often were.[14]

There is nothing in this aspect of the story that requires any particular explanation – or verdict. The purpose of this paper is, rather, to relate the vignette to the *longue durée* of the history of houses for the sick, of hospitals; more especially, those of them that included, or indeed were exclusive to, the insane. Since Dudden's acerbic notice, to look no further back, Gregory's anecdote has occasionally been registered in passing, usually for other purposes.[15] It has hardly ever been discussed. Nor has it been acknowledged in the way that I should like to characterize it here – as the earliest clear attestation in European history, if not exactly of a lunatic asylum, then of a hospital in which a lunatic was based; that is, as a progenitor of those fully-fledged madhouses which will loom so large in the social history of mental illness from the 'classic age' defined by Foucault to the decarceration of the 1960s.[16]

II

For any defence of that view, the first subject must be the nature of the affliction at the centre of the vignette. In one of her fundamental articles on the *Dialogues*, Sofia Boesch Gajano pointed up the intimate connection in them between sickness, sin, and possession, and observed briefly of the Amantius episode that the techniques of his cure resembled those of exorcists.[17] Granted that Gregory's world is full of demons – even on a nun's salad – and that sinners are vulnerable to them, and to illness.[18] Granted also that the patient's mad outburst is seemingly induced by the proximity of the healer, much as demons start to shout and argue in the presence of an exorcist or a saint's relics.[19] Still, the technique of Amantius – prayerful laying-on of hands – is not in fact the common mode of demon-taming in the *Dialogues*. More obviously, neither sin nor demonic intrusion is so much as hinted at in this scene from hospital life.[20] Gregory can be observed changing register, from supernatural to natural causation, and from exorcism to prayer, in the preceding narrative of Eleutherius. Eleutherius's cure of the boy is explicitly an exorcism; quite different from Amantius's response to the frenetic. But then we move to Gregory's own respite from *syncope*, another Greek technical term – although his use of it is somewhat removed from any of our dictionary definitions.[21] The respite is earned by prayer in an oratory, and that success prepares the way for the account of the frenetic's happy release. As Gregory's discourse turns from the boy's demon to his own stomach, he 'goes medical'. His disease aetiology becomes naturalistic and remains so for the Amantius episode. And this is not the only reference to natural insanity in the *Dialogues*. Earlier on, in the miracles of St Benedict, we have been introduced to the 'recent' case of a *mulier mente capta* who had completely lost her senses – cause unspecified.[22] She wandered the countryside until she stumbled unthinkingly into Benedict's grotto at Subiaco, wherein she was cured of her madness simply by spending the night.

There should be no surprise at such tales. Like virtually everyone else in his time, and later, in Europe – perhaps until the decline of the 'witch craze' – Gregory operated with an extremely pluralist aetiology of disease. Demons, magical powers, and natural substances – pre-eminently the four humours of the Hippocratic-Galenic tradition – all had interrelated roles. Possession, in the sixth century as before and for long after, lay on a spectrum of ways to categorize sharply abnormal speech and behaviour.[23] There were, of course, ambiguous cases, such as the one recorded in a much-cited passage (that Gregory presumably knew) from Augustine's Literal Commentary on Genesis.[24] In a house with which Augustine was familiar, there was a man thought to be possessed. He encouraged this diagnosis by predicting the approach, at a twelve-mile range, of the priest who, alone it seems, could calm him and induce him to take food. Was he really possessed? Augustine observes sceptically that his *mentis alienatio sive daemonium* responded to the priest's presence only after the accompanying fever had abated – as is usual with frenetics (*sicut phrenetici sanari solent*).[25]

Gregory shows none of Augustine's uncertainty with respect to his own frenetic. He used the word elsewhere, as a loose simile, without emphasizing its Greek origin.[26] Ambiguous cases, if such there were for him, occupied only a narrow band on the spectrum of possibilities. The civil and canon legal traditions within which he operated presuppose an entirely naturalistic set of mental afflictions. It was a letter from Gregory on persuading a mad bishop (*mente alienata*) to resign during one of his lucid intervals that would be repeated by Gratian in the *Decretum*.[27]

Behind the legal tradition of course lay the medical.[28] Gregory's is perhaps the first 'medicalized pontificate'. He clearly had some vernacular understanding of the psychosomatic view of mental illness prominent in the

Galenic tradition – a tradition that endured longer and more vigorously in Italy, especially Ravenna, than anywhere else in western Europe during the early Middle Ages.[29] The wrong emotions could make one physically ill, and physical illness – a humoral imbalance – could be manifested in mental abnormality. That was because, to echo the title of one of Galen's treatises, 'the faculties of the soul follow the mixtures of the body'. As Carole Straw writes, 'the connection of body and soul is altogether real in Gregory'.[30] His chronic intestinal pains and fevers clouded his intellect, as he affirms in a prefatory letter describing the composition of the *Moralia in Job*.[31] The health-harming traffic between mind and body ran in the other direction too. Both Gregory and the Patriarch Eutychius were made ill by the stress of their controversy in Constantinople, the latter fatally so.[32] Writing after the Lombard Ariulf's advance on Rome in the summer of 592, Gregory reported to the bishop of Ravenna that his melancholy at the turn of events brought on a stomach ache.[33] In part, the *Dialogues* were composed virtually as a remedy for that recurrent melancholy.[34]

All of this is wholly in keeping with the psychosomatic interpretation of insanity that Gregory could have derived from a Greek doctor in his entourage.[35] Did he also have written sources? There is no evidence that Gregory knew the medical writings of Alexander of Tralles, author of a letter on intestinal worms as well as a substantial medical compendium, and the first to prescribe rhubarb as a remedy for constipation. Alexander was born in Tralles (modern Aydın) in Lydia, but reportedly moved to Rome and is traditionally, although on no clear authority, held to have died there in 605. His compendium was translated into Latin, perhaps in Rome or Ravenna.[36] Alexander gives a variety of treatments – principally diet and bloodletting – for phrenitis, the disease of Amantius's patient, which Gregory, here describing a miracle, would have felt no need to mention. Alexander also, however, dwells on the frenetic's insomnia, *fantasiae*, and threatening behaviour and manic talk – as well as the deep sleep into which he falls after an episode of this madness. These aspects of the disease all seem to tally with Gregory's briefer 'non-technical' account, even though for him phrenitis may have been a chronic rather than an acute condition.[37]

III

Alexander specifies the type of room in which the frenetic patient should be kept, and the amount of air and light that he should be permitted. He was not thinking of a hospital. Like all the medical writers of his time, he ignored the one development in institutional health care that, for historians today, marks out late from classical antiquity and provides a novelty to counterpoise the seamless continuity of Galenism.[38] Gregory in contrast sets his anecdote of Amantius firmly in a hospital, a house of the sick with (apparently) 'round-the-clock' monitoring of the inmates. Because of his somatic view of

117

mental disorder, he sees no incongruity between the frenetic and the other patients. Each of them endures a *vehemens aegritudo*. The frenetic is not in a different category from the others, still less in a different room. He is noisier than they, but that is not represented as a reason for ejecting him from the hospital or indeed for having refused to admit him in the first place. Because he disturbs the minds of the others, depriving them of sleep, he makes them all more ill in body – the converse of the aetiology of his own affliction. Apart from that, he blends into the general scene. Gregory does not portray himself as having selected the frenetic in advance as Amantius's test case. Rather, he seems to take it as axiomatic that a varied collection of seriously ill people fit to challenge a charismatic is to be found in this house of the sick, and not, for example, at a saint's shrine or in a church portico. And he presents the frenetic as a chance opportunity, not a special case in obvious need of miraculous intervention when all else has failed.[39]

Where was this hospital? Gregory does not say. Sections of the *Dialogues* either side of the story of Amantius are set in Gregory's own monastery of St Andrew on the Caelian. Moreover, *domus infirmorum* would become a standard designation of the monastic infirmary,[40] and it is hardly significant that there is no mention of such an infirmary in what little evidence we have of Gregory's foundation.[41] And yet neither the inmates nor their carer are referred to as brothers, and Gregory is not interested in specifying the character of this *domus*. The oratory on the floor above does not necessarily imply a monastic setting, because most of the Roman hospitals attested in this period were associated with oratories.[42] Nor does Gregory give any clues as to its location, perhaps because they were not needed. The initial monastic-clerical audience of the *Dialogues* might have been able to place this *domus* in the topography of Rome, most likely near the pope's Lateran palace or within the larger papal quarter on the Caelian. For Gregory, however, the precise location was irrelevant: the point of the story was simply to demonstrate Amantius's healing power to his, and his audience's, satisfaction. For us, in a different but not unrelated way, the interest of the story is in its effects rather than its causes. We want to know, not whether it was true, or can be anchored in one of the Roman hospitals we happen to know about, but whether it was plausible. We want to know, that is, whether a madman in a hospital (of whatever kind) would have been perceived as extraordinary or, on the contrary, lay comfortably above the 'horizon of expectation' of Gregory's audience.

In our approach to that question, it is essential to appreciate the rarity and even the novelty, in Gregory's time, of that charitable, overnight care of the sick and needy that is the ancestor of the modern biomedical hospital. Such establishments, as Peter Brown has reminded us,[43] began in Byzantium. Yet they had not been evident there until around the middle of the fourth century. They arose in quite specific circumstances, having much to do with the Church's need for 'conspicuous expenditure', and had few direct forerunners. The 'hospital idea' was a particular conception of how to organize charity, urban topography, and ecclesiastical or monastic building. It was an ideological, much more than an architectural, development – and, as I now think, was conceived partly in opposition to the louche late antique inn or *pandocheion*, a point I hope to develop elsewhere.[44] It spread quite quickly across Byzantine territories and thence, later, to the 'land of Islam'. Diffusion westwards was generally much slower. There are no signs of such hospitals in Frankish territory until the early sixth century,[45] and in Britain, monastic infirmaries apart, until after the Norman Conquest.[46]

Italy seems, however, to have been more quickly receptive. Jerome's correspondence documents what was probably the first hospital in Rome, and perhaps the first one in Italy.[47] His *Letter* 77, an encomium on the Lady Fabiola written in the spring of 400 when news of her death reached him, attributes to her this distinction:

> And first of all [upon selling her immense property; *primo omnium* – meaning 'this was the first thing she did', or 'she was the first to do this'?] she established a *nosokomion* [in support of the latter translation of *primo*, Jerome gives a Greek word for hospital, in Greek characters, which his Latin-speaking audience would not previously have encountered and which was virtually a neologism in Greek] into which she gathered the sick from off the streets [*in quo aegrotantes colligeret de plateis*] . . .[48]

Jerome goes on to describe their dreadful appearance and her tender personal care. In another letter, he attributes to Pammachius the recent foundation of a hospital at Portus.[49]

With this evidence as starting point – all allowance made for its rhetorical patterning, its demonstrable exaggeration of the ascetic founder's financial sacrifices – it would be easy to gather the references to early Italian hospitals and create an impression of widespread and sustained activity.[50] The temptation to do so must be resisted. The evidence of these foundations, stretched out in real time and space rather than clustered in dense footnotes, is actually quite meagre and sporadic. Nor are the hospitals in question clearly all of one kind. Their Byzantine originals were mostly called *xenodocheia*, houses for strangers, not *nosokomeia*, houses for the sick – with 'strangers' being taken (I suspect) in a broad theological sense rather than a narrow demographic one.

The *domus infirmorum* that Gregory describes cannot therefore be related to a stable and flourishing tradition. First, Gregory did not, despite his fondness for Greek technical terms, call his hospital a *xenodochium* or (à la Jerome) a *nosokomion*. His inmates were expressly the sick rather than 'strangers'. Second, it was not obvious that a bishop in a major city should be much concerned to found or maintain hospitals. Basil of Caesarea is the great prototype; but Augustine did not establish a hospital of his own in his massive episcopal complex – he left that to another. Nor is Ambrose credited with a hospital – his concern for the poor, sick, and possessed was differently conveyed.[51] Gregory himself has always been known for his intense and wide-ranging charitable concerns, particularly his direction of the food supply of the famine-prone Roman population and his support for hospitals both in the city and far afield.[52] Yet, unlike his predecessor Pelagius, he was not recalled as an originator of philanthropic institutions, just as, outside St Peter's, he was overall not 'a building pope'.[53]

Against what background, then, can we project Gregory's account? From his time there are a few familiar pieces of evidence about hospitals explicitly intended for the sick. In Arles, much earlier in the sixth century, Caesarius had reportedly set up a *spatiosissima domus* for the *infirmi* beside his cathedral so that they would hear Mass being celebrated and be instructed and comforted by the liturgy.[54] This report has some bearing on the position of the oratory above the sick ward in Gregory's hospital. In Visigothic Mérida, Bishop Masona, more or less Gregory's contemporary, set up a *xinodocium* with *ministri vel medici* for the sick and for pilgrims – but no mention of the mad in his biography.[55]

IV

These are not close enough analogues. We need to look in different directions – and we need to extend our 'rules of engagement' (as, on this occasion, Gregory did not) to the possessed as well as the 'naturally' insane. Because the texts thus brought into play hint at the unexpected presence of the possessed in hospitals, this broadening of scope perhaps makes the hospitalization of the insane more rather than less likely. Of course, if we followed the implicit argument of the hagiographers, the possessed should go to the tomb of a dead saint or the presence of a living holy man to participate in the 'psychodrama' of exorcism.[56] Moreover nothing could be less conducive to the therapeutic calm of a hospital 'ward' than the violent ravings of such unfortunates. But suppose the possession was often long-lasting – unrelieved by 'psychodrama'. Suppose too that possession was often an idiom for a variety of genuinely psychosomatic problems, many of them far milder than the fever that beset Augustine's clairvoyant in the Commentary on Genesis. In that case, the long-term gathering of the possessed round a shrine could make of the setting a quasi-hospital. Elsewhere, using Byzantine evidence and building on the work of Michael Dols and others, I have tentatively developed that train of thought. I have argued that looking after the chronically possessed, and by extension the mentally ill, at shrines as well as in monasteries, was perhaps more frequent than we had thought – more so than has been implied by accounts that eliminate the insane and possessed from medieval hospital historiography.[57] After all, any hospital might be turned into a house of the possessed by a demonic invasion:

> For there are also many others of our group [say the demons to Saint Theodore of Sykeon less than a generation after Gregory] who suspect you are coming to shut us up here; on the pretext of illness the creatures made themselves to lie down in bed in the hospitals so as to hide; but some are also in houses . . . [58]

Sometimes the activities of an individual at a shrine could virtually create a private charitable clinic. To paraphrase one seventh-century miracle story: a woman called Martha had enjoyed a wild youth; but, having abandoned debauchery, she came to the 'clinic' [iatreion] of Cosmas and Damian [in Constantinople] when she developed an illness 'coming from her cranium'. She stayed at the shrine seeking a cure, giving her goods to the poor. If she saw women who had fallen under the domination of 'the Enemy', but were recovering their reason after being tortured in spirit, she invited them to her lodging within the atrium of the shrine and looked after them.[59]

The similarity of shrine and hospital could be close enough to strike those writing up the saint's deeds:

> A certain sailor for many years had problems with his testicles and he approached the holy martyr [Artemius, again in seventh-century Constantinople]. His name was Isidore and he was about fifty-three years old. But he was unaware that he was being agitated by an evil spirit. Now in the aisle at the left, the saint is accustomed to make his rounds as if he were a chief physician in charge of a hospital [hos epi xenonos], just as many have often been convinced by experience, and to be sure one night the saint in full view approached the man, while many of those awaiting the cure looked on, at the very place where the possessed man [pneumatoumenos] was lying down.[60]

Other Byzantine evidence suggests that some much-frequented shrines really did become hospital-like. The Church of St Anastasia in Constantinople, known to hagiographers as the *Anastaseion*, seems to have had a wide reputation as a virtual asylum.[61] It features prominently in two fictitious saints' Lives of the tenth century, those of Andrew the Fool and Basil the Younger, as an institution for healing victims of demonic possession, sorcery, and mental illness. When the young slave Andrew first began to act out his 'folly for Christ's sake', his master despatched him to the 'venerable church of the Holy and Glorious Martyr Anastasia . . . giving orders that he should be chained and sending a generous sum of money to the sacristan for his treatment.'[62] Andrew and the other sick persons incubating in the shrine received a nocturnal visitation from the martyr and her companions, making the rounds of the patients. Pausing to speak to Andrew, the martyr declined to 'heal' him, but confirmed him in his choice of a life of holy folly. Discharged as incurable, Andrew roamed the streets of Constantinople.

The *Anastaseion* is mentioned twice in the *Life of Basil the Younger* in connection with cases of possession. In the first case, Basil is presented with a possessed woman who has run away from the *martyrion* of St Anastasia, with 'attendants of the sick' from the church in hot pursuit.[63] The second case concerns a eunuch named John, the victim of a *pharmakon* – a spell, or poison – who has lost his mind.[64] His servants are shown discussing the possible forms of treatment for their master. One suggests the hostel (*katagogion*) of the Apostle Andrew; another insists, 'not there, but let us take him to the reverend temple of the all-praiseworthy martyr Anastasia who unbinds spells [*ta pharmaka*], and she will overshadow him.' John eventually resorts, successfully, to St Basil. Neither of Basil's two clients has actually been cured at the *Anastaseion*, but of course have to appeal, finally, to him. The clear implication, however, is that this church was a very obvious provider of supernatural therapy in cases of possession or madness, and that it had developed clear procedures for helping sufferers (at a price – recall that Andrew the Fool's master gave a substantial sum to the sacristan).

Western shrines of the early Middle Ages also naturally attracted the chronically possessed. Around 400, Sulpicius Severus writes of St Martin of Tours:

> The monastery of the blessed [Martin] lay two miles from the city; but whenever he was coming to the church there, he had only to set foot outside the threshold of his cell for one to hear the possessed roaring throughout the whole church [*per totam ecclesiam energumenos rugientes*] and the bands of guilty ones trembling as if their judge were approaching, so that the groans of the demons announced the approach of the bishop to the clerics, who were not previously aware that he was coming.[65]

Gregory of Tours describes a resident shrine madman in Gaul two centuries later. Perhaps not possessed, he is presented as in part the agent of his own recovery, through diet:

> Principius was a good man and a citizen of Périgueux. He was thought to have suffered some unknown madness [*amentiam nescio quam incurrisse putabatur*], and he was sometimes in such pain that he seemed to have lost his senses [*de sensu videretur excedere*]. After he endured this for many months, he went to the church of the blessed bishop. He remained there for four months, I think,

and abstained from eating meat and [drinking] wine. After he was benefited by the assistance of the blessed confessor, he returned to his own home in good health.[66]

Perhaps the oddest literary depiction of institutionalized anguish from the Merovingian world involves a 'real' hospital rather than a shrine. It comes in a work scarcely noticed in this context, the apocryphal *Acts of Simon and Jude* from the *Apostolic History* which pretends to have been written by Abdias, one of the seventy-two disciples and the first bishop of Babylon. Despite the author's claim that the work was originally written in Hebrew, these *Acts* quote the Vulgate and the *Ecclesiastical History* of Rufinus, and are now normally given a likely provenance in later sixth-century Francia. There is a contest between apostles and magicians in Babylon.[67] As M. R. James usefully paraphrases:

> [The wizards] were enraged and called in a host of snakes. The apostles were hastily summoned, and made the snakes all turn on the magicians and bite them: they howled like wolves. Kill them outright, said the king; but the apostles refused, and instead made the serpents suck out all their venom, which hurt still more. And for three days in the hospitals [*depositati sunt ad hospitalia*], the wizards continued screaming. When they were on the point of death, the apostles healed them, saying: Our God does not ask for forced service; if you will not believe, you may go free. They wandered about Persia, slandering the apostles and telling the people to kill them when they came.

If *hospitalia* is to be translated as hospitals, then a later sixth-century date, a time when these establishments were still new and rare and the vocabulary of them not settled, seems plausible. The text invokes neither demons nor insanity. But its image of the hospital as a place in which screaming magicians submit to miraculous 'counter-magic' not only reminds us of Amantius and the Roman frenetic. It shows how little we know about the ways in which early hospitals were perceived, and how mutable their future was in Gregory the Great's time.

V

Such material provides a context for Gregory. It makes his vignette more explicable. And yet it also throws his naturalistic, somatic, view of psychological disorder into sharper relief. For out and out naturalism, however, naturalism which would not allow much scope to visiting charismatic healers, our yardstick must be neither western European nor Byzantine, but Islamic. The hospitals founded by caliphs, viziers, and notables in major

Islamic cities, from the ninth century onwards, came rapidly to include the mad alongside – sometimes to the exclusion of – other patients.[68] The best explanation for this development was offered by Michael Dols. These hospitals were epiphenomenal to the translation movement that had been initiated so as to bring Greek philosophy, science, and medicine into Arabic. The hospitals were Galenic in ethos – staffed by learned and expensive physicians for whom, as for Galen, the varieties of insanity were fundamentally humoral, and thus as somatic as any other illness.

Here, by way of illustration, are two pieces of evidence brought into the discussion by Peter E. Pormann.[69] The first is from the newly discovered medical *Compendium* of Al-Kaskarī:[70]

> This is a summary of what Rufus [of Ephesus] discussed in his book *On the Ailment of Melancholy*. I for my part consider valid [only] those things which I have used and proved by experience while I was treating this disease, that is melancholic delusion, in the hospitals in which I served, such as the hospital of Sā'id – God have mercy upon him –, the hospital of Badr – God have mercy upon him –, and the hospital of Our Lady, the Mother of the Commander of the Faithful [the Caliph] al-Muqtadir [r. 908–30] – may God give strength to both of them.

The second piece of evidence is the testimony of the better-known judge and poet at-Tanūhī (d. 994):

> Abū al-Hasan Muhammad ibn Gassān, the physician, told me the following: 'With us in Basra in the hospital [*bīmāristān*] was a madman [*ragul muwaswas*], known as al-Hasan ibn 'Aun, who belongs to the children of the scribes [*kuttāb*]. He was locked up for treatment in the hospital in the year 342 AH [953–4 CE]. His sojourn lasted many years, and he recovered. He subsequently worked in the hospital as an orderly, until his recovery was complete. I frequented the hospital in order to study medicine, and was therefore seeing him regularly.'[71]

That is not of course Gregory's medical world. He is no secular Galenist in his view of the scope of hospital treatment. His infirmary does not even come across as another Vivarium, deploying the limited medical arsenal that Cassiodorus recommended.[72] Yet Gregory's hospital is not wholly dissimilar to the Islamic model either. After all, the implication of his story about Amantius is that, but for his presence, the frenetic would have gone on suffering in the hospital, being looked after by the attendants, perhaps (given Gregory's affectation of medical know-how) being put on a special diet prescribed by the pope himself.[73]

Juxtaposing sixth-century Rome and tenth-century Baghdad is not meant to imply some hitherto undetected cultural connection. It is simply an attempt to place Gregory's anecdote on the larger historical map of institutionalized insanity. If the older historiography of lunatic asylums reached back before the French Revolution, it conventionally began with fifteenth-century Spain.[74] Then, when more became known of the medieval Islamic *bimaristan* and its mad inmates, Spain became the conduit through which the idea of segregating the insane passed to Christendom.[75] After all, in the Middle Ages hospital founders and regulators had plentiful reasons for excluding the mad, the possessed, and other categories such as lepers and plague victims – and many did so.[76] The last two were to go into specialist houses. The others had to shift for themselves. In general such people would spread disease, whether of the body or of the soul. They would disrupt the liturgy and pollute the sacraments of the hospital's chapel. They would place inordinate demands on its staff, of either care or restraint. Even at the end of the Middle Ages, when institutional care for the insane had, for various reasons still far from clear, become more acceptable, in Spain and indeed across Europe, such care remained patchy and small in scale.[77] The 'medicalization' of later medieval society had its limits. Even in the most medically sophisticated and lavishly endowed hospital in Renaissance Florence, Santa Maria Nuova, a harbinger of the modern hospital if ever there was one, the insane were simply chained up in a cell and purged or given the occasional sedative. 'We have set apart another place for those who have lost their minds through illness, where they are kept in chains.'[78] And this brief, grim, notice (in a version of the hospital statutes prepared in order to impress Henry VII of England) follows pages of detail about how the other patients are to be received and treated.

For all these qualifications, medieval Europe (like medieval Byzantium) did have a history, however tenuous or intermittent, of putting its insane in hospitals. Gregory gives us a preface to this history. He expands its chronological range, and re-emphasizes its independence from Islamic example. Slowly, on all fronts, the insane are being freed from the narrow and simplified institutional history that once fettered them. Victorian 'asylumdom'? Greatly exaggerated; the history of madness 'outside the walls' and within the family is just as important.[79] Foucault's earlier 'great confinement' of the insane? It did not happen.[80] Gregory prompts us also to reconsider the other end of the story: its apparent beginning in late antiquity, only two centuries after the Christian hospital was invented. By showing how he wanted to test a healer's reputation, the pope gives no more than a hint of a possibility – of what was imaginable by and acceptable to an audience in late antique Rome. Yet, as Peter Brown has taught us throughout his oeuvre, evidence of what was thinkable can be as illuminating, and as extensive in its ramifications, as evidence of what happened.

Acknowledgements

I am grateful to Klaus-Dietrich Fischer, Clare Pilsworth, and Chris Wickham for indispensable comments on a draft of this paper.

Notes

1 Frederick Homes Dudden, *Gregory the Great: His Place in History and Thought*, 2 vols (London, 1905), vol. I, p. 343.
2 *Grégoire le Grand, Dialogues*, ed. Adalbert de Vogüé, trans. Paul Antin, SC 251, 260, 265, 3 vols (Paris, 1978–80), pp. 404–407, III.35 (hereafter cited only by book and section number). The translations of this work that follow are my own unless otherwise noted, although I have consulted that by Odo John Zimmerman, *Saint Gregory the Great, Dialogues*, The Fathers of the Church (Washington, DC, 1959). On Gregory in general and the *Dialogues* in particular, a massive literature can be captured, and the most recent and best of it sampled, in John C. Cavadini (ed.), *Gregory the Great: A Symposium* (Notre Dame, IN, 1995); R. A. Markus, *Gregory the Great and his World* (Cambridge, 1997); Conrad Leyser, *Authority and Asceticism from Augustine to Gregory the Great* (Oxford, 2000), pp. 131–159. [See now also Bronwen Neil and Matthew Dal Santo (eds), *A Companion to Gregory the Great* (Leiden, 2013).]
3 Dudden, vol. I, pp. xv, v.
4 Ibid. p. 343.
5 1874–1955. Fellow of Lincoln College Oxford (1898–1914), he migrated as Master to Pembroke in 1918. He also served as vicar of fashionable Holy Trinity, Sloane Street, London, and as chaplain to Kings George V and VI. There are three likenesses in the National Portrait Gallery, yet Dudden is omitted from the *Oxford Dictionary of National Biography*. I have not located any relevant personal papers.
6 H. Hensley Henson, 'Spiritual Healing', *Hibbert Journal* 23 (1925): 385, quoted by Stuart Mews, 'The Revival of Spiritual Healing in the Church of England, 1920–26', *Studies in Church History* 19 (1982): 301.
7 Dudden, vol. I, p.15.
8 *Dialogues*, III.33.
9 Ibid. 33.2–7.
10 Ibid. 33.7.
11 Ibid. 35.1–5.
12 Dudden, vol. I, p. 34.
13 See esp. William D. McCready, *Signs of Sanctity: Miracles in the Thought of Gregory the Great* (Toronto, 1989); Joan M. Petersen, *The 'Dialogues' of Gregory the Great in their Late Antique Cultural Background* (Toronto, 1984) [, Matthew Dal Santo, *Debating the Saints' Cult in the Age of Gregory the Great* (Oxford, 2012)]. Brown's most recent published thoughts on Gregory are to be found in *The Rise of Western Christendom*, 2nd edn (Oxford, 2003), ch. 8, esp. pp. 213–214. See also, for his interpretation of an earlier phase in Roman history, 'Dalla "*plebs Romana*" alla "*plebs Dei*": aspetti della cristianizzazione di Roma', in Brown et al., *Governanti e intellettuali: popolo di Roma e popolo di Dio (I–VI secolo)* (Turin, 1982), pp. 123–145.
14 McCready, pp. 112–113; Petersen, pp. 1–15.
15 Petersen, pp. 14, 53; McCready, pp. 203–204; Peregrine Horden, 'Responses to Possession and Insanity in the Earlier Byzantine World', *Social History of Medicine* 6 (1993): 177–194 (at 189 n. 63), an expanded version of 'Possession Without

Exorcism: The Response to Demons and Insanity in the Earlier Byzantine Middle East', in Evelyne Patlagean (ed.), *Maladie et société à Byzance* (Spoleto, 1993), pp. 1–19. [See now Achim Thomas Hack, *Gregor der Grosse und die Krankheit* (Stuttgart, 2012), pp. 203–205, outlining the Amantius episode, with bibliography, including an article by one P. Horden.]

16 Michel Foucault's *Folie et déraison* (Paris, 1961) is for the first time fully translated: *History of Madness* (London, 2006).

17 Sofia Boesch Gajano, 'Demoni e miracoli nei "Dialogi" di Gregorio Magno', in *Hagiographie, cultures et sociétés IVe–XIIe siècles* (Paris, 1981), pp. 263–281, esp. 268.

18 Barbara Müller, 'The Diabolical Power of Lettuce, or Garden Miracles in Gregory the Great's *Dialogues*', *Studies in Church History* 41 (2005): 46–55; *Dialogues*, I.4.7, with de Vogüé, vol. III, p. 359.

19 *Dialogues*, I.10.2.

20 de Vogüé, vol. III, p. 355.

21 See also *Dialogues*, IV.16.3, for the analogous use of 'paralysis'.

22 Ibid. II.38.1.

23 Horden, 'Responses', pp. 186–187. See also e.g. Ronald C. Finucane, *Miracles and Pilgrims: Popular Beliefs in Medieval England* (London, 1977), p. 109; Christian Krötzl, *Pilger, Mirakel und Alltag* (Helsinki, 1994), pp. 248–249; the classic of Michael MacDonald, *Mystical Bedlam: Madness, Anxiety, and Healing in Seventeenth-Century England* (Cambridge, 1981), esp. App. D, including the incidence of 'frenzy'; and now also David Lederer, *Madness, Religion and the State in Early Modern Europe: A Bavarian Beacon* (Cambridge, 2006).

24 XII.17.35–6; *PL* 34, col. 468. For the mutual aggravation of physician and frenetic as an analogy, see Augustine, *Contra Cresconium*, IV.51.61, *PL* 43, col. 580.

25 See also Cam Grey, 'Demoniacs, Dissent, and Disempowerment in the Late Roman West: Some Case Studies from the Hagiographical Literature', *Journal of Early Christian Studies* 13 (2005): 39–69 at p. 45, kindly shown to me by the author in advance of publication. Compare the multiple conflicting diagnoses of the fictitious Byzantine madness-feigning saint, Andrew, in his *Life*, ed. Lennart Rydén, *The Life of St Andrew the Fool*, 2 vols (Uppsala, 1995), vol. 2, lines 262–271, 1251–1257; and of a real late medieval painter as recorded by a monastic infirmarer in the 1480s: Peter Murray Jones, 'Music Therapy in the Later Middle Ages: The Case of Hugo van der Goes', in Peregrine Horden (ed.), *Music as Medicine: The History of Music Therapy since Antiquity* (Aldershot, 2000), p. 128: 'concerning the nature of the sickness of this convert different people held different opinions. Some said it was a kind of phrenitis magna. Others asserted that he was surely in the power of a demon. Some signs of either kind of misfortune were present. Nevertheless from all sources I heard that throughout the entire period of his indisposition he never wanted to injure anyone except himself. This is not heard about phrenetics or people under the power of demons; therefore I believe that God alone knew what the trouble was' (trans. Jones).

26 *Homiliae in Evangelia*, II.33.4, *PL* 76, col. 1241 ('quasi phreneticus').

27 *Letters*, XIII.6, *S. Gregorii Magni registrum epistularum*, ed. Dag Norberg, *Corpus Christianorum* 140, 140A, 2 vols (Turnhout, 1982), pp. 1000–1001 (see also XIII.5, pp. 998–999); I have also consulted *The Letters of Gregory the Great*, trans. John R. C. Martyn, Pontifical Institute of Mediaeval Studies Medieval Sources in Translation 40, 3 vols (Toronto, 2004). Gratian, *Decretum*, C. VII, q. 1, c. 14, in *Corpus iuris canonici*, ed. Emil Friedberg, vol. I (Leipzig, 1879), pp. 572–573; R. Colin Pickett, *Mental Affliction and Canon Law* (Ottawa, 1952), p. 40 (see also p. 38).

28 For background see Fabio Stok, 'Follia e malattie mentali nella medicina dell'età romana', in Wolfgang Haase (ed.), *Aufstieg und Niedergang der römischen Welt*, II.37.3 (New York, 1996), pp. 2282–2410.

29 Pierre Riché, *Education and Culture in the Barbarian West Sixth through Eighth Centuries* (Columbia, SC, 1976), esp. pp. 142–143; Lawrence I. Conrad et al., *The Western Medical Tradition 800 BC to AD 1800* (Cambridge, 1995), pp. 82–86. Medicine perhaps associated with Ravenna can be sampled in Agnellus of Ravenna, *Lectures on Galen's De sectis* (Buffalo, NY, 1981). For context see Innocenzo Mazzini and Nicola Palmieri, 'L'école médicale de Ravenne', in Philippe Mudry and Jackie Pigeaud (eds), *Les écoles médicales à Rome* (Geneva, 1991), pp. 285–310. Stanley W. Jackson, 'Unusual Mental States in Medieval Europe, I: Medical Syndromes of Mental Disorder: 400–1100 A.D.', *Journal of the History of Medicine* 27 (1972): 262–297, is a convenient summary of the late antique Galenic and 'Methodist' traditions; see esp. pp. 268–274 on phrenitis. For Galen himself the standard collection is Paola Manuli and Mario Vegetti (eds), *Le opere psicologiche di Galeno* (Naples, 1988); see now also John P. Wright and Paul Potter (eds), *Psyche and Soma: Physicians and Metaphysicians on the Mind-Body Problem from Antiquity to the Enlightenment* (Oxford, 2006), esp. the contribution of Heinrich von Staden.

30 Carole Straw, *Gregory the Great: Perfection in Imperfection* (Berkeley, CA, 1988), p. 41. This medical aspect of the emotions is missed by Barbara H. Rosenwein, *Emotional Communities in the Early Middle Ages* (Ithaca, NY, 2006), ch. 3 (on Gregory).

31 *PL* 75, col. 515B, not in Norberg's edn; *Letters*, V.53a, in the numbering of the Martyn trans., following *MGH, Epp* 1–2, ed. Paul Ewald and Ludo Moritz Hartmann, 2 vols (Berlin, 1877–99).

32 Dudden, vol. 1, pp. 142–4; Richards, pp. 38–39. [See now Hack, *Gregor der Grosse*, pp. 37–77, for an 'illness biography' of the pope.]

33 *Letters*, II.38, ed. Norberg, pp. 122–123.

34 *Dialogues*, I.1–10.

35 *Letters*, XIII.42, ed. Norberg, p. 1046; Peter Llewellyn, *Rome in the Dark Ages* (London, 1971), p. 102; Richards, p. 47. See also *Dialogues*, IV.57.8, for the physician brothers Justus and Copiosus.

36 *Alexander of Tralles*, ed. and trans. Theodor Puschmann, 2 vols (Vienna, 1878–9, repr. with addenda Amsterdam, 1963), now much in need of revision. See Barbara Zipser, 'Die *Therapeutica* des Alexander Trallianus: ein medizinisches Handbuch und seine Überlieferung', in Rosa Maria Piccone and Matthias Perkams (eds), *Selecta colligere*, vol. II (Alexandria, 2005), pp. 211–234, discussing at pp. 217–219 the oldest witness, a tenth-century manuscript of southern Italian or Sicilian provenance. The Latin translation, really a reworking with an admixture of other material, has been printed only in Lyon in 1504 (*Practica Alexandri yatros Greci*); David Langslow is at work on an edition. I am very grateful to him for a preview of the relevant part of the text, from an eleventh-century MS in Angers (457), corresponding to Puschmann, vol. I, pp. 509–527. See meanwhile D. R. Langslow, *The Latin Alexander Trallianus: The Text and Transmission of a Late Latin Medical Book* (London, 2006), prolegomenon to the edition, esp. pp. 1–2 on how little we know about Alexander's dates and career, and p. 36 on the equally uncertain dating and provenance of the Latin version.

37 The relevance of Alexander to other passages in the *Dialogues* is noted by Boesch Gajano, 'Demoni', nn. 51, 55. There is no reason to conjecture the diffusion in Gregory's Italy of the fullest surviving ancient discussion of phrenitis: book I of Caelius Aurelianus, *On Acute and Chronic Diseases*, ed. and trans. I. E. Drabkin

(Chicago, 1950), or ed. Gerhard Bendz and trans. Ingeborg Pape, *Corpus medi-corum latinorum* (Berlin, 1990, 1993).

38 Peregrine Horden, 'The Earliest Hospitals in Byzantium, Western Europe, and Islam', in Mark Cohen (ed.), *Journal of Interdisciplinary History*, special issue, 'Poverty and Charity: Judaism, Christianity, Islam', 35 (2005): 361–389 [reprinted as Ch. 2 this volume].

39 As Clare Pilsworth points out to me, the narrative resembles the model of cure as social reintegration that Raymond Van Dam discerns in Gregory of Tours' *Miracles* of St Martin: see his *Saints and their Miracles in Late Antique Gaul* (Princeton, NJ, 1993), ch. 3.

40 Though not used in *Rule of St. Benedict*, cap. 36.

41 Anna Maria Giuntella, 'I monasteri', in Letizia Pani Ermini (ed.), *Christiana loca: lo spazio cristiano nella Roma del primo millennio* (Rome, 2000), pp. 181–182.

42 Eva Margareta Steinby (ed.), *Lexicon topographicum urbis Romae*, vol. V (Rome, 1999), s.v. 'Xenodochium', pp. 215–218. See also Francesca Romana Stasolla, '*Xenodochia*', in Pani Ermini (ed.), pp. 198–191. For context see now Neil Christie, *From Constantine to Charlemagne: An Archaeology of Italy AD 300–800* (Aldershot, 2006), pp. 98–107, and for background, William V. Harris (ed.), *The Transformations of* Urbs Roma *in Late Antiquity*, Journal of Roman Archaeology supplementary series 33 (Portsmouth, RI, 1999), esp. Beat Brenk, 'La cristianizzazione della Domus dei Valerii sul Celio', pp. 69–84.

43 *Poverty and Leadership in the Later Roman Empire* (Hanover, 2002), pp. 33–44. For what follows see also Horden, 'The Christian Hospital in Late Antiquity: Break or Bridge?', in Florian Steger and Kay Peter Jankrift (eds), *Gesundheit–Krankheit: Kulturtransfer medizinischen Wissens von der Spätantike bis in die frühe Neuzeit* (Cologne, 2004), pp. 2–24; id., 'The Earliest Hospitals', to the references in which add now Andrew T. Crislip, *Christian Monasticism and the Transformation of Health Care in Late Antiquity* (Ann Arbor, MI, 2005).

44 On the *pandocheion*, see Olivia Remie Constable, *Housing the Stranger in the Mediterranean World: Lodging, Trade, and Travel in Late Antiquity and the Middle Ages* (Cambridge, 2003), ch. 1.

45 Thomas Sternberg, *Orientalium More Secutus: Räume und Institutionen der Caritas des 5. bis 7. Jahrhunderts in Gallien*, Jahrbuch für Antike und Christentum Ergänzungsband 16 (Münster, 1991).

46 Audrey Meaney, 'The Practice of Medicine in England about the Year 1000', *Social History of Medicine* 13 (2000): 221–237, at 224–227; Sethina Watson, 'The Origins of the English Hospital', *Transactions of the Royal Historical Society* 16 (2006): 75–94, of which the author kindly allowed me a preview.

47 For the nearly contemporary foundation of Paulinus at Nola see Sternberg, *Orientalium More Secutus*, p. 187; Sigrid H. Mratschek, '*Multis enim notissima est sanctitas loci*: Paulinus and the Gradual Rise of Nola as a Center of Christian Hospitality', *Journal of Early Christian Studies* 9 (2001): 511–533, at 514–516.

48 Jerome, *Letter* 77.6, in *Sancti Eusebii Hieronymi epistulae*, ed. Isidorus Hilberg, *Corpus Scriptorum Ecclesiasticorum Latinorum* 55, new edn (Vienna, 1996), p. 43. The context has now been reconsidered by Stephen Lake, 'Fabiola and the Sick: Jerome, *epistula* 77', in Barbara Feichtinger and Helmut Seng (eds), *Die Christen und der Körper: Aspekte der Körperlichkeit in der christlichen Literatur der Spätantike* (Leipzig, 2004), pp. 151–172; see esp. 156–160.

49 *Letter* 66.11, ed. Hilberg, p. 661; though compare 77.10 (p. 47). For context see Philip Rousseau, *Ascetics, Authority, and the Church in the Age of Jerome and Cassian* (Oxford, 1978), pp. 116–117.

50 Walther Schönfeld, 'Die Xenodochien in Italien und Frankreich im frühen Mittelalter', *Zeitschrift der Savigny-Stiftung für Rechtsgeschichte, Kanonistische Abteilung* 12 (1922): 1–54.

51 For Basil see Brown, *Poverty*, pp. 38–42. For Augustine see his *Sermon* 356.10, in *PL* 39, col. 1578, with Horden, 'Christian Hospital', p. 97. On Ambrose see Alfred Breitenbach, 'Ambrose von Mailand: ein Bischof für die Kranken? Eine Beurteilung anhand des *Lukaskommentars* und der Schrift *De officiis*', in Feichtinger and Seng (eds), *Die Christen und der Körper*, pp. 101–150.

52 Dudden, vol. 1, pp. 53, 247–251, 301, 316–320; Richards, pp. 88–89, 95–97; Richard Krautheimer, *Rome: Profile of a City, 312–1308* (Princeton, NJ, 1980), pp. 76–78. See esp. John the Deacon's *Life*, ii.51–3, *PL* 75, cols 109–110. It is instructive to note how much of the information in Steinby, *Lexicon topographicum*, s.v. 'Xenodochium', and Stasolla, '*Xenodochia*', derives from Gregory's correspondence.

53 *Liber pontificalis*, ed. Louis Duchesne, 2 vols (Paris, 1886–92), vol. I, p. 309 (Pelagius II); Richards, p. 97; Krautheimer, p. 87.

54 *Vita*, I.20, *Sancti Caesarii Arelatensis opera varia*, ed. Germain Morin, vol. 2 (Maretioli, 1942), p. 303, trans. William Klingshirn, *Caesarius of Arles: Life, Testament, Letters* (Liverpool, 1994), p. 18. For this and what follows see also Lake, 'Fabiola', pp. 166–169.

55 *Vitas Sanctum Patrorum Emeretensium*, V.3, ed. A. Maya Sánchez, *Corpus Christianorum* 116 (Turnhout, 1992), pp. 50–51; trans. A. T. Fear, *Lives of the Visigothic Fathers* (Liverpool, 1997), pp. 74–75.

56 Brown, *The Cult of the Saints* (Chicago, 1981), p. 111.

57 Horden, 'Responses', to the references in which add now Sergei A. Ivanov, *Holy Fools in Byzantium and Beyond* (Oxford, 2006). Michael W. Dols, '*Majnūn': The Madman in Medieval Islamic Society* (Oxford, 1992). What follows generally builds on the dossier in my 'Responses'.

58 *Life of Theodore* §161, ed. André-Jean Festugière, *Vie de Théodore de Sykéôn*, 2 vols (Brussels, 1970), vol. I, p. 143.

59 *Miracles of Cosmas and Damian*, §12, ed. Ludwig Deubner, *Kosmas und Damian* (Leipzig, 1907), pp. 128–129; trans. André-Jean Festugière, *Saint Thècle . . .* (Paris, 1971), pp. 120–121.

60 *Miracles of St Artemios*, §6, ed. Athanasios Papadopoulos-Kerameus, *Varia graeca sacra* (St Petersburg, 1909), repr. and trans. Virgil S. Crisafulli and John W. Nesbitt, *The Miracles of St. Artemios* (Leiden, 1997), pp. 86–89.

61 First pointed out by Lennart Rydén, 'A Note on Some References to the Church of St. Anastasia in Constantinople in the Tenth Century', *Byzantion* 44 (1974): 198–201. See further Jane Baun, *Tales from Another Byzantium* (Cambridge, 2007), pp. 115–117, to which I am indebted in what follows.

62 For the quotation and what follows see *The Life of St Andrew the Fool*, ed. Rydén, vol. II, lines 96–129.

63 *Life of Basil the Younger*, ed. A. N. Veselovskii, 'Razyskaniia v oblasti russkogo dukhovnogo stikha', *Sbornik otdeleniia russkogo iazyka i slovesnosti Imperatorskoi akademii nauk* 46 (1890): supplementary pp. 68–69.

64 Ibid. pp. 69–72; quotation following at p. 70. I am very grateful to Jane Baun for guidance around this frustrating edition, ed. and trans. Denis F. Sullivan et al. (Washington DC, 2014). For a further testimony to the *Anastaseion*, see also *The Life of Irene Abbess of Chrysobalanton*, §49, ed. Jan Olof Rosenqvist (Uppsala, 1986), p. 62. For St Anastasia performing an equivalent role in sixteenth-century Bavaria, see Lederer, p. 44.

65 Sulpicius Severus, *Dialogues*, III.6, ed. Carolus Halm, *Sulpicii Severi libri qui supersunt* (Vienna, 1866), p. 204.

66 *De virtutibus S. Martini*, IV.44, in *Gregorii episcopi Turonensis miracula et opera minora*, ed. Bruno Krusch, *MGH, SRM*, 1.ii (Hanover, 1885), p. 210; trans. Van Dam, *Saints and their Miracles*, p. 302. Compare Brown, 'Learning and Imagination', in his *Society and the Holy in Late Antiquity* (London, 1982), p. 18: 'the possessed were a recognized category grouped round the shrine. They would be given their meals, were blessed once a day – and were set to scrubbing the paving of the church.'

67 *Acts of Simon and Jude*, from the *Apostolic History of pseudo-Abdias*, VI.16–17, in *Codex apocryphus Novi Testamenti*, ed. Johann Albert Fabricius, 2 vols (Hamburg, 1703, 1719), vol. II, p. 674, paraphrased in Montague Rhodes James (trans.), *The Apocryphal New Testament* (Oxford, 1924), p. 465. For some context, though dealing with earlier material, see Jan N. Bremmer, 'Magic in the *Apocryphal Acts of the Apostles*', in Bremmer and Jan R. Veenstra (eds), *The Metamorphosis of Magic from Late Antiquity to the Early Modern Period* (Leuven, 2002), pp. 51–70. The text is noted in passing by Valerie I. J. Flint, *The Rise of Magic in Early Medieval Europe* (Oxford, 1991), p. 29.

68 Dols, ch. 6 (A); Horden, 'Earliest Hospitals', p. 370.

69 Peter E. Pormann, 'Medical Methodology and Hospital Practice: The Case of Fourth-/Tenth-Century Baghdad', in P. Adamson (ed.), *In the Age of al-Farabi: Arabic Philosophy in the Fourth/Tenth Century* (London, 2008), pp. 95–118. I am very grateful to the author for allowing me to draw upon this paper in advance of publication. See also Pormann, 'Theory and Practice in the Early Hospitals in Baghdad: Al-Kaškarī on Rabies and Melancholy', *Zeitschrift für Geschichte der Arabisch-Islamischen Wissenschaften* 15 (2002/2003): 197–248.

70 MS Aya Sofya 3716, fol. 125a.10–14. A facsimile of the MS including this difficult text was published by Fuat Sezgin*, Book on Medicine* (Frankfurt, 1985), but its value for hospital history remained unappreciated until Pormann's study. On Kaskarī (the transliteration he now prefers to Kaškarī), see Pormann, 'Theory and Practice', pp. 204–205. [Quotation from revised translation in Peter E. Pormann (ed.), *Rufus of Ephesus: On Melancholy* (Tübingen, 2008), p. 192.]

71 [Trans. Pormann, *Rufus*, p. 193.] See also Dols, pp. 117–119, for the madman's verses.

72 Cassiodorus, *Institutes*, §31, ed. Roger A. B. Mynors, *Cassiodori senatoris institutiones* (Oxford, 1937), pp. 78–79, trans. James W. Halporn, *Cassiodorus, Institutions of Divine and Secular Learning and On the Soul* (Liverpool, 2004), pp. 165–166 (see also the comprehensive introduction by Mark Vessey).

73 Gregory's earliest (English) biographer records the story that the pope influenced a Lombard king (Ariulf?) to withdraw from Rome, mollifying his *fervidum pectus* (seething – almost frenetic – heart). The pope then prescribed a milk diet that, by returning the king to the habits of his pastoral infancy, cured his stomach ailment: *The Earliest Life of Gregory the Great*, ed. and trans. Bertram Colgrave (Lawrence, KS, 1968), §23, pp. 114–116; Richards, pp. 184–185. We have seen that Gregory knew all about stomach problems.

74 For this and what follows see Dols, p. 112 with notes; Dora B. Weiner, 'The Brothers of Charity and the Mentally Ill in Pre-Revolutionary France', *Social History of Medicine* 2 (1989): 321–337, at 325.

75 H. C. Erik Midelfort, 'Madness and Civilization in Early Modern Europe: A Reappraisal of Michel Foucault', in Barbara C. Malament (ed.), *After the Reformation: Essays in Honor of J. H. Hexter* (Philadelphia, 1980), p. 253; Roy

Porter, 'Madness and its Institutions', in Andrew Wear (ed.), *Medicine in Society: Historical Essays* (Cambridge, 1992), pp. 279–280.

76 See e.g. Nicholas Orme and Margaret Webster, *The English Hospital 1070–1570* (New Haven, CT, 1995), p. 58; also Jean Imbert, *Les hôpitaux en droit canonique* (Paris, 1947), p. 126.

77 George Rosen, *Madness in Society: Chapters in the Historical Sociology of Mental Illness* (Chicago, 1968), pp. 138–142, relies heavily on older secondary authorities, as does Weiner, p. 324. For Spain see James W. Brodman, *Charity and Welfare: Hospitals and the Poor in Medieval Catalonia* (Philadelphia, 1998), pp. 69, 85–6; Michael McVaugh, *Medicine before the Plague: Practitioners and their Patients in the Crown of Aragon 1285–1345* (Cambridge, 1993), pp. 233–234. For England, see Jonathan Andrews et al., *The History of Bethlem* (London, 1997), ch. 9. Other areas, with allegedly long histories of institutional care for the insane, such as Geel in Flanders (Porter, 'Madness', p. 280; Weiner, p. 324 n. 5) are urgently in need of fresh scholarly study. The best modern study of madhouses in Germany begins in the sixteenth century: H. C. Erik Midelfort, *A History of Madness in Sixteenth-Century Germany* (Stanford, CA, 1999), pp. 356–381; see also Lederer, pp. 267–271, for Bavaria.

78 Katherine Park and John Henderson, '"The First Hospital among Christians": The Ospedale di Santa Maria Nuova in Early Sixteenth-Century Florence', *Medical History* 35 (1991): 183. For context see now Henderson, *The Renaissance Hospital* (New Haven, CT, 2006), esp. pp. 312–313.

79 Peter Bartlett and David Wright (eds), *Outside the Walls of the Asylum: The History of Care in the Community 1750–2000* (London, 1999); Roy Porter and David Wright (eds), *The Confinement of the Insane: International Perspectives, 1800–1965* (Cambridge, 2003); Akihito Suzuki, *Madness at Home: The Psychiatrist, the Patient and the Family in England, 1820–1860* (Berkeley, CA, 2006).

80 Roy Porter, *Mind-Forg'd Manacles: A History of Madness in England from the Restoration to the Regency* (London, 1987).

6

THE SICK FAMILY IN THE EARLY MIDDLE AGES

The evidence of Gregory of Tours

'As Gregor Samsa awoke one morning from uneasy dreams, he found himself transformed in his bed into a gigantic verminous insect . . .' The opening of Franz Kafka's story 'Metamorphosis'. However we interpret that text, it is hard to avoid the conclusion that the transformation which Gregor undergoes is at least partly a symptom or an expression of the tensions, the suppressed hostilities, within the Samsa family. And, at the end of the story, when Gregor has died, it also seems that some kind of healing has been wrought for others. The whole family had been sick, lifeless, dependent on Gregor's unremitting toil – an aspect well brought out in Steven Berkoff's stylized dramatization (Berkoff 1988). Now the family is better: 'Then they all three [parents and sister] left the apartment together, which was more than they had done for months, and went by tram into the open countryside outside the town . . . Leaning back comfortably in their seats they canvassed their prospects for the future, and it appeared on close inspection that these were not at all bad . . .' (Kafka 1961: 9, 62). Although only one member of a family may exhibit symptoms, the whole family is sick and needs treatment.

This interpretation of Kafka's emblematic story, only one among many possible, hardly strikes an unfamiliar note. Still, before coming to the medieval material advertised in my title, it is worth taking time to muster some comparative evidence and bring the phenomenon into sharper focus. It has been suggested that to 'psychosomatic' we add 'sociosomatic' as a term for disease aetiologies that involve social relationships. Perhaps we can go on to coin, as a subdivision of the sociosomatic, the 'oico-' or 'oecosomatic', from the Greek *oikos*, household (although there is the problem that this term sounds as if it has something to do with ecology).

The intimate link between familial and individual wellbeing comes at us from the literature of medical anthropology with great regularity, not least from the literature dealing with Africa. Here are some examples, reported in the 'ethnographic present' although of course much may have changed since the time of the original field work. 'Traditional' healers in Labadi, a Ghanaian coastal town, bring their chronic and mysterious ailments, and their cases of witchcraft and sorcery, to healers whose job is to restore lineage solidarity just as much as individual wellbeing. These healers try to involve all members of an afflicted individual's lineage in diagnosis and treatment – and in remuneration for their efforts at cure. Kin are consulted at every stage. And all of them must, on pain of being suspected of ill-will, visit the patient. The real unit of treatment is indeed the lineage and not the individual (Mullings 1984). Among the Ganda of east Africa, a folk illness or type of pollution called *obuko*, the symptoms of which include swelling of the cheeks, limbs, and genitals, is held to be caused by the breach of certain taboos – for instance the sharing of prepared food by parents-in-law and their children-in-law (Robertson 1996: 601–602). Among the Ndembu, now classics in the anthropology since the 1950s, thanks to Victor Turner, all misfortunes, including illness, have their perceived cause in tensions between different members of the tribe. These induce the ancestors to sink their incisor teeth, *ihamba*, into the individual source of tension. But the resultant pain is merely a symptom of a collective sickness. The *ihamba* must be ceremonially removed in front of the entire village, each member of which has previously aired his or her grievances against the patient. The healing is again corporate (Turner 1968).

Africa does not give all the best examples. Among the families of the Indian state of Maharashtra studied by Vieda Skultans, for instance, women, through trance, take on the mental illness of other members of their families:

> The most frequent movement of illness is away from husbands and sons towards wives and mothers. The indigenous theory underlying such beliefs is that families rather than individuals are the target for malevolent spiritual attacks . . . The disappearance of symptoms in one individual does not signal the end of the history of illness. The family anticipate further manifestations of the original affliction in some other guise in other family members . . . Usually the affliction follows in the wake of a dispute over land or property involving members of the extended family . . . There is a fatalistic acceptance of family feuding. One informant neatly summed up the attitude by saying that one could plead with God but not with an angry relative. (Skultans 1987: 670)

These examples have, of course, many counterparts in a variety of modern western psychotherapeutic traditions. To mention only the psychoanalytic one: in *The Family as Patient*, first published (in German) in 1974, Horst Richter wrote: 'Rapidly though the literature on the relationship between family dynamics and psychogenic disturbances is growing, we still lack a discriminative, convincing model for understanding the process of interchange between individuals and the forms of its [that is, the family's] disturbance, such as we have, thanks to Freud, for the intra-individual process' (1974: 39). I am not sure quite how far that remains true – for those who preserve a faith in any form of psychoanalysis. Richter was already able confidently to delineate 'the anxiety-neurotic family', 'the paranoid family', and 'the hysterical family', and to provide grim case histories which at the very least showed the need for some type of familial therapy. The literature of psychoanalytic family therapy certainly proliferates (e.g. Davies 2010), as does that of therapies of other theoretical persuasions, as witness the *Journal of Family Therapy*.

What evidence is the medical historian to offer under this heading? At the conference for which the first version of this paper was written, submissions had been invited on the theme of 'the family as a generator of disease'. Mine turned out to be the sole contribution. Why is it that we still tend to think in individualistic terms, of individual sick people and individual healers? And what kind of evidence *might* have been included under that heading of 'the family'? The point of the present paper is to provoke others to make good the lack of historical discussion, especially by medievalists, of 'the family as generator of disease'. The first question I put to myself in preparing this paper was: what is the equivalent in pre-modern European history of these anthropological and psychoanalytic perceptions of family malaise which I have just used to open up the subject? What healers most often, or most influentially, operated with the family, rather than the isolated individual or the wider social or material environment, as a unit of diagnosis and healing? Even to begin to address that would of course involve a lengthy investigation. So, to be brief and selective I offer the medieval saint as at least one type of family therapist. The saint's miraculous power that accrued to him or her in virtue of a special relationship to God, psychological penetration, and capacity for taking what we would now call a holistic view of individual frailty – these mark out the saint as a healer of this familial kind. The *saint*, not the ordinary parish priest or confessor, who doubtless often acted as such a therapist but whose pastoral ministry in such matters is scarcely documented. The closest we can reach to it is usually the literature of penance, that 'medicine of the soul' as it was in medieval tradition; and this literature is generally individualistic in emphasis. It only occasionally refers to the dis-ease or pollution that can affect the group or community as the result of an unresolved quarrel (e.g. McNeill and Gamer 1938: 167: the monastic 'Old Irish Penitential', clauses 12–16; on the text see Meens 2014: 62). The *saint*, again, not the physician with a humoral aetiology of both the oeco- and the somatic elements in illness.

My contention is, then, simply that the biographies of saints, together with the records of the miracles that they performed whether during their lifetimes or posthumously, may give us the best and largest corpus of evidence for something approximating to family therapy in pre-modern Europe. The material has not usually been approached in this way, and it is easy to see why. Much of the medieval hagiography supplies abundant detail of healing miracles, so that one obvious course for the medical historian is to tabulate the ailments involved – paralysis, mutism, fevers, and so on. It also demonstrates that saints, their clients, and their hagiographers subscribed to aetiological pluralism: diseases could have natural, personal, demonic, and divine origins. This means that the obvious thing for historians to do with the information is to use it to knock down some stereotype, such as the notion that medieval illness was consistently attributed to sin. On the other hand, if the evidence is apparently so informative about sickness beliefs and behaviour, it nonetheless presents huge problems of interpretation. Much energy has therefore been devoted to classifying the functions and purposes of hagiography. The effect of this can be to make the writing seem so caught up in its own poetics, so far removed from the everyday reality of suffering and healing, that to extract particulars of individual cases from it becomes hazardous. There is no medical detail that may not be serving some large metaphorical purpose and can therefore be separated from its literary context. For all these reasons, the familial dimension of these sources has been relatively neglected.

Help is at hand, though, from medical anthropology. We do not have to worry so much about what nosological reality, if any, might lie beneath the surface of a miracle story, seeing in the cure either an instance of the faith healing of a psychosomatic condition or the spontaneous remission of an organic disease. We can, instead, attend with a clear conscience to the surface of the text, and treat it as an interpretation, an ascription of meaning to disease. This interpretation is as much a fact of the past as any action of the saint (living or dead) or of those he or she is described as curing. It is not a mere gloss on some primary biological or behavioural reality that we have to try to remove. Of course, it is perhaps, in some cases, only the hagiographer's *parti pris* interpretation; in other cases, there is enough evidence that saint and client, hagiographer and audience participated in a common medical culture – in which saints conformed to an established model, and their clients were influenced in their sickness behaviour by the hagiography that they had read or, more likely, heard.

The writings of the sixth-century aristocratic bishop Gregory of Tours (late 530s–594) do, I think, open up such a common culture to us (on him see now e.g. Murray 2016). I shall try to illustrate my suggestions principally by reference to him, though with some excursions to other medieval sources. Gregory is an early medieval figure, and an influential one in hagiographical terms: he therefore shows that the phenomenon of family therapy, to the extent that we find it in his writings, is not some late medieval peculiarity. I say 'to the extent that we find it' because it is by no means necessarily to the hagiographer's purpose to give us the sort of detail we want.

First let me present some illustrations. The typical family in Gregory's writings is given as nuclear: parents and one or two children. Occasionally there is a reference to, for instance, co-resident brothers. Among the wealthy and powerful, both clerical and lay, servants and slaves are, if present, for the most part inarticulate. It is worth beginning with that preliminary because demographers have sometimes used such material unsystematically for evidence (admittedly indirect) of family and household; too much has revolved around a few colourful vignettes. There are no extended households or tightly knit kin groups here, but that is partly no doubt because Gregory wishes to uphold what modern politicians have referred to as 'core family values' (see further Réal 2001).

Even so, we should not expect Gregory's idea of the sick family to be entirely familiar to modern therapists. For him, epidemics such as plague can proceed house by house, but not because of the population biology of rodents and fleas or interpersonal transmission. The context is important, and reveals the way Gregory conceptualizes the disease. Saints looking down from heaven protect certain areas of a city, especially its shrines – or in one case protect a whole city from plague's ravages (VP 17.4; GC 78).[1]

Gregory wrote from early experience or close family recollection. 'When that plague of the groin that the prayer of Saint Gallus [Gregory's uncle, a bishop] eventually repulsed was approaching Clermont, signs and marks appeared on the walls of homes and churches [vaguely cross-shaped; a sign of protection]. My mother had a vision during the night in which it seemed that the wine in our cellars had been changed to blood. She wept and said "Woe am I, for our house has been marked for the plague."' Fortunately a man, name and origin unspecified, reminded her of the approaching anniversary feast of a martyr. His mother went and kept vigil all night at his shrine. Gregory concludes: 'Although the houses of our neighbours were marked [and presumably stricken by plague] our home remained untouched [*inviolata*]' (GM 50).

If one pious action could save a household, a single impious one could bring it down. Again Gregory knew what he was talking about. He has no qualms about offering us his own family history as exemplary of the household therapy of saints.

One of my servants was motivated by his faith and brought back venerable wood from the railing around the holy Martin's tomb in Tours and kept it in his cottage for protection. I was unaware of this. But his family began to be severely ill – I think because this wood was not honoured or respected as was appropriate. And since the man was completely ignorant about what was happening, and since the situation did not improve but even deteriorated, in a vision during the night he saw a terrifying personage who said to him: 'Why are you suffering this way?' The man replied: 'I am completely ignorant about the reason for what has happened.' The personage said to him: 'you have suffered these misfortunes because you thoughtlessly keep with you this wood that you took from the bed of Lord Martin. But go now, bring this wood to the deacon Gregory, and let him keep it in his possession.' Immediately the man brought the wood to me. With the greatest reverence I took it and put it in an appropriate place. Then the entire family [*omnis familia*] in his home was cured, with the result that thereafter no one there suffered any misfortune. (VM 1.35)

Such stories were not confined to Gregory's own circle.

As some monks were transporting the relics of St Saturninus into another region, the path of their journey led them to pass the boundary of the village of Brioude, in the territory of Clermont. Since the sun was setting, they turned aside to the cottage of a poor man and requested the lodging they needed. Once the man took them in, they told him what they were delivering. Advised by human intuition and the fear of God, the man took the reliquary with its relics to his storeroom and set it on top of the grain that was kept in a container [elevating it as if on an altar; but also superimposing it on his chief source of food]. At daybreak, the travellers took back their relics, thanked the man, and resumed their journey. But the next night the poor man received a warning from a dream in which an old man said to him: 'Do not stay in this place, because it has been sanctified by the relics of the martyr Saturninus.' The poor man thought little of this vision; as is characteristic of rusticity [country-bumpkin boorishness, meaning, for Gregory, lack of reverence for his saints] the man remembered nothing of these warnings [or could not afford to remember them and abandon his farm]. But soon he fell into misfortune. His small possessions began gradually to diminish and his wife to waste away from another illness. [Notice the equation of material and biological misfortune, familiar to medical anthropologists.] Within a year he had been reduced to such poverty that he possessed nothing and could not feed or house himself. After thinking to himself he said to his wife: 'I have sinned before God and his saints, because I did not leave this cottage as I was warned. I know that the misfortunes we now suffer have come upon us for this reason. Now, however, let us obey the vision that we saw and let us remove the cottage from this place, so that we might be saved.' After he tore down the cottage he built an oratory out of wooden planks. Every day he prayed in this oratory and requested the assistance of the blessed martyr. Finally his misfortunes ceased ...

– and, presumably, his wife recovered her health (GM 47).

Here, of course, the family dis-ease is consequent upon the actions of a saint rather than being cured by him. But the narrative does show how illness as the result of sin, the sin of irreverence, could be passed around within a family in a manner that would not be wholly strange to the Maharashtrians mentioned earlier. From husband to wife, for instance. A negligent count (*comes*) of Clermont (the local royal official; a 'lord lieutenant') failed to repair the lid of the sarcophagus of a saintly girl after some of the church vaulting had collapsed on it. The count lived with the consequences of this neglect in a way that Gregory does not specify. When he died, moreover, his widow became seriously ill and went blind. No medicine availed, of course, until she did the obvious thing and provided a new lid for the sarcophagus, thus in a way moving the barrier from in front of her own eyes to cover those of the saintly girl (GC 34).

The most obvious way in which sin and the illness which is its expression can be seen to move around within a family is from parents to children. The saint as family therapist interprets the child's affliction in the light of its parents' behaviour, and gets them to mend their ways as well as curing the child. Gregory had a story to tell in this vein. It is to be found in the abridged and reworked Latin version that he made of the Acts or Miracles of the Apostle Andrew, and thus has a predominantly classical and pagan setting. A man's son bathed in the women's bath and was seized by a demon. His father wrote to Andrew for help – help for the whole family. He, the father, also had a fever and his wife suffered from a condition that sounds like dropsy. The apostle exorcised the boy, rebuked the father for his loose living and the wife for her infidelity, also curing both (AA 5, pp. 579–581).

A broader view of the effects of the 'sins of the fathers' comes from a later (eleventh-century) Byzantine source, Michael Psellus's reworking of the *Life* of St Auxentius. The saint meets on the road a mother with a baby whose eyes are bloodshot, and whose face is all twisted, its hands failing to hold on to its mother and forgetting to suckle. The saint looked at the baby for a long time, then gave his diagnosis: 'it is not in the new-born baby that one should look for the cause of this, but in ourselves. Faced with the sins of adults God often spares them and punishes and punishes incomplete beings instead, just as he stirs up the elements to bring us to our senses through their devastation. God will heal this infant. You take care that the evil does not increase and bring harm to you as well' (*Life of Auxentius* 19, ed. Joannou 1971: 96–70).

Byzantine evidence also shows aspects of the saint that Gregory does not bring out so well. First the living saint as counsellor and therapist, an all-purpose source of healing wisdom. In the fifth-century *Life of Hypatius*, we meet a priest who married and received half his wife's dowry. He wanted to claim the other half but his wife seemed infertile. Even before the marriage, the woman's parents had been angry with her, presumably for her poor match. When they heard about the lack of little ones, moreover, not only would they not complete the dowry, they also refused to make their peace with her. Both parties came to see the saint. He failed to persuade the parents to soften their hearts. Indeed, they said that if their daughter died childless they wanted back the portion of the dowry that they had already handed over. Eventually, in the presence of all involved, like a good African healer restoring lineage solidarity, the saint summoned the girl, placed her symbolically in the middle of her family, and told her, in the name of Our Lord Jesus Christ, that she would conceive and bear a son. She was to name him Personas, after the child's [paternal] grandfather. Which, it need hardly be added, she did. The parents made peace with her and handed over the rest of the dowry (ed. Bartelink 1971: 93–95).

Hypatius was clearly remembered as an effective counsellor. But the most versatile and best-documented Byzantine therapist of this kind was the sixth-century St Theodore of Sykeon (his Life ed. and trans. Festugière 1970; trans. Dawes and Baynes 1977). He operated indeed at every level of inclusiveness from the individual to the entire village community, the latter in one instance riven by a property dispute between an enterprising kulak and the rest, and therefore subject to an epidemic of possession (sections 114, 116). 'Did husband and wife come to hate each other,' his biographer writes, 'they would go to him and he would pray over them and the hatred was dispelled' (section 145). Theodore also took on the entire possessed household of one of the emperor's grooms. 'Both the groom's servants and his beasts were bewitched by unclean spirits, and when members of the household were at breakfast or dinner, stones would be thrown at the tables . . . they also broke the women's looms. The whole house, too, was filled with mice and snakes [clearly diabolical in species] which terrified the inhabitants and made the house quite uninhabitable' (section 131). (Compare Gregory, AA 29, p. 641, for a possessed household.)

Many other stories that might be relevant to the theme of the sick family are less explicit than these. Much can only be inferred. Perhaps the hagiographer does not know the circumstances of the case he reports. Perhaps they seem irrelevant to his purpose of proclaiming, and trying to enforce, reverence for his particular saints. Stories that bring together the ailments of parents and children, that date the onset of an affliction such as blindness from the death of a parent, or that merely show that a quarrel of some kind was an opportunity for the Devil to do his work – these hint at social or familial dynamics which are pertinent to the illness, but they do no more than that. To return to Gregory: he, like the other hagiographers quoted, does not always want sinful failings in personal relations to be shown as the causes of sickness. For one thing, many of the sick people he mentions are described as pious, therefore relatively free from sin. For another thing, he recalls John chapter 9: 'And as Jesus passed by, he saw a man which was blind from his birth. And his disciples asked him, saying, Master, who did sin, this man, or his parents, that he was born blind? Jesus answered,

Neither hath this man sinned, nor his parents: but that the works of God should be made manifest in him'. Sometimes, that is, as Gregory interprets it, the context in which to understand the illness is not the immediate family (the sins of the fathers) but the whole of local society. If he could have read Michael Herzfeld on 'tropes in the exploration of bodily and social disorder', and grasped the terminology, he might well have endorsed the conclusion: 'what is recognized as illness . . . is a model of the [social] disorder rather than the disorder itself' (Herzfeld et al. 1986: 107).

We have then to approach the topic of the family in Gregory's thinking by always keeping in mind the wider social context. It is no use blotting out all but explicit references to household ills. An example. A poor man of Le Mans was napping in his garden under the midday sun and woke to find that his fingers were doubled up into his palms and very painful – a 'model', presumably, of aggression or tension. He slipped into unconsciousness and had a vision of a man dressed in black who turns out to be the great St Martin of Tours. The saint's message anticipates those of so many later apparitions: 'your disability reveals the anguish that awaits sinful men . . . Go now through the villages and proclaim that everyone is to abstain from perjury and usury . . . For the anger of the Lord is causing the hatreds and ailments of the people. Therefore be prompt in announcing that people are to reform, lest they die a cruel death as a result of their own crimes . . .' The man did as he was told and eventually, of course, his hands were healed. No specific familial aspect there but an emphasis on the connection between individual and communal malaise, the sickness of one figure and the sinfulness of others (VM 2.40).

Sickness in Gregory is often a model of social disorder in a slightly different way. Illness is equivalent to separation – from family, from wider community. The sick are unable to work, sometimes unable to marry. They have no resources, often (it seems) no supportive family, and they join the ranks of the local Church's approved beggars, the *matricularii* (VM 2. 22, 24). Their cure is not only bodily and spiritual, it is their reintegration into the community and often, in the process, into their family as well. A sign of this can be their renewed participation in the liturgy. Gregory tells us a Kafkaesque story. 'Excessive swelling combined with a fever had frozen a woman's mouth open so that she was unable to control her tongue [a metaphor literalized?]; because she was unable to speak like a human, she instead only bellowed like an animal.' The additional detail needed here, which Gregory artfully withholds until the end of the narrative, is that the woman was then a slave. Like Gregor Samsa, her physical condition reflected her household role. Cure came to her, as to a number of others in Gregory's writings, as a concomitant of emancipation from slavery. And the cure arrived, significantly, while she was standing in the middle of the congregation, during the recital of the Lord's Prayer. 'She too opened her mouth and began to chant the prayer with the other people' (VM 2. 30). Recovery of speech equals freedom and reintegration.

I should conclude. But I have no argument or conclusion to offer beyond the deliberately provocative one stated earlier: that the medieval saint is the nearest we can find to a pre-modern family therapist, and that his or her activities under this heading deserve fuller consideration than I have been able to give in a short paper. Gregory would have known how to conclude, however, since the foregoing was originally read at a conference on a Sunday morning. He would have repeated the warning that can be found in a number of his anecdotes: those whose *rusticitas* is so great that they work on a Sunday suffer contraction of the fingers, burning in the feet, and blindness. A warning to weekend workaholics.

Acknowledgements

I am most grateful for help and advice to David Harley, Claire Trenery, and the late Patrick Wormald.

Note

1 References to Gregory's hagiographical writings are generally given using the abbreviations expanded in the reference list under his name, followed by the section number common to the edition of the Latin and the translations.

References

Bartelink, G. J. M. (ed. and trans.) (1971). *Callinicos. Vie d'Hypatios.* Sources chrétiennes 177. Paris: Cerf.

Berkoff, S. (1988). *The Trial; Metamorphosis; In the Penal Colony: Three Theatre Adaptations from Franz Kafka.* Oxford: Amber Lane.

Davies, H. A. (2010). *The Use of Psychoanalytic Concepts in Therapy with Families: For All Professionals Working with Families.* London: Karnac.

Dawes, E. A. S., and Baynes, N. H. (1977). First published 1948. *Three Byzantine Saints: Contemporary Biographies.* London: Mowbray.

Festugière, A.-J. (ed. and trans.) (1970). *Vie de Théodore de Sykéon.* Subsidia hagiographica 48. 2 vols. Brussels: Société des Bollandistes.

Gregory of Tours, *Acts of Andrew* [AA]: ed. J.-M. Prieur (1989). *Acta Andreae.* Corpus christianorum series apocryphorum 5. 2 vols (pp. 551–651). Turnhout: Brepols.

Gregory of Tours, *Glory of the Confessors* [GC]: ed. B. Krusch (1885, new edn 1969). *De gloria confessorum.* MGH SRM 1.2 (pp. 294–370). Hanover: Hahn. Trans. R. Van Dam (1988). *Gregory of Tours. Glory of the Confessors.* Liverpool: Liverpool University Press.

Gregory of Tours, *Glory of the Martyrs* [GM]: ed. B. Krusch (1885, new edn 1969). *De gloria martyrum.* MGH SRM 1.2 (pp. 34–111). Hanover: Hahn. Trans. R. Van Dam (1988). *Gregory of Tours. Glory of the Martyrs.* Liverpool: Liverpool University Press.

Gregory of Tours, *Life of the Fathers* [VP]: ed. B. Krusch (1885, new edn 1969). *De vita patrum*. MGH SRM 1.2 (pp. 211–294). Hanover: Hahn. Trans. E. James (1985). *Gregory of Tours. Life of the Fathers*. Liverpool: Liverpool University Press.

Gregory of Tours, *Of the Miracles of Saint Martin* [VM]: B. Krusch (ed.) (1885, new edn. 1969). *De virtutibus sancti Martini*. MGH SRM 1.2 (pp. 134–211). Hanover: Hahn. Trans. R. Van Dam (1993). *Saints and their Miracles in Late Antique Gaul* (pp. 200–303). Princeton, NJ: Princeton University Press.

Herzfeld, M. et al. (1986). Closure as Cure: Tropes in the Exploration of Bodily and Social Disorder [with Comments and Replies]. *Current Anthropology* 27.2: 107–20.

Joannou, P.-P. (1971). *Démonologie populaire, démonologie critique au XIe siècle: la vie inédite de S. Auxence* (Wiesbaden: Harrassowitz).

Kafka, F. (1961). *Metamorphosis and Other Stories*, trans. Willa and Edwin Muir. London: Penguin

McNeill, J. T. and Gamer, H. M. (1938). *Medieval Handbooks of Penance: A Translation of the Principal Libri Poenitentiales and Selections from Related Documents*. New York: Columbia University Press.

Meens, R. (2014). *Penance in Medieval Europe 600–1200*. Cambridge: Cambridge University Press.

Mullings, L. (1984). *Therapy, Ideology, and Social Change: Mental Healing in Urban Ghana*. Berkeley: University of California Press.

Murray, A. C. (ed.) (2016). *A Companion to Gregory of Tours*. Leiden: Brill.

Réal, I. (2001). *Vies de saints, vie de famille: représentation et système de la parenté dans le royaume mérovingien (481–751) d'après les sources hagiographiques*. Turnhout: Brepols.

Richter, H. E. (1974). *The Family as Patient: The Origin, Nature, and Treatment of Marital and Family Conflicts*. London: Souvenir Press.

Robertson, A. F. (1996). The Development of Meaning: Ontogeny and Culture. *Journal of the Royal Anthropological Institute* 2.4: 591–61.

Skultans, V. (1987). The Management of Mental Illness among Maharashtrian Families: A Case Study of a Mahanubhav Healing Temple. *Man*, n.s. 22.4: 661–79.

Turner, V. W. (1968). *The Drums of Affliction: A Study of Religious Processes among the Ndembu of Zambia*. Oxford: Clarendon Press.

7

WHAT'S WRONG WITH EARLY MEDIEVAL MEDICINE?

Introduction

If one surveys the state of medical knowledge in late antiquity and in the early Middle Ages in Western Europe, it is deplorable.[1]

How to tell if a sick person will die? One possible way was copied by a scribe from an older exemplar, probably in a religious house somewhere in the territory of modern France, perhaps Burgundy, around the year 800.[2] First the scribe wrote a heading: 'signa si eger moriturus est aut uitalis' ('signs whether the sick man [*aeger* in classical Latin] is about to die or has life left in him'). Then comes the crucial information. 'Take the tick of a black dog in the left hand [*in sinextra manu tetu*] and go into the sick room, and if, when the sick man sees you, he turns himself towards you, *non euadit* [he's 'a goner']'. Several alternative techniques immediately follow, presumably to make sure. One of them requires wiping the sick man from head to toe with a lump of lard and throwing it to a dog in an unfamiliar neighbourhood (or an unfamiliar dog: the Latin is ambiguous). If the dog eats the lard, the man will live.

What is wrong with early medieval medicine? Admittedly, such material might perpetuate the 'eye-of-newt' image of medieval medicine among the general public.[3] But why does it elicit epithets like 'deplorable' from scholars of the period? In the essay which opens with the exasperated verdict quoted above, Gerhard Baader's exposition is dotted throughout with epithets such as 'primitive' and 'unsophisticated', and with references to 'low standards'. The deprecatory tone is obviously felt necessary because the author is being faced with 'anonymous Vulgar Latin texts' (though, perhaps mercifully, not the one just summarized) 'full of superstition and folk medicine'. Baader is only a few degrees milder in his vocabulary than those medical historians of the first half of the twentieth century who saw, in early medieval medical texts with their (as they supposed) mindless copying of sterile formulae, clear signs of intellectual decline and cultural deliquescence.[4]

The quick rejoinder to judgements of this kind was famously given by Ranke. Every age is 'immediate to God'. Each should be evaluated on its own terms, rather than those of a later time.[5] We should add 'place' and 'earlier time' to Ranke's concern about supposed progress in history, because Baader, like many other scholars, is implicitly upbraiding the early medieval West for not being sufficiently Eastern and also for not being sufficiently classical. A proper defence of early medieval medicine will, however, have to be a little longer than Ranke's dictum.

To begin with definitions. By early medieval medicine I mean here the medicine, and wider therapeutic culture, of western Europe in the period c.700–1000; that is, predominantly, Carolingian and post-Carolingian Europe. It is a medicine that, in its representative texts, comes to us overwhelmingly in Latin. With the important exception of the Old English, the vernacular material is negligible in size – though not, of course, in scholarly interest.[6] Among the Latin texts are our canine oracles. Any discussion of early medieval medicine must face up to the interpretative challenges that they, and their kind, present – newts and all.

Those challenges take three main forms: textual, sociological, conceptual. The main one is thrown down by the surviving manuscripts – well over 160 of them for the period under review[7] – and the medicine-related texts that they contain. These manuscripts seem to be the fullest representation that we have of the medicine of the age. Moreover, the vast majority of them have been surveyed. A map, at least, of their contents is readily accessible.[8] And yet, as we shall see, their texts so often resist our attempts to work with them as individuals, and still more to generalize about them as a corpus. Unsurprisingly, then, we do not quite know how to edit them (proliferating editions notwithstanding).[9] Nor do we know how to read them, even though (as I shall suggest at the close) they are, in character, very much texts of our own time as well as their own.

This is, secondly, because it is very hard to reconstruct the conditions in which the manuscripts were produced and read and the people involved. We cannot readily supply any given text with a clear personal context in the wider history of medicine and healing. We mostly lack that kind of 'sociological' evidence.

The third challenge is conceptual. The most basic terms we want to deploy – such as 'work', 'text', 'use', even (or especially) 'medicine' – are all severely problematic. In addition, what we read often raises in acute form (at least as acute as the medicine of any other period from ancient Babylon to Renaissance Italy) such vexed categories as 'magic', 'science', 'religion', and their interrelations.[10]

The outcome of all these difficulties is a field in which probably fewer scholars are at work than in those of classical antiquity or the later Middle Ages and Renaissance; a field (I shall suggest) somewhat detached from wider currents in the cultural and intellectual historiography of the period;

above all, a field that has no master narrative, however provisional, except a very negative one defined (as by Baader) in such prejudicial terms as 'decline' or 'lack', and coloured by nostalgia. This is a speciality in which there has been no general accessible synthesis since 1937, despite some major synoptic articles.[11] In such an invertebrate world it is easy to feel disorientated.

What follows is not a replacement narrative. But it is an attempt to face some of the problems of interpretation. My inspiration has been the work of Anglo-Saxonists. The contrast between the concentrated vigour of work on medicine surviving in the Old English vernacular and the inevitably more diffused efforts of those dealing with continental European Latin medicine is instructive. Stray remedies and glosses apart, Anglo-Saxonists have to work with a substantial corpus of around 500 folios but embodying only five major works, three of which survive in unique manuscripts. I certainly do not mean to suggest that interpretative difficulties are much reduced, but the focus is at least clear. And the result has been a coherent set of revisionist interpretations. In contra-distinction to earlier scholarly talk of deliquescence and superstition, these interpretations have recalibrated the magical and quasi-pagan elements that had loomed far too large in older historiography.[12] The medicine in the vernacular has been shown to have widespread roots in continental Latin writings, although this implied validation of the vernacular by reference to the Latin reads ironically in the light of what is said by other specialists about the Latin material itself.[13] The elves that populate some of the medical texts have also been given a cultural context.[14] And even a 'wild and woolly' (and comparatively insular) text such as *Lacnunga* ['Remedies'] has been domesticated (perhaps excessively so?) into a working physician's *vade mecum*.[15] The plant remedies in the herbal material have been shown to represent thoughtful adaptations to local conditions.[16] And Old English *materia medica* has in general been defended as biologically rational and efficacious, with the magical and religious aspects glossed simply as contributors to the placebo effect.[17] In short, Anglo-Saxon medicine has been made to seem like real medicine rather than scribal ignorance or perversity.

That line of defence, which relies on invoking modern biology and herbalism, has been applied to the early medieval Latin writings as well.[18] Yet it is not the one that I shall adopt here. Rather, at the risk of producing a cabinet of curiosities, I want to look at a selection of texts or particular moments in texts. These will exemplify the interpretative challenges that are too quickly sidestepped by the proclamation of plain herbal remedies as the essence of early medieval medicine, and by the (as I see it) over-confident application to them of biochemistry.[19] I shall come back to the introductory example and the uses of dogs in the sickroom. First let us try a topic on which modern pharmacological evidence has little bearing. We must stare the newt in the eye – or rather, on this occasion, the vulture.

Vulture medicine

Around the same time as our opening example, another scribe somewhere in the Carolingian world was faced with a blank page in a large manuscript.[20] The page fell not between texts but towards the end of only book 1 of the great five-book treatise by Dioscorides (*floruit c.*65 CE), *De materia medica.* We might guess that the blank was a mistake discovered only after the lengthy text was complete, but there could have been some interruption to the copying. Whatever the circumstances, a blank page was too rare and expensive to leave. How to fill it? There was no shortage of herbal remedies in circulation.[21] Yet, instead, our scribe copied out, quite neatly and in the same double columns that characterize the Dioscorides text, an epistle on vulture medicine.[22] This was not veterinary material, but the remedies to be derived from the body of a newly captured vulture. 'Here begins the Letter of the Vulture' is the heading, in not altogether standard Latin. The text purports to be a letter from the king of Rome to the province of Alexandria and Babylon (presumably the Babylon in Egypt).[23]

'The human race does not know how much efficacy [*virtus*] the vulture has in it and how much it promotes health.'[24] No explanation of this *virtus* is given, no preference expressed for types or ages of vulture. But we are told that the bird should be killed with a sharp reed instead of a sword, and within an hour of being captured. The killer should act alone (?) [*singulos*]. Before he decapitates the vulture, he should say: 'Angelus Adonai Abraham, on your account the prophecy is fulfilled.' These words should be repeated when the bird is cut open to begin the harvest of remedies: its head bones, wrapped in deer skin, for migraine; eyes wrapped in wolf skin for eye problems; heart in lion or wolf skin against possession; spleen dried and mixed with bitumen of sulphur and oil of copper and old axle grease as an ointment against paralysis. The vulture does not only promote health in these ways; it can aid social wellbeing and economic prosperity too. Put its tongue in your right shoe and all your enemies will adore you. Rub its grease into a traction animal that you are trying to sell and on that day you will receive the asking price. There ended the list from which the scribe was copying. He wrote 'finit finit' so as to leave no doubt. He had filled only the top third of the right-hand column on his blank page, but the remainder of that column is empty. Overleaf, Dioscorides resumes.

What to make of this? Conceptual questions immediately loom. 'Angelus adonai abraham': such a ritual utterance, with its implied coercive force, its air of mechanical efficacy, bears the often- supposed hallmarks of the magical. Yet how then do we interpret the biblical character of the invocation? Is this Christianized magic or 'magicalized' Christianity, some unorthodox outgrowth of proper observance? Or does more depend on the way that the text might have been used than on the words on the page? The invocation could be enunciated in a prayerful way, as ideally was the liturgy, rather than in a mechanical way that paid no attention to the words.[25]

The only path through these difficulties is surely to be found in respecting local definitions and categories, so far as we can establish them. For early medieval sufferers, the real contrast was less between incompatible systems of ideas – religion, medicine, magic – or between the orthodox and the deviant, than between different authorities.[26] Few disputed that ritual words and gestures had power over invisible forces, which could reside mysteriously in substances. That was seen by most Christians in our period in the mass. The question was: whose words, and which forces.[27] Our vulturologist presumably thought he knew. So perhaps did the scribe who copied his work.

Who, though, was that scribe? Did he copy the material expecting to apply it and achieve practical results? His setting is likely to have been a monastery, but is this monastic medicine? Monastic labourers might be interesting in selling an animal for a good price. Yet what about the following passage? 'You dry and beat [the vulture's] tiny kidneys and testicles and give it with wine to him who is unable to have intercourse with his wife; he will find it a remedy.' Useful general information? For future 'pastoral' advice to the laity? Would it in any case have been easy to implement the recommendations, whether inside or outside a religious house? Vultures can, I assume, be caught, but how easily? Or was it that the mere possession of the information, without any headless vultures around, conferred a certain potential advantage? That raises the larger question of whether the epistle is to be taken as medicine at all or as a 'secret of nature', a species of occult knowledge, tucked (if not quite hidden) away in a manuscript the sheer size of which (over 320 folios) would make it more a work of reference than a book for any bedside.[28]

In default of a personal setting for our vulture lore, we can look only to the context supplied by the manuscript. First, how should we conceptualize this short text's relationship to the much longer surrounding medicine of Dioscorides? Are 'magic' and 'science' (on our definitions) here rubbing shoulders? It is best to begin by acknowledging our subconscious preferences. Dioscorides is 'the real thing', ancient science or medicine that we can respect; vulture medicine is not. Dioscorides's work is full (nearly 600 species of plants) and systematic. His 'drug affinity' classification bears comparison with modern pharmacognosy.[29] The Latin translation in our manuscript is not quite up to the original. Nonetheless we can see it, in its original form and then in an alphabetical rearrangement, as cleaving a path from antiquity, through the Renaissance, and into the early seventeenth century as an authority on, above all, herbal medicaments.[30] Some of its remedies doubtless still find adherents today. That is why it is almost always the plants that are discussed and the medieval botanical illustrations that are reproduced in modern scholarship, not the significant minority of remedies from animals in book 2 or those from minerals in book 5. 'Real medicine', biomedicine, comes from flora but not, for the most part, from fauna – or from stones. It is thus privileged in discussions of pre-modern medicine.

Pre-modern preferences differed. To begin with Dioscorides himself: first, his work is hardly free of elements that some scholars want to label superstitious and magical.[31] Second, among his animal-derived prescriptions in the old Latin translation is the deployment of the entrails of the bearded vulture in remedies for colic and stones.[32] He is not, however, especially eccentric in that. Vulture medicine has a long if convoluted and obscure history in ancient and medieval writings, including those of Alexander of Tralles, the sixth-century Byzantine author who is also represented in Latin in our manuscript.[33] I shall not go through the texts here; they were assembled by MacKinney as long ago as 1942,[34] showing that over 35 vulture-based remedies thread their way through ancient and late antique medical literature and out into the Middle Ages. And the point is not to engage in the familiar philological pastime of source-hunting,[35] but to guess at the meaning of the text as it emerges around the year 800.

Pursuing that meaning, we have to reckon with another way in which early medieval values were the converse of our own. We prefer the complete Dioscorides, albeit here in Latin (along with fairly full texts of other significant authorities, Alexander and the fourth-century Oribasius). In this monumental company the vulture text, even though its 'animal magic' is not nearly as outlandish as we might have supposed, might still seem an intrusion. So too might the formula of exorcism that is interpolated in the Alexander (although the author himself was not averse to including magical remedies).[36] Yet the early Middle Ages, as will emerge more fully below, preferred the short work, often in epistolary form, to the larger treatise. The manuscripts transmitting the (more or less) full Latin versions of Dioscorides, Oribasius, and Alexander are relatively few in number. To that extent, our manuscript with the vulture letter is hardly representative. What the producers and, by implication, the users of Carolingian medical manuscripts liked were shorter versions. Some of these handier texts were ascribed to Dioscorides but not actually written by him. They displayed novel and only superficially clear classifications. For instance, 'Dioscorides', in pseudonymous, truncated, and creatively reworked form, was held to have written 'on feminine herbs', in contrast to the second-century Apuleius, author of *The Golden Ass*, to whom, falsely, was attributed a work on masculine ones.[37]

Our vulturologist was therefore interpolating his short text into a quite special collection; and we may hypothesize that he perceived it as special because of the very length and thus completeness of the other texts. Whatever our scribe had as an exemplar for his vulture letter, it was 'ancient', for him probably at least as ancient as Dioscorides since it was a letter from the 'king of Rome'. It was not that the authoritative and 'scientific' setting of Dioscorides validated the intrusion of the vulture lore but the other way round. The vulture material was more authoritative. And its epistolary form, far from being a sign of fakery, as it is for modern scholars, made it seem more real, almost guaranteeing its authenticity.

Questions about the scope and definition of magic, religion, and medicine, and especially of *materia medica*; about the social setting and use of therapies; about the nature of medical authorship; about the boundaries between ancient and medieval medicine – all these seem implicated by our dead vulture. No amount of contextualizing can, or indeed should, 'normalize' such material. It perhaps partakes of that medicine of the excremental and the generally repulsive of which the German word *Dreckapotheke* is so evocative. Its power derives from its outlandishness, which we should be careful not to analyse away.[38]

Now, for a second example, from towards the end of our period, let us turn from treatment back to medical prediction, and initially to one of its main vehicles in medieval medicine, not at all repulsive.

Urine

Around the year 1000 one of the most famous doctors – and artists, and composers – in Europe was Notker, a monk of St Gall in Switzerland (d. 1022). Stories circulated of his knowledge of medical aphorisms, his learning in medicines and antidotes, and in 'Hippocratic prognostications'.[39] There was no perceived conflict between monastic and medical callings. The duke of Bavaria, presumably having decided to consult him, first tried to catch him out. As a test, he sent him some urine, not his own but that of a servant girl. On examining the specimen Notker proclaimed a miracle. In thirty days the duke would give birth to a son. And the girl did indeed give birth. As with the vulture, no explanation is offered in the monastic history (by his younger contemporary Ekkehard) that reports on Notker's skill. Notker was 'instructus', but that is all we are told here.

The first aspect of the story to register is its witty, literary quality. Notker's extraordinary, quasi-divinatory talent is being shown off.[40] Most prognosticating, like the canine variety in our opening example, was an attempt to answer the stark question of whether an illness was terminal. Predicting birth rather than death was presumably held to require quite unusual sensitivity. It would be nice to think that the great Galen, the Holmes-like diagnostician depicted in his autobiographical treatise *On prognosis*,[41] would have recognized in Notker a kindred artist, though worlds separate them, and though Galen was a virtuoso of pulse, not urine.[42] Secondly, the story helps create the impression that the post-Carolingian world was rather bereft of trustworthy healers, for St Gall was some 150 miles distant from the Bavarian court. Yet, then as now, the elite will travel, or send a specimen, any distance to secure the very best in treatment, ignoring local but, as they see them, inferior alternatives.

Notker apart, moreover, St Gall was still quite notable as a medical centre. It was hard to supply a context for our vulture medicine, or the opening vignette involving a dog. In contrast, St Gall can be given a quite 'thick' medical description. So I want to use that example to bring out a number of aspects of the period and area in which Notker shone. His house became the home of the St Gall plan, a famous ninth-century blueprint for the ideal monastery, including a sizeable infirmary and herb garden.[43] It was also the home of what specialists now reckon an important manuscript of the sixth-century monastic Rule of St Benedict, in which the abbot's pastoral role is likened to that of 'a wise physician', some testimony to the esteem in which the best doctors were held.[44] The ninth-century library catalogue of St Gall lists 264 codices, six of them medical in content, and two more were added later.[45] Manuscripts survive that can be associated with the library or scriptorium and that include prognostic material and uroscopy as well as a basic exposition of the theory of the humours.[46] Finally, the contents of some manuscripts brought to St Gall from Italy attest the vigour of trade with the eastern Mediterranean in the Carolingian period, and the arrival, in western Europe, of exotic culinary/medicinal ingredients such as pepper – well before European medicine is generally supposed to have been invigorated by Islamic remedies.[47] One manuscript was also originally folded for greater portability before being brought north across the Alps and later bound in with another collection to form a single codex. That folding could suggest practicality, either in the field for collecting plants or at the bedside.[48] So also could the small size of another St Gall manuscript, a ninth-century collection of texts including chunks of Oribasius and genuine excerpts from Galen.[49]

New drugs, herb gardens, humours, uroscopy, Hippocrates, Galen: it all seems very sane and rational. Here is a centre of educated yet practical, Greek-inspired healing, which we can, if only through the highly coloured vignette of Notker, witness in action. Not all monasteries will have been anything like as 'medicalized' in our period, outside the 'super league' of large and wealthy houses.[50] Still, even on its own St Gall does seem to challenge the stereotypes of the early Middle Ages.

And yet, once again, there is a more perplexing side to the evidence. First, one of the codices that perhaps came to St Gall from Italy included a version of our vulture text, in a miscellany that also embraces writings ascribed, mistakenly, to Hippocrates and Galen (among them 'Galen' on urine), material on prognostic technique, and the *herbarium* of 'Apuleius'.[51] Thus, both at the level of the whole culture of this monastery and again at that of a single codex, we find arresting juxtapositions.

The same codex that includes all this has in addition a version of the introduction to humoral medicine just mentioned. This is a variable cluster of very short items. In some manuscripts it is grandly entitled 'The Wisdom [*Sapientia*] of the Art of Medicine', but here is given, Pauline-style, as

'The First Epistle of Hippocrates'.[52] We should not be surprised to find a modicum of humoral aetiology here in Latin texts, just as we do in their Old English counterparts.[53] The start of the collection, moreover, reassures.[54] The four humours are immediately placed in cosmological context: four winds, four seasons, four corners of heaven. Yet later on we are also given the four parts of the body and the four angles at which the head can be placed (with a fifth as the normal upright position). And the humours are not quite the classical ones: they are assigned to specific places within the body. 'Yellow bile resides in the right-hand part of the body under the liver, black bile in the left, under the spleen.' This is all somewhat more specific than the main detectible source for this odd treatise, a medical epistle ascribed to the fourth-century African physician Vindicianus.[55]

In a final part of the collection, present in only two manuscripts, a 'question-and-answer session' explains a number of conditions and ailments in one sentence each. Here the humours are in contrast very loosely defined: 'from which humour does frenzy arise? From too much wine . . .', which is not strictly an answer to the question. Far more detail is given on the *numbers* of cures available for each body part or illness, rather than on what those cures are. And in a sentence on anatomy we are told that women have two fewer bones than men but, in very garbled Latin, that eunuchs only one fewer (the difference was probably thought to be in the teeth).[56] Should we reckon this strange humoral vocabulary and this zeal for enumeration to be part of a grounding in 'natural philosophy', or of a rhetorical training in how to impress patients at the bedside?[57]

Writing like this resists all attempts at categorizing. So, in a different but equally frustrating way, does the final set of material from St Gall that I want to look at.

Womb conjuring

'That a woman may conceive. Item, that you may bring about an abortion.' That is the sort of heading that we find in a group of medical receipts in a ninth-century manuscript quite possibly copied in the St Gall scriptorium.[58] In another manuscript, which may have been assembled at St Gall (even if one or both of its constituent parts were produced elsewhere), we find two contrasting kinds of gynaecological material.[59] The larger (almost 150 pages) occupies most of the second part of the codex.[60] It is a version of a medical digest also preserved elsewhere. In the St Gall copy, uniquely, it is given the imposing if undiscriminating title, 'Acute and Chronic Diseases of [i.e. according to] Hippocrates, Galen and Soranus'. It ends with some detailed chapters on women's health, especially suffocation of the womb, and adds that 'in bringing on menstruation it is very useful for a woman to go riding [*caballizare*]'. A few folios earlier, though originally in a separate volume, perhaps again filling up blank pages right at the end, we find a different approach to the wandering, and thus suffocating, womb: a formula of exorcism:[61]

> I conjure you, womb, by our Lord Jesus Christ, who walked on the water with dry feet, . . . resuscitated the dead, . . . by whose wounds we are cured, . . . by him I conjure you not to harm the maidservant of God . . . not to hold on to her head, neck, throat, chest, ears, teeth, eyes, nostrils, shoulders, arms, hands, heart, stomach, liver, spleen, kidneys, back, sides, joints, navel, viscera, bladder, thighs, shins, ankles, feet, or toes, but to remain quietly in the place which God delegated to you, so that this handmaiden of God, . . . may be cured.

No surviving ancient medical writer thought that the womb wandered as far as the strikingly full list of body parts would suggest.[62] But, as with the vulture letter and Dioscorides, no one involved in creating the single codex still in St Gall thought the conjuration unfit to consort with a treatise travelling under the names of the great triumvirate of ancient learned medicine, Hippocrates, Galen, and Soranus. That still leaves the bigger question: what did monks have to do with gynaecology, and even with abortion?[63] This is not a question to address only to the St Gall evidence. A number of other codices must derive from a similar milieu.[64] Discarding the notion of collective monastic lewdness, which the rather public nature of the evidence – large and expensive codices, library catalogues – will hardly sustain,[65] we are left with five possibilities. First, the material was copied alongside other types of medicine because its sources were just as ancient. It was an act of preservation, although not an unthinking one. Second, there is no reason for surprise: the literature on women's bodies had almost always been and would remain, indeed in increasing measure, a male matter – for husbands, fathers, physicians.[66] There was no sudden monastic takeover. There had been some literate midwives in antiquity but we hear nothing of any early medieval descendants of them. Women assisted at births using orally transmitted and practically acquired techniques, in almost total separation from the written tradition. Third, some of the scriptoria that copied texts on gynaecology, as on medicine generally, could have belonged to religious houses of women.[67] The role of nunneries in Carolingian 'scriptomania' is likely to have been greater than the direct evidence of codices suggests. We are not necessarily looking at a strictly male intellectual domain. Fourth, what now looks to us like medicine was seen by monastic copyists and librarians of either sex as natural history (equivalent to what would later be called natural philosophy), not least because of the unquestionable importance of its underlying subject matter, the generation of life. On the other hand, fifth, some of the brief items of information at least read as if they were intended as practical advice: 'if the woman's milk dries up, celandine is to be drunk with wine. That is beneficial.'[68]

What woman? Early medieval monasteries in the West were not like Mount Athos. They witnessed the comings and goings of royal and aristocratic patronesses; of the mothers, sisters, daughters, and former wives of monks; of labourers on the monastery's estates. Perhaps it was with patronesses in mind that the recommendation about riding seemed worth recording. Perhaps those to benefit from drinking celandine included servant girls such as the one whose urine Notker so impressively 'read'.

There is something in all these possibilities. Overall, we can perhaps conclude that there was nothing especially monastic about what has often been called monks' medicine. It is simply that it comes to us mostly from monastic manuscripts. Moreover, if we were going to find traces of the way in which this medicine was shaped by Christian ethics, the domain of gynaecology is surely among those where we would have found them. But we do not. The 'problem' of monastic gynaecology is ours, not the monks'.

The black dog

To round off the collection of examples, we should return to the ones with which we began: those two forms of 'cynomancy'. What is going on in them? Again, we may want to ask: are they in any sense medicine? No treatment seems to be in prospect, let alone a cure. Unlike the challenge to Notker, the question is simply whether the patient will live. Why can dogs and their ticks be used in the ways described? As with the vulture, no explanation is given. The general form of these, like other techniques recorded in the manuscripts, is 'for this, do that (and don't ask questions)'. We might want to gloss the second canine technique as an example of disease transference, from the sick person to the dog in the ingested lard. That sort of magic (as it is perhaps too easily labelled) is common enough in the medicine of this period, indeed of almost all periods.[69] In trying to establish a rationale, it is tempting also to resort to the label 'folklore' and to search the encyclopedias and motif-indexes. Doing so seems to help with the first technique mentioned. The association of black dogs with death is common enough in 'folk' traditions – as in literature, e.g. the hound of the Baskervilles.[70] In turning towards the dog's tick, held in the visitor's inauspicious left hand, the sick man turns towards death: *non euadit*. But leaving it at that is really an admission of defeat because folklore is a catch-all for what cannot otherwise be explained historically. Attempts to rationalize its products must of necessity rely on notions of symbolism that are far too generalised to elucidate any particular historical context. Even at its best, folklore reveals traditions but tells us little about meanings, whether those of the Middle Ages or of the nineteenth century, when so much of the lore was first recorded.

Our 'cynomancer' and copyist probably did have some sense that these techniques were part of a tradition. But it did not derive from 'popular' or 'folk' practice. Consider the following examples of disease transference. For a cough, spit into the mouth of a tree-climbing frog and release it. For spleen complaints, apply a live fish and then return it to the sea. And, closer to our dog procedures, for pain in any of the body's major organs, apply a sucking puppy to the affected part; the puppy must be killed and if subjected to an autopsy its organs, washed with wine, will reveal through their diseased aspect the exact source of the human patient's pain.[71] There is hardly an apparent 'superstition' for which some source or analogue cannot be found in the voluminous information assembled by the Elder Pliny (d. 79 CE) in his *Natural History* (*Historia naturalis*). A *historia* is an enquiry – with, often, a chronological dimension – into what is notable or unusual. Vulture medicine is both of those. So it should be no surprise that Pliny offers some sixteen vulture remedies and 'magical' precautions, several of which find their way, however indirectly, into that Carolingian epistle.[72]

We could note here also, for comparison, another example that again resists our desire to separate flora and fauna as sources of medicine. A strange collection of remedies survives in at least two manuscripts of our period, where it keeps company with herbals of 'Apuleius' and 'Dioscorides'. It ranges across the therapeutic (not just prognostic) virtues of human urine, of women's hair and milk, and even, despite the ancient tradition warning of its dangerous effects, of menstrual blood. A little of the strangeness is removed when the text emerges as a probably late antique reworking of consecutive sections of Pliny's books 28–30.[73]

It is Pliny who, by now predictably, supplies a clue to the first of our two canine puzzles, involving the dog's tick:

> The Magi say that the gall of a black male dog . . . acts as a talisman protecting a house from evil medicines entirely. It is the same if the inner walls are sprinkled with the dog's blood or his genital organ is buried under the threshold of the front door. People would wonder less at this if they knew how highly the Magi extol that very loathsome animal the tick . . . a tick from the left ear of a dog, worn as an amulet, relieves all pains. The Magi also consider the tick an augury of life or death, for if the patient responds when he who has brought in with him a tick, standing at his feet, enquires about the illness, there is sure hope of recovery; if no reply is made the patient will die. The Magi add that the tick must be taken from the left ear of a dog that is black all over.[74]

Pliny is good at both having and eating his cake. Earlier on in his work he has more than once denounced the fraudulent *vanitates* of the Magi.[75] Yet he continues to report their prescriptions and to lend them credibility by the rhetorical device of playing off what he sees as their most extravagant claims against relatively plausible ones. Note that all this ironic detachment has disappeared from our early medieval version of the tick oracle. So has its purported source in Persian magic, the other uses of black-dog parts and fluids, and the importance of taking the tick from the dog's left ear (although the participant's left hand must be used to introduce the insect into the sick-room). Above all, at some point between the Roman and the Carolingian empires, the outcomes have been reversed. In c.800, turning towards the tick signifies the inevitable. Yet in Pliny, as we might have intuited – even without the benefit of Persian wisdom – the responsive patient is the one who will survive. He shows that he has enough life in him to answer an enquiry about his state of health, and that is at least promising. Our scribe – or his exemplar, or whoever was directing his work – was not deliberately bowdlerizing. To judge by the paucity of surviving manuscripts, he is unlikely to have been working from anything like an extensive, let alone a complete, copy of the *Natural History*, or even of a full text of its medical sections. For the most part, Pliny's medical 'enquiries' travelled from antiquity into the early Middle Ages in Europe in highly selective digests from the medical books that were assembled in late antiquity – digests in which this authorship was by no means necessarily preserved and into which extraneous material was freely interpolated.[76]

Danger of death

The question of categories obtrudes once more. Is 'cynomancy' medicine? We are being offered means of prognosis, and medical historians, many of them beneficiaries of modern biomedicine with its interventionist bias, may find it hard to recapture the extent to which pre-modern (certainly ancient and medieval) doctors said much more than they did and concentrated on predicting the course of the illness.[77] Prognosis and diagnosis were inextricable, as the example of Notker has already begun to show. The former was impossible without some attempt at the latter, and prognosis often followed diagnosis to the exclusion of treatment. To judge very crudely by the contents of surviving medical manuscripts of the early Middle Ages, prognosis was at least as important as therapy and dietetics.[78] The rationale for its prominence had been made clear centuries before in the opening lines of the Hippocratic text *Prognosis*.[79] Successful prognosis fills in the gaps in the patient's own account and increases the doctor's reputation (compare Galen's self-advertisement in his *On Prognosis*). Foretelling the course of the disease makes curing it easier. Alternatively, it absolves the doctor from blame should the condition be pronounced incurable. That sounds balanced, but the rest of *Prognosis* is often about signs of death, starting with those on the face, and such was the emphasis carried forward into the early Middle Ages.

Again, as with Pliny, the transmission is partial and indirect.[80] The Hippocratic text was translated into Latin more than once in the fifth or sixth centuries CE, and it was probably available at some centres of textual production in the time when our 'canine' scribe was active. Yet far more widely disseminated, in un-classical Latin, were various much shorter pieces of writing (hardly 'works'). These circulated under the names of Hippocrates, Galen, or Hippocrates's contemporary, Democritus. Distant refractions of chapter 2 of the Hippocratic treatise, many of them described the facial *signa mortifera*, literally the death-bearing signs, as if the signs themselves were active: small eyes, sunken cheeks, dryness of the face, sharpening of the nose, distortion of the earlobes, insomnia, diarrhoea, and vomiting. Among these texts was the so-called *capsula eburnea* or 'ivory casket'. This was a piece of advice about the (mostly dermatological) signs of death. The casket was the container in which Hippocrates (or in some traditions Democritus) had the text buried with him in his tomb. There, 'Caesar' would later discover it and pass it to his personal physician.

Such forms of prognostication can be adjudged medical because they depend on the interpretation of the patient's body. But other, rather different techniques circulated in the Carolingian world. Some, called *lunaria*, involved crisply (i.e. entirely without explanation) predicting the outcome of the disease according to the day of the thirty-day lunar cycle on which the patient fell sick: 'who falls ill on day 2 will quickly recover', and so forth.[81] Others required converting the sufferer's name into a numerical value (onomancy), a technique that can be traced back to Babylonia.[82]

The available forms of prognosis thus spanned what we might nowadays categorize as clinical observation, astrology, and divination. Our black dog's ticks are (so far as I know) found nowhere else among surviving early medieval codices. Yet they were hardly an irrational aberration from the medical mainstream. Nor was their deployment for prognosis a 'folk' invention. (Far earlier than Pliny, we find another, not too dissimilar, piece of Babylonian prognostics, from the mid-eleventh century BCE: if the learned 'exorcist' sees a multi-coloured pig on his way to visit the sick person, the patient is suffering from dropsy and to go near him is dangerous.)[83] In the early Middle Ages, the different texts and techniques were in no way seen as mutually exclusive. One manuscript might contain prognostics attributed (mistakenly) to Democritus, Hippocrates and Galen. Another might juxtapose the genuine Hippocratic *Prognosis* and the fancifully 'packaged' *capsula eburnea*.[84] The manuscript containing our dog material includes a *lunare*, but its collection of prognostic techniques also follows up the one requiring lard with some characterizations of the moribund person's face – such as sunken eyes and sharpened nose – that are reminiscent of their Hippocratic original.[85]

The triumph of the miscellany

Seen as a whole, that same 'canine' manuscript has more to tell us.[86] It gives a wider intellectual context for its various prognostic recommendations. For these are only a few parts of a quite extensive miscellany. The codex is quite small in dimension (232 × 133 mm), which suggests portability and practicality rather than the library and only occasional reference. Yet its 126 folios contain over 25 different pieces. One purports to represent the basic teachings of Hippocrates, Galen, and Soranus. It thus, like that St Gall tract mentioned earlier, yokes together two quite different schools of ancient medical thinking, the Galenic 'rationalist' and the 'Methodist', although this part of the collection soon turns into a series of remedies with no particular theoretical slant.[87] There is a dietetic calendar that tells the reader what to eat and drink month by month. There is the spurious third book of the introductory text on therapeutics attributed to Galen; an extract from Isidore of Seville's *Etymologies* on the ages of man; some lines on medicinal weights and measures; some gynaecological information of a kind which we have already encountered; material in letter form on such matters as blood-letting; the short epistle of Vindicianus which was the partial source for that 'Wisdom of the Art of the Medicine' described above; an equally short, supposed dialogue between Plato and Aristotle on the soul; and much else besides. And, at the head of all this, we find an account of the lives and deaths, a *passio*, of the physician-saints Cosmas and Damian, with a message of comfort that has relatively little to do with secular healing. 'To whoever is sick and has this passion read over him, the Lord will show pity.'[88]

That may be some clue to the milieu in which the whole collection took shape: the monastic infirmary. There, divine and saintly medicine complemented prescriptions and blood-letting. And, in serious cases, nothing was of greater clinical importance than predicting the hour of death. Forewarned of a brother's imminent demise, the rest of the community could gather round in prayerful support, and could conduct, without hurry, the rites for the dying that were being elaborated in the eighth and ninth centuries, exactly the period during which our manuscript was put together.[89]

A general view of early medieval medicine

After looking at an array of particular examples, there must be some attempt to generalize. I return to the three headings with which I started: concepts, texts, sociology. On the conceptual front, the point to make is simple. We have to blur boundaries, even abandon categories. Magic, religion, science; theological, scientific, practical; diagnosis and prognosis; monastic and 'lay'; even plants and animals – these are none of them helpful distinctions to impose on our evidence. Again and again we have seen them confounded.

As for the texts: the miscellany, not the full-scale treatise, is the characteristic product – a mixture of letters, lists, and excerpts. Very little attention is given to anatomy and aetiology. The philosophical underpinnings of medicine have been dropped. Humoral theory, though quite often mentioned, is only briefly set out and takes unexpected forms. Pharmacy, *materia medica*, dietetics, and diagnosis/prognosis predominated. There is very little surgery apart from blood-letting. By classical standards the Latin can be very poor. These manuscripts are probably the work of scribes who know little medicine and less Greek, and who are thus baffled by transliterated technical terms. With each generation of copying, the chances of error multiply exponentially.[90]

Even the manuscripts that to medical historians most resemble the systematic treatise are still essentially anthologies on the standard model. The so-called 'Lorsch Book of Medicines', put together in the early ninth century at that recently founded abbey, begins with a celebrated 'defence of medicine'.[91] It sets out at some length (seven folios) to demonstrate the compatibility of Christianity and healing, and the place of medicine, as a subdivision of *physica*, within the hierarchy of the 'sciences'. It is nonetheless an often poorly written patchwork of biblical and patristic quotations. And in keeping with that, after its lofty opening it still turns to the miscellaneous types of writing that we have seen above in the manuscript of those canine oracles: a *lunare*, month-by-month dietetics, weights and measures, and remedy lists.

The Lorsch 'defence' and the relative orderliness of its collection are, moreover, both highly unusual. More representative is 'The Wisdom of the Art of Medicine'. Overall, it is easy to see why excerpting, compressing, and reworking into miscellanies seemed necessary. As papyrus ceased to be available north of the Alps around 700, and parchment became the only writing medium, so the cost of copying, measured now in animal skins and the labour of their preparation, may well have increased.[92] Only what was perceived to be really worth preserving justified the expense of the medium and the time in copying. Medical philosophy seldom cleared that hurdle. Nor were there any institutions of sufficient prestige and influence to impose common form on what did make it through the scriptorium. There was no Carolingian Renaissance in medicine at all comparable to those that, for example, tried to reformed and standardize liturgy or impose on monasteries the Benedictine Rule.[93] The interest shown in medicine at the centre of the Carolingian world comes from learned 'amateurs', not reforming practitioners implementing some imperial policy.[94] No medical work is known to have found a place in Charlemagne's library, the beacon of the Renaissance. And his important early commissioning of a copy of Quintus Serenus's *Liber medicinalis* (which incidentally contains seven vulture formulae) probably owed more to the interest of its verse than to its medical content.[95]

Far from being standardized, the 160–200 surviving medical manuscripts of the Carolingian world are each unique.[96] The Carolingian achievement was to increase the volume, and thus diversity, of manuscript production and render earlier copies redundant (so that many of them are no longer extant). No one of the numerous available anthologies – the majority of them copied and assembled in the ninth century – exactly reproduces another. Some texts were copied in clusters, but again often with some variations in content and arrangement and, as we have seen several times now, in ascribed authorship. As Faith Wallis has powerfully shown, that makes them very hard to edit, except by imposing on them alien notions of authorial 'original' and later 'recension'.[97] This is a textual world in which each manuscript is the best, because sole, witness to its particular content, and the only appropriate kind of 'editing' may thus be transcription. To generalize about the manuscripts is therefore very hard. There are no clear evolutions in the relative popularity of one component text over another (although the surviving manuscripts may be a very oblique guide to the range of what once existed). Perhaps, as we have already noted, some new *materia medica* was introduced, as the Carolingian world opened itself up to the comparative riches of the eastern Mediterranean. Dietary advice came to be organized by month rather than by season.[98] Beyond that, it cannot be said that any one kind of philosophy or approach came to dominate. There were no such philosophies, theory having largely been bled out of the material.

'Sociology' is no easier a heading than 'texts'. The manuscripts can quite often be associated with particular centres of production, and in a very few cases with particular patrons.[99] Yet of no Carolingian codex can we say specifically why it was copied or for what purpose or readership. The books that survive come almost entirely from the institutions best able to preserve them: monasteries and, in the later part of the period, cathedral schools. We should not infer from that, however, that this is all monkish or 'nunnish' medicine. Some of the codices, we have already noted, may have originated in female scriptoria. Second, some may have been intended for 'lay' (non-monastic and non-clerical) households or at least have been copied in whole or part from lay compilations.[100] Our canine prognoses that require tossing lard to an unknown dog or bringing a dog's tick into the sickroom do not immediately evoke the monastic infirmary, even though the preoccupation in the texts with 'death-bearing signs' on the face might be thought essentially monastic.

Perhaps the intended audience of such information was much wider. Priests needed to have some knowledge of the Christian calendar, not only for the date of Easter but for all other feasts. And the *computus* manuscripts that diffused such information often came encrusted with medical and dietetic information.[101] A manual produced by the abbey of Lorsch *c*.900, perhaps for parish priests being sent out onto some of its estates newly carved from the forest, includes, alongside pastoral and computistic material, the 'Egyptian days', on which one should not be bled or given any medicine, and a *lunare*.[102] It also has one of those tables for predicting the outcome of illness from the numerical equivalent of the letters in the patient's name, and lists preventive regimes for each month of the year. The emphasis is on prognosis, so as to offer appropriate ritual and pastoral support to the terminally ill. And we should not imagine that priests routinely acted as unofficial community doctors.[103] Nonetheless, the only lightly Christianized rural world in which some parish priests were moving in the early tenth century could still have required them to compete for attention with local 'magicians' or 'witch-doctors' (probably more numerous than priests were).[104]

There was, then, a wider therapeutic world beyond the monastic precinct. The problem for us is that we can say so little about it, and its nature and scale can be matters for no more than conjecture.[105] We know of only a small number of identifiable individual doctors. Hagiography provides our best evidence for the 'everyday life' of the period, and thus for healing practices, but does not take us beyond didactic vignettes.[106] We do not have the inscriptions and papyri that elucidate some of the lower reaches of the medical 'profession' in the classical world, or the archives that reveal a number of their later medieval successors. Legal texts, charters, penitentials, and historical narratives offer only glimpses. Sorcerers and other 'magical' healers are yet more obscure. Overall, indeed, the relative numerical importance that we can attribute to each type of healer is in inverse proportion to the volume of evidence available. Saints, so well documented, can have catered, at their shrines, for only a minority of the sick. At the other end of the spectrum, the 'informal' sector of self-help or reliance on family and neighbours for basic nursing was presumably the largest. Yet this sector is seldom documented, although texts survive that are explicitly for the self-medication of those without access to doctors.[107]

The special case of healing saints apart, how exactly any of these various healers behaved – monks, priests, lay doctors, magicians, domestic therapists – is lost to us. All we can say with reasonable confidence is that little of it took place in schools.[108] Some gentlemen amateurs among the episcopacy or at the Carolingian court will have derived most of their medical knowledge from reading. But, overall, taking in practitioners of all kinds, most skills were transmitted orally and through clinical experience. The role of texts was limited and oblique, even in the most literate setting that the age could boast, the monastery. The texts we have been looking at nearly all required completion by the reader, as an active, not passive user.[109] They furnished reminders of how to proceed, aspects of knowledge and practice already in part assimilated orally. That, of course, imposes very severe limits on how much these texts can now tell us about the healer's formation or clinical behaviour.

For all these reasons, medical historians have found it exceedingly hard to develop any sort of overall narrative picture of early medieval medicine. The only narrative available seems to be one of lack, with a scarcely disguised nostalgia for a classical past or nostalgia for a future of which the early Middle Ages could have no inkling: a future of university medicine as the gold standard of medical education and practice. In this narrative, the medicine we have been looking at is not Greek; it is not ancient; and it is not medieval, because it lacks stable texts and syllabuses, philosophical underpinning, a body of students, and a clear succession of masters within the appropriate institutional setting.[110]

Period pieces?

In questioning such negativity, it is worth remarking first that in few other areas of scholarship concerning the early Middle Ages is there so much pessimism or nostalgia. The historiographies of, for example, law or agriculture do not seem to be comparably afflicted by the great difficulty of reconstructing practice on the basis of the recalcitrant surviving texts. Indeed, the pendulum has swung away from a Gibbonian narrative of 'decline and fall', in favour of an emphasis on the creative novelty of late antiquity and the early Middle Ages – so much so that Bryan Ward-Perkins has reasserted the older view (to which many medical historians, not only Baader, still implicitly adhere) that 'the fall of Rome' entailed 'the end of civilisation'.[111]

A second point to make in our period's favour is that, put bluntly, early medieval medicine is, in fact, ancient medicine. That is, it derives for the most part from ancient sources. But these sources do not usually belong to the Hippocratic-Galenic tradition. Translations of Hippocrates and Galen from Greek into Latin were very limited by comparison with the extent of their originals.[112] The usual sources are themselves either older Roman writers such as Pliny or late antique epitomizers of the fourth to fifth centuries. The early medieval textual tradition of the excerpt and the anthology is really the ancient tradition that goes back to Pliny. It is as if, in the early Middle Ages, the tide of Greek learning receded to expose a half-forgotten but still recognizable shore.

Of course, with the exception of northern Italy (and there only until c.700) the early Middle Ages in the West lacked the urban institutions that could sustain secular schooling, in medicine as in other subjects. But the West had always been the poorer, less urbanized half of the Roman world, and in antiquity its medical practitioners had been poor and obscure by comparison with those of the East.[113] Medical historians sometimes write as if all ancient doctors were like Galen or were educated in Alexandria. But most healers were self-taught or informally apprenticed, knew little about medical philosophy, and cared less. The early medieval tradition of oral training in medicine is also hardly different from the ancient one. 'Galen's wealthy friends could arrange to have copies made of his discourses . . . But *most doctors* [in the Roman empire] *may have owned at best a few brief handbooks or digests of earlier doctrines to supplement what they had learned by word of mouth or simply by watching others . . .*'[114] The words in italics aptly describe the early Middle Ages too.

Differences between the two periods remain, but they should not be exaggerated. The same applies to the presumed synchronic contrast between East and West in the early Middle Ages. Let us not overestimate Byzantine medicine. It continued to be composed and copied in learned Greek tinged with philosophy – up to a point. Its great encyclopedias and compendia are more even in coverage and systematic in organization than anything being produced in the contemporary West.[115] Yet it too had its 'deplorable' aspects. Some of Galen's more theoretical writings survive only in translation into Syriac and Arabic, and that is presumably because they were no longer thought worth copying in Greek. At the other end of the spectrum of sophistication, the medical writings associated with hospitals or with 'small-town' private practice are hardly lacking in confusion and obscurity, and in their limited aetiology bear comparison with western remedy lists.[116]

Even the relevance here of the sophisticated Galenism of medicine newly translated into Arabic in the 'land of Islam' should not be overestimated. As in Byzantium so in medieval Islam, theory and practice could diverge. What we find in elegant philosophical treatises was not necessarily what the patient experienced at the 'sharp end'.[117]

Brave new world?

In the eyes of its critics, the major contrast with early medieval western medicine is that of the later Middle Ages in Europe, between medicine without schools and post-Salernitan, university medicine, with its regular syllabi and its philosophical underpinning in new translations from the Arabic.[118] The supposed fault of early medieval texts is not just that they stem from a culture that has lost its knowledge of Greek. They are measured against a yardstick provided partly by medical writings from antiquity, but still more by post-Salernitan medicine.

What exactly is the contrast between pre- and post-Salernitan medicine supposed to have been? Is it that the first did not work but the second did? Let us admit at once that early medieval medicine did not work. It is, to borrow David Wootton's title, 'bad medicine', usually no more effective than a placebo, sometimes worse.[119] To say that is to deny the claims made by the 'biological realists' (as they might be labelled) for whom early medieval remedies were copied and recopied because they were proven by trial and error to be anti-microbially efficacious, for reasons that modern pharmacology and chemistry can supply although they were of course unavailable at the time. Laboratory tests on Od English remedies fail to confirm this optimism.[120] Rather than looking for biomedical efficacy we should think, as anthropologists do, in terms of therapeutic success.[121] And on that score there is no strong reason to deny the early Middle Ages its successes, even if achieved with the aid of a dog's tick or a headless vulture.

What changes with Salerno? The medicine of the later Middle Ages was also bad medicine. It too would fail the test of biological efficacy. What has been held to make the difference is the 'discourse' or 'rhetoric' of the 'rational and learned doctor', the ideal type offered us by Roger French, the doctor who has his Aristotle as well as his Galen with which to impress his clients.[122] This new medicine took a long time to establish itself, far longer than standard accounts of the contrast between pre- and post-Salerno would suggest. At first the invigorating translations from the Arabic appeared in manuscript anthologies alongside older material, as if there were no essential difference between them.[123] And the enormous increase in the production of medical books during the 'long' twelfth century diffused Salernitan-type medicine to only quite specific parts of Europe, notably England and northern France.[124]

Undeniably, during the thirteenth century and after, there was a growing demand for medical learning of the kind to be derived from the new translations. And it had a wide social reach.[125] In 1304, a 'wise woman' living near Barcelona was arraigned by her bishop for irregular medical practice. Asked if she knew anything of the art of medicine, 'she said no, except that she could diagnose a patient's illness from his urine'. Asked how she could do this, she replied that 'citrine urine indicates a continued fever, *vermeyla* a tercian fever, *rubia* the first stages of a quartan fever . . . and that white spumous urine indicates an aposteme'. She added that she had learned this from a foreign doctor. There is one of the furthest ripples created by the impact of a bookish, scholastic medicine that had first gained acceptance in courts and universities. This woman's uroscopy was hardly different from that of her monarch's physicians, who appraised the royal water each morning; and it derived ultimately from a substantial technical literature that included a treatise ascribed to the great Arnau de Vilanova. If her bravura terminology was meant to impress clients, then she was also, however unwittingly, endorsing Arnau's advice to doctors unable to interpret a urine specimen: diagnose obstruction of the liver and use the word *opilatio*, 'because they do not understand what it means'.

But was such pretentious mystification inevitably superior to the different (and for us irrecoverable) rhetoric of the early medieval physician – whether the quasi-divinatory Notker or the humbler rural practitioner? For many of the wealthier high medieval patients, patrons of university masters and recipients of their *consilia* (letters of advice), it clearly was. And yet very little of early medieval medicine was judged so deficient that it was entirely superseded by all the philosophically orientated material. To recall an early example: the therapeutics of menstrual blood seems to have had only a limited future after the early Middle Ages.[126] But in most cases the manuscripts of the Carolingian era that we have been looking at were not the end of codicological trail. Similar texts reappear in thirteenth- to fourteenth-century compilations and then, in some cases, in Renaissance editions as part of the humanist recovery of antiquity (in this case late antiquity). Vulture medicine, for instance, continues to circulate throughout the Middle Ages, not least in the vernacular. One thirteenth-century German text affords us the crucial information that we must catch our vulture unawares. Forewarned, it may, pre-emptively, swallow its own brain.[127]

The major point is this. Early medieval medicine is not only (late) antique medicine. It is also medieval medicine.[128] Especially in the wake of the Black

Death and the renewal of interest in astrological and other forms of 'occult' medicine, and as medical writings in the European vernaculars multiplied, many of the varied techniques that we have found in early medieval manuscripts recur.[129] A Latin version (taken from the Arabic) of the genuine Hippocratic *Prognosis* may have been part of the *Articella*, the standard introductory 'textbook' in the universities. But other forms of prognostication were not forgotten:

> Take the name of the patient, the name of the messenger sent to summon the physician, and the name of the day upon which the messenger came to you; join [the numerical values of] all their letters together, and if an even number result the patient will not escape.[130]

The priest-physician and medical encyclopedist John Mirfield reported this technique with some sceptical detachment, but he reported it none the less.[131] He died in 1407, a learned man though not university educated, long associated with St Bartholomew's Hospital, London. We no longer think that only good things come from universities or that good things, intellectually speaking, come only from universities. Anyone tempted to set medieval university medical education on a pedestal should read Cornelius O'Boyle's reconstruction of the mindless formalism of introductory lectures on the *Articella* in fourteenth-century Paris.[132]

In our post-postmodern age, the open-ended, fragmented, conceptually labile, intertextual aspects of early medieval medical writing ought to appeal rather than repel.[133] Early medieval medicine deconstructs itself before our eyes as we turn the manuscript pages. Early medieval medicine is just premodern medicine in one of its many possible guises. We should get used to it.

Acknowledgements

Research for this paper was generously supported by the Wellcome Trust, grant reference numbers 044962, 082296. For advice and references I am grateful to Patricia Baker, Eliza Glaze, Monica Green, Peter Murray Jones, Clare Pilsworth, Nicholas Purcell, Faith Wallis, and Linda Voigts. My greatest debt is to Klaus-Dietrich Fischer and Monica Green for their thorough scrutiny of this paper in draft.

Notes

1 Baader 1984, p. 251.
2 Beccaria 1956, pp. 161–166 (no. 34), item 24 (p. 165); Wickersheimer 1966, pp. 100–112, at p. 110 (item 29). Klaus-Dietrich Fischer kindly sent me an unpublished lecture in which he briefly discusses this passage. See also Paxton 1993, p. 646. I hope that the present paper (which in part develops themes in Horden 2000) is accessible to non-specialists. Footnotes have been kept to a minimum,

favouring recent works in which further bibliography may be found. I also omit manuscript call numbers, referring simply to the fundamental catalogues of Wickersheimer and, especially, Beccaria, in which most of the surviving medical manuscripts of the period are described in detail.

3 Van Arsdall 2007, p. 195; Glaze 1999, p. 1.
4 References in Voigts 1979, p. 252; discussion in Van Arsdall 2005.
5 von Ranke trans. e.g. in Iggers and von Moltke 1983, p. 52.
6 E.g. Falileyev and Owen 2005.
7 To judge by Beccaria 1956, which is not complete and starts in the ninth century. Wickersheimer 1966 adds a good few for French libraries alone but has more inclusive terms of reference. See also Contreni 1990, p. 269. For indications of earlier manuscripts see Glaze 1999, pp. 66–68.
8 Again Beccaria 1956, Wickersheimer 1966.
9 Wallis 1995b. For potted introductions to and editions of the medical writings referred to below, see Sabbah et al. 1987, and Fischer 2000 with supplements.
10 I return to these themes throughout, narrowing the focus from a wider sketch of the period in Horden in Noble and Smith 2008.
11 For the call to synthesise see Sigerist 1934, p. 37. MacKinney 1937, the most recent published monograph, is essentially the text of lectures. Glaze 1999 is a masterly thesis, the book of which is eagerly awaited. I am much indebted to it, as also to Wallis 1995b, Fischer 1994, and the older study, Riddle 1974.
12 Meaney 2000, pp. 29–36; Pettit 2001, vol. I, p. xlvii.
13 Cameron 1983a, 1983b.
14 Hall 2007.
15 Pettit 2001, vol. I, pp. xlvi, li–liv. See also Nokes 2004, p. 74, for the emergence, though his study of Bald's *Leechbook*, of 'a portrait of a body of professional leeches'.
16 Voigts 1979.
17 Cameron 1993, pp. 117–158; Riddle 2007; Van Arsdall 2007. For a different approach to the magic see Jolly 1996.
18 Riddle 1974, 2007.
19 See also, in this vein, Glaze 1999, pp. 5–6. Retrospective biochemistry poses as many problems as retrospective diagnosis. Fischer 1986 performs a similar exercise to those I shall undertake with a literally hare-brained remedy, showing its sources in Galen and others.
20 Beccaria 1956, pp. 157–159 (item 4); Wickersheimer 1966, p. 93.
21 Wallis 1995b, p. 112 n. 30, offers some approximate statistics for the contents of the surviving manuscripts; pharmacology is the largest single category.
22 The text is transcribed and translated from this manuscript in MacKinney 1943. Möhler 1990 includes an edition based also on later witnesses.
23 Möhler 1990, p. 180, with discussion pp. 230–238, 'straightens out' the text into a letter from Alexander the Great. But I am interested here in what our scribe wrote, not the presumed original. For the pairing of Alexandria and Babylon-in-Egypt in a ninth-century travel narrative, see McCormick 2001, p. 134.
24 All translations, slightly modified, from MacKinney 1943, pp. 45–46.
25 Jolly 1996, pp. 115–116.
26 Flint 1991; Olsan 2003.
27 I paraphrase Jolly 2002, p. 16.
28 For some context see Eamon 1994, pp. 15–30, although his outlook on the period has much in common with Baader's.
29 Riddle 1985.

30 E.g. Riddle 1984; Stannard 1999; Collins 2000, pp. 32–35, 148–154.
31 Riddle 1981, p. 63.
32 Stadler 1899, p. 193.
33 We await the first modern edition of the Latin Alexander from David Langslow; see meanwhile Langslow 2006.
34 MacKinney 1942a, 1942b.
35 On the difficulties of which see Möhler 1990; also Barb 1950.
36 Beccaria 1956, p. 159 (item 5). For Alexander's magic see e.g. Duffy 1984, pp. 25–26.
37 Riddle 1981; Collins 2000, pp. 154–156.
38 See e.g. von Staden 1992. The classic, to the German translation of which Freud wrote a preface, is Bourke 1891; for vulture dung see p. 235.
39 For what follows, Haefele 1980, pp. 238–240; also Duft 1972.
40 On this aspect of prognosis, and some comments on Notker, see Wallis 2000, pp. 277–278.
41 Nutton 1979.
42 Nutton 2004, pp. 237–238.
43 Most recently discussed by D'Aronco 2007.
44 Probst 1983, pp. 79–81.
45 Glaze 1999, pp. 71 n. 23, 270–271. For wider context, McKitterick 1989, pp. 169–196.
46 Beccaria 1956, pp. 364–383 (nos. 129–134).
47 Voigts 1979, pp. 259–261; McCormick 2001, pp. 711–712.
48 Bischoff 1966, p. 99.
49 Glaze 1999, p. 271 n. 11; Beccaria 1956, p. 386.
50 Glaze 1999, p. 103.
51 Beccaria 1956, p. 379 (item 32).
52 Ibid. p. 380 (item 36).
53 Meaney 1992; Ayoub 1995. Wallis 1995b, pp. 117–124, argues that such naturalistic theory was progressively eliminated on theological grounds. Glaze 1999, with whom I agree, emphasizes practical constraints.
54 For what follows see Wlaschky 1928, pp. 104–106, 108–109, with the comments on his editorial method of Wallis 1995b, p. 111. For a manuscript that Wlaschky did not use, see Glaze 1999, p. 132 n. 45.
55 For some context see Klibansky et al. 1963, pp. 60–66.
56 Fischer 1985. For a helpful summary of contemporary medical views of eunuchs see Ringrose 2003, pp. 51–66.
57 Wallis 1995b, pp. 121–122, relates it to *computus*, to which I return below; Glaze 1999, p. 132 n. 45, disagrees. I am more concerned here with reception than with sources.
58 Beccaria 1956, p. 370 (item 2a).
59 Ibid. p. 381.
60 Ibid. p. 383 (item 8). See also Fischer 2000, p. 240.
61 Beccaria 1956, pp. 382–383 (item 1b), trans. Green 1985, pp. 170–171.
62 For brief general summaries of early medieval Latin gynaecology and its ancient sources, see Cadden 1993, pp. 42–49; Green 2001, pp. 14–17, and for the wandering womb, King 1998, pp. 214–238.
63 Perhaps also contraception, although the arguments of Riddle (e.g. 1997) on this score are controversial.
64 Fischer 2000, pp. 240–242.
65 Glaze 1999, p. 282.
66 Green 2008b, for what follows pp. 34–36 especially. I am also very grateful to Monica Green for discussion of this issue.

67 McKitterick 1992, 1989.
68 Green 1985, p. 169, citing Jörimann 1925, p. 19 = Beccaria 1956, p. 367 (item 26).
69 Though for some critical comments on such imputed 'folk' theories, see Gordon in van der Eijk et al. 1995.
70 Bächtold-Stäubli 1927–42, vol. 4, cols 470–472.
71 Pliny, *Natural History*, e.g. XXX.42 (14), Jones 1963, pp. 304–305, with other examples in French 1994, p. 244.
72 MacKinney 1942a, pp. 1263–1264.
73 See Ferraces Rodríguez 2006. I am again grateful to Monica Green, who alerted me to the charms of this text.
74 Pliny, *Natural History*, XXX.82–3 (24), Jones 1963, pp. 330–332.
75 Pliny, *Natural History*, XXX.1 (1), Jones 1963, pp. 278–279. Beagon 1992, pp. 101–113, 202–239, is a searching discussion of Pliny on magic and medicine.
76 Önnerfors 1963.
77 Demaitre 2003.
78 Wallis 1995b, p. 112 n. 30.
79 Lloyd 1978, p. 170.
80 For what follows see esp. Paxton 1993.
81 Wallis 1995a, p. 116, translation modified.
82 Ibid. pp. 126–127; Wallis 2000, p. 274.
83 Heeßel 2004, p. 102.
84 E.g. Beccaria 1956, pp. 169 (item 23), 171 (31), 365 (9, 10).
85 Paxton 1993, p. 646.
86 For what follows, Beccaria 1956, pp. 161–166; Wickersheimer 1966, pp. 100–112.
87 See Nutton 2004, chs 13, 14, 16.
88 See also Paxton 1993, p. 645, and, for what follows, 631–632.
89 Paxton 1990b.
90 Fischer 1994; Glaze 1999, pp. 122–143.
91 Stoll 1992; Glaze 1999, pp. 80–87, contrasting with Wallis 1995b, p. 124. I am additionally indebted to Klaus-Dietrich Fischer for discussion of this manuscript.
92 McCormick 2001, pp. 704–708.
93 For what follows see Glaze 1999, pp. 69–92 (though with perhaps a more optimistic interpretation than mine); Riché 1976, pp. 404–444; Contreni 1995, esp. p. 747.
94 Contreni 1990.
95 Bullough 1985, p. 280; MacKinney 1942a, p. 1266.
96 Glaze 1999, p. 78; Contreni 1990, p. 269.
97 Wallis 1995b.
98 Groenke 1986.
99 Glaze 1999, e.g. pp. 79, 100.
100 Pilsworth unpublished, on Beccaria 1956, p. 217 (no. 57), as a manuscript for a lay household; compare Bricout 2006.
101 Wallis 1995a.
102 Paxton 1990b.
103 Paxton 1995.
104 Flint 1991, pp. 114–116; Murray 1992.
105 For more detail and bibliography on what follows, see Horden 2008.
106 Flint 1989.
107 Fischer 1986.
108 Baader 1972.
109 Voigts 1979, p. 252; Wallis 2000, pp. 272 (drawing an analogy with connoisseurship), 278; Van Arsdall 2007, pp. 201–202 (offering comparison with modern *curanderos*).

110 Even such masterly and sympathetic students of the period as Wallis and Glaze are not, I believe, immune to this nostalgia for the future.
111 Ward-Perkins 2005.
112 Baader 1984; Fischer 2003.
113 Nutton 1992.
114 Nutton 2004, p. 4, italics added.
115 Nutton 1984, and for what follows Nutton 2004, pp. 5–7.
116 Bennett 2000, 2003; Zipser 2009, kindly shown to me in 'typescript' by the author.
117 Horden 2000, p. 218. Álvarez-Millán 2000; Savage-Smith 2000; Pormann and Savage-Smith 2007, ch. 4.
118 Of which a convenient and authoritative sketch is Siraisi 1990, ch. 3.
119 Wootton 2006.
120 Brennessel, Drout, and Gravel 2006.
121 Hsu 2002, pp. 9–10.
122 French 2003, chs 3 and 4.
123 Glaze 1999, p. 163.
124 Green 2008a, kindly shown me by its author in advance of publication.
125 For what follows see McVaugh 1993, pp. 139–142.
126 Green 2005.
127 Brévart 2008, p. 40 (no. 2). See also Stürmer 1982.
128 Riddle 1974 includes a provocative swipe at scholastic medicine.
129 I am grateful to Linda Voigts for discussion. See also Voigts 2008 and Olsan 2003.
130 Cited from Rawcliffe 1995, p. 100.
131 On Mirfield see Getz 1998, pp. 49–52.
132 O'Boyle 1998.
133 Cooter 2007.

Bibliography

Álvarez-Millán, C. 2000. 'Practice versus Theory: Tenth-Century Case Histories from the Islamic Middle East', *Social History of Medicine* 13: 293–306.

Ayoub, L. 1995. 'Old English *wæta* and the Medical Theory of the Humours', *Journal of English and Germanic Philology* 94: 332–346.

Baader, G. 1972. 'Die Anfänge der medizinischen Ausbildung im Abendland bis 1100', *Settimane di studio del Centro italiano di studi sull'alto medioevo* [Spoleto] 19: 679–718.

Baader, G. 1984. 'Early Medieval Latin Adaptations of Byzantine Medicine in Western Europe', *Dumbarton Oaks Papers* 38: 251–259.

Bächtold-Stäubli, H. (ed.) 1927–42. *Handwörterbuch des deutschen Aberglaubens*. Berlin: de Gruyter.

Barb, A. A. 1950. 'The Vulture Epistle', *Journal of the Warburg and Courtauld Institutes* 13: 318–322.

Beagon, M. 1992. *Roman Nature: The Thought of Pliny the Elder*. Oxford: Clarendon Press.

Beccaria, A. 1956. *I codici di medicina del periodo presalernitano (secoli IX, X e XI)*. Rome: Edizioni di Storia e Letteratura.

Bennett, D. 2000. 'Medical Practice and Manuscripts in Byzantium', *Social History of Medicine* 13: 279–291.

Bennett, D. 2003. 'Xenonika: Medical Texts Associated with *Xenones* in the Late Byzantine Period', PhD thesis, University of London.

Bischoff, B. 1966. 'Über gefaltete Handschriften, vornehmlich hagiographischen Inhalts', in Bischoff, *Mittelalterliche Studien*, vol. 1, 93–100. Stuttgart: Anton Hiersemann.

Bourke, J. G. 1891. *Scatalogic Rites of All Nations. A Dissertation upon the Employment of Excrementitious Remedial Agents . . . in All Parts of the Globe*. Washington, DC: W. H. Lowdermilk.

Brennessel B., Drout, M. D. C., and Gravel, R. 2006. 'A Reassessment of the Efficacy of Anglo-Saxon Medicine', *Anglo-Saxon England* 34: 183–195.

Brévart, F. B. 2008. 'Between Medicine, Magic and Religion: Wonder Drugs in German Medico-Pharmaceutical Treatises of the Thirteenth to Sixteenth Centuries', *Speculum* 83: 1–57.

Bricout, S. 2006. 'Note sur deux laïcs carolingiens et la médecine au IXe siècle', *Latomus* 65: 458–461.

Bullough, D. 1985. '*Aula renovata*: The Carolingian Court Before the Aachen Palace', *Proceedings of the British Academy* 71: 268–301.

Cadden, J. 1993. *Meanings of Sex Difference in the Middle Ages*. Cambridge: Cambridge University Press.

Cameron, M. L. 1983a. 'The Sources of Medical Knowledge in Anglo-Saxon England', *Anglo-Saxon England* 11: 135–155.

Cameron, M. L. 1983b. 'Bald's *Leechbook*: Its Sources and their Use in Its Compilation', *Anglo-Saxon England* 12: 153–182.

Cameron, M. L. 1993. *Anglo-Saxon Medicine*. Cambridge: Cambridge University Press.

Collins, M. 2000. *Medieval Herbals: The Illustrative Traditions*. London and Toronto: British Library and University of Toronto Press.

Contreni, J. J. 1990. 'Masters and Medicine in Northern France during the Reign of Charles the Bald', in M. T. Gibson and J. L. Nelson (eds), *Charles the Bald: Court and Kingdom*, revised edn, 267–282. Aldershot: Ashgate.

Contreni, J. J. 1995. 'The Carolingian Renaissance: Education and Literary Culture', in R. McKitterick (ed.), *The New Cambridge Medieval History*, vol. 2, 709–757. Cambridge: Cambridge University Press.

Cooter, R. 2007. 'After Death/After-'Life': The Social History of Medicine in Post-Postmodernity', *Social History of Medicine* 20: 441–464.

D'Aronco, M. A. 2007. 'The Benedictine Rule and the Care of the Sick: The Plan of St Gall and Anglo-Saxon England', in B. Bowers (ed.), *The Medieval Hospital and Medical Practice*, 235–251. Aldershot: Ashgate.

Demaitre, L. 2003. 'The Art and Science of Prognostication in Early University Medicine', *Bulletin of the History of Medicine* 77: 765–788.

Duffy, J. 1984. 'Byzantine Medicine in the Sixth and Seventh Centuries: Aspects of Teaching and Practice', *Dumbarton Oaks Papers* 38: 21–27.

Duft J., 1972. *Notker der Arzt: Klostermedizin und Mönchsarzt im frühmittelalterlichen St. Gallen*. St Gallen: Fehr'sche Buchhandlung.

Eamon W., 1994. *Science and the Secrets of Nature: Books of Secrets in Medieval and Early Modern Culture*. Princeton, NJ: Princeton University Press.

Falileyev, A., and Owen, M. E., with McKee, H. 2005. *The Leiden Leechbook: A Study of the Earliest Neo-Brittonic Medical Compilation*. Innsbruck: Institut für Sprachen und Literaturen der Universität.

170

Ferraces Rodríguez, A. (ed. and trans.) 2006. 'Antropoterapia de la antigüedad tardía: *Curae quae ex hominibus fiunt*', *Les études classiques* 74: 219–252 (with French trans. of text by C. Petit, 253–259).

Fischer, K.-D. 1985. 'Ein weiteres spätantikes Zeugnis für die Zahnzahl der Eunuchen', *Medizinhistorisches Journal* 20: 261–262.

Fischer, K.-D. 1986. 'Anweisungen zur Selbstmedikation von Laien in der Spätantike', in *Akten des 30. Internationalen Kongresses für Geschichte der Medizin*, 867–874. Düsseldorf: Düsseldorf University.

Fischer, K.-D. 1994. 'Überlieferungs- und Verständnisprobleme im medizinischen Latein des frühen Mittelalters', *Berichte zur Wissenschaftsgeschichte* 17: 153–165.

Fischer, K.-D. 2000. 'Dr Monk's Medical Digest', *Social History of Medicine* 13: 239–251.

Fischer K.-D. (ed.) 2000. *Bibliographie des textes médicaux latins: antiquité et haut moyen âge. Premier supplément, 1986–1999*. Saint-Étienne: Publications de l'Université de Saint-Étienne. Second supplement 2000, and Addendum 2002, http://www.biusante.parisdescartes.fr/histoire/medicina/documents/fischer2002.php, last accessed 10 Aug. 2018.

Fischer, K.-D. 2003. 'Neues zur Überlieferung der lateinischen Aphorismen im Frühmittelalter', *Latomus* 62: 156–164.

Fischer, K.-D. unpublished. 'Von Wunden und Wundern'.

Flint, V. I. J. 1989. 'The Early Medieval *medicus*, the Saint – and the Enchanter', *Social History of Medicine* 2: 127–145.

Flint, V. I. J. 1991. *The Rise of Magic in Early Medieval Europe*. Oxford: Clarendon Press.

French, R. 1994. *Ancient Natural History: Histories of Nature*. London: Routledge.

French, R. 2003. *Medicine before Science*. Cambridge: Cambridge University Press.

Getz, F. M. 1998. *Medicine in the English Middle Ages*. Princeton, NJ: Princeton University Press.

Glaze, F. E. 1999. 'The Perforated Wall: The Ownership and Circulation of Medical Books in Medieval Europe, ca. 800–1200', unpublished PhD thesis, Duke University.

Gordon, R. 1995. 'The Healing Event in Graeco-Roman Medicine', in P. J. van der Eijk, H. F. J. Horstmanshoff, and P. H. Schrijvers (eds), *Ancient Medicine in its Socio-Cultural Context*, vol. 2, 363–376. Amsterdam: Rodopi.

Green, M. H. 1985. 'The Transmission of Ancient Theories of Female Physiology and Disease through the Early Middle Ages', unpublished PhD thesis, Princeton University.

Green, M. H. (ed. and trans.) 2001. *The Trotula: A Medieval Compendium of Women's Medicine*. Philadelphia: University of Pennsylvania Press.

Green, M. H. 2005. 'Flowers, Poisons, and Men: Menstruation in Medieval Western Europe', in A. Shail and G. Howie (eds), *Menstruation: A Cultural History*, 51–64. Basingstoke: Palgrave Macmillan.

Green, M. H. 2008a. 'Rethinking the Manuscript Basis of Salvatore de Renzi's *Collectio Salernitana*: The Corpus of Medical Writings in the "Long" Twelfth Century', in D. Jacquart and A. Paravicini Bagliani (eds), *La 'Collectio salernitana' di Salvatore de Renzi*, 15–60. Florence: SISMEL/Edizioni del Galluzzo.

Green, M. H. 2008b. *Making Women's Medicine Masculine: The Rise of Male Authority in Pre-Modern Gynaecology*. Oxford: Oxford University Press.

Groenke, F.-D. 1986. *Die frühmittelalterlichen lateinischen Monatskalendarien*. Berlin: Institut für Geschichte der Medizin der Freien Universität Berlin.

Haefele, H. F. (ed. and trans.) 1980. Ekkehard IV, *Casus Sancti Galli: St. Galler Klostergeschichten*. Darmstadt: Wissenschaftliche Buchgesellschaft.

Hall, A. 2007. *Elves in Anglo-Saxon England: Matters of Health, Belief, Gender and Identity*. Woodbridge: Boydell Press.

Heeßel, N. P. 2004. 'Diagnosis, Divination and Disease: Towards an Understanding of the Rationale behind the Babylonian Diagnostic Handbook', in H. F. J. Horstmanshoff and M. Stol (eds), *Magic and Rationality in Ancient Near Eastern and Graeco-Roman Medicine*, 97–116. Leiden: Brill.

Horden, P., 2000. 'The Millennium Bug: Health and Medicine around the Year 1000', *Social History of Medicine* 13: 201–219.

Horden, P., 2008. 'Sickness and Healing', in T. F. X. Noble and J. M. H. Smith (eds), *Early Medieval Christianities, c.600–c.1100*, 416–432. Cambridge: Cambridge University Press [reprinted as Ch. 4 in the present volume].

Hsu, E. 2002, 'Medical Anthropology, Material Culture, and New Directions in Medical Archaeology', in P. A. Baker and G. Carr (eds), *Practitioners, Practices and Patients: New Approaches to Medical Archaeology and Anthropology*, 1–15. Oxford: Oxbow.

Iggers, G. G., and von Moltke, K. 1983 (eds) [1973]. *Leopold von Ranke: The Theory and Practice of History*. New York: Irvington.

Jolly, K. L. 1996. *Popular Religion in Late Saxon England: Elf Charms in Context*. Chapel Hill: University of North Carolina Press.

Jolly, K. L. 2002. 'Medieval Magic: Definitions, Beliefs, Practices', in K. L. Jolly, C. Raudvere, and E. Peters (eds), *The Athlone History of Witchcraft and Magic in Europe*, vol. 3: *The Middle Ages*, 1–71. London: Athlone Press.

Jones, W. H. S. (ed. and trans.) 1963. Pliny, *Natural History*, Loeb Classical Library, vol. 3. London and Cambridge, MA: Heinemann and Harvard University Press.

Jörimann, J. (ed.) 1925. *Frühmittelalterliche Rezeptarien*. Zürich: Hoenn.

King, H. 1998. *Hippocrates' Woman: Reading the Female Body in Ancient Greece*. London: Routledge.

Klibansky, R., Panofsky E., and Saxl, F. 1964. *Saturn and Melancholy: Studies in the History of Natural Philosophy, Religion, and Art*. London: Nelson.

Langslow, D. R. 2006. *The Latin Alexander Trallianus: The Text and Transmission of a Late Latin Medical Book*. London: Society for the Promotion of Roman Studies.

Lloyd, G. E. R. (ed.) 1978. *Hippocratic Writings*. Harmondsworth: Penguin.

MacKinney, L. C. 1937. *Early Medieval Medicine with Special Reference to France and Chartres*. Baltimore, MD: Johns Hopkins University Press.

MacKinney, L. C. 1942a. 'The Vulture in Ancient Medical Lore', *Ciba Symposia* 4: 1258–1271.

MacKinney, L. C. 1942b. 'The Vulture in the Medieval World', *Ciba Symposia* 4: 1272–1286.

MacKinney, L. C. 1943. 'An Unpublished Treatise on Medicine and Magic from the Age of Charlemagne', *Speculum* 18: 494–496.

McCormick, M. 2001. *Origins of the European Economy: Communications and Commerce A.D. 300–900*. Cambridge: Cambridge University Press.

McKitterick, R. 1989. *The Carolingians and the Written Word*. Cambridge: Cambridge University Press.

McKitterick, R. 1992. 'Nuns' Scriptoria in England and Francia in the Eighth Century', *Francia* 19: 1–35.

McVaugh, M. R. 1993. *Medicine Before the Plague: Practitioners and their Patients in the Crown of Aragon, 1285–1345*. Cambridge: Cambridge University Press.

Meaney, A. 1992. 'The Anglo-Saxon View of the Causes of Illness', in S. Campbell, B. Hall, and D. Klausner (eds), *Health, Disease and Healing in Medieval Culture*, 12–33. London: Macmillan.

Meaney, A. 2000. 'The Practice of Medicine in England about the Year 1000', *Social History of Medicine* 13: 221–237.

Möhler, R. 1990. *'Epistula de vulture': Untersuchungen zu einer organotherapeutischen Drogenmonographie des Frühmittelalters*. Pattensen: H. Wellm.

Murray, A. 1992. 'Missionaries and Magic in Dark Age Europe', *Past and Present* 136: 186–205.

Nokes, R. S. 2004. 'The Several Compilers of Bald's *Leechbook*', *Anglo-Saxon England* 33: 51–76.

Nutton, V. (ed. and trans.) 1979. Galen, *On Prognosis*, Corpus medicorum graecorum. Berlin: Akademie.

Nutton, V. 1984. 'From Galen to Alexander: Aspects of Medicine and Medical Practice in Late Antiquity', *Dumbarton Oaks Papers* 38: 1–14.

Nutton, V. 1992. 'Healers in the Medical Market Place: Towards a Social History of Graeco-Roman Medicine', in A. Wear (ed.), *Medicine in Society*, 15–58. Cambridge: Cambridge University Press.

Nutton, V. 2004. *Ancient Medicine*. London: Routledge.

O'Boyle, C. 1998. *The Art of Medicine: Medical Teaching at the University of Paris, 1250–1400*. Leiden: Brill.

Olsan, L. T. 2003. 'Charms and Prayers in Medieval Medical Theory and Practice', *Social History of Medicine* 16: 343–66.

Önnerfors, A. 1963. *In medicinam Plinii studia philologica*. Lund: Gleerup.

Paxton, F. S. 1990a. *Christianizing Death: The Creation of a Ritual Process in Early Medieval Europe*. Ithaca, NY: Cornell University Press.

Paxton, F. S. 1990b. *'Bonus liber*: A Late Carolingian Clerical Manual from Lorsch', in L. Mayali and S. A. J. Tibbetts (eds), *The Two Laws: Studies in Medieval Legal History dedicated to Stephan Kuttner*, 1–30. Washington, DC: Catholic University of America Press.

Paxton, F. S. 1993. *'Signa mortifera*: Death and Prognostication in Early Medieval Monastic Medicine', *Bulletin of the History of Medicine* 67: 631–650.

Paxton, F. S. 1995. 'Curing Bodies – Curing Souls: Hrabanus Maurus, Medical Education, and the Clergy in Ninth-Century Francia', *Journal of the History of Medicine* 50: 230–252.

Pettit E. (ed.) 2001. *Anglo-Saxon Remedies, Charms, and Prayers from British Library MS Harley 585: The Lacnunga*. 2 vols. Lewiston, VA: Edwin Mellen Press.

Pilsworth C., unpublished. 'Medical Miscellanies and Karlsruhe, Badische Landesbibliothek MS 172', paper for colloquium 'The Monk, the Muse and the Matrona: Medical Texts, Moral Advice and Gender in Early Medieval Alemannia', University of Manchester, May 2004.

Pormann, P. E., and Savage-Smith, E. 2007. *Medieval Islamic Medicine*. Edinburgh: Edinburgh University Press.

Probst, B. (ed.) 1983. *Regula Benedicti, de codice 914 in bibliotheca monasterii S. Galli servato.* St Ottilien: EOS.

Riché, P. 1976 [1962]. *Education and Culture in the Barbarian West, Sixth through Eighth Centuries.* Columbia: University of South Carolina Press.

Riddle, J. M. 1974. 'Theory and Practice in Early Medieval Medicine', *Viator* 5: 158–184.

Riddle, J. M. 1981. 'Pseudo-Dioscorides' *Ex herbis feminis* and Early Medieval Medical Botany', *Journal of the History of Biology* 14: 43–81.

Riddle, J. M. 1984. 'Byzantine Commentaries on Dioscorides', *Dumbarton Oaks Papers* 13: 95–102.

Riddle, J. M. 1985. *Dioscorides on Pharmacy and Medicine.* Austin: University of Texas Press.

Riddle, J. M. 1997. *Eve's Herbs: A History of Contraception and Abortion in the West.* Cambridge, MA: Harvard University Press.

Riddle, J. M. 2007. 'Research Procedures in Evaluating Medieval Medicine', in B. Bowers (ed.), *The Medieval Hospital and Medical Practice*, 3–17. Aldershot: Ashgate.

Ringrose, K. M. 2003. *The Perfect Servant: Eunuchs and the Social Construction of Gender in Byzantium.* Chicago: University of Chicago Press.

Sabbah, G., Corsetti, P.-P., and Fischer, K.-D. (eds) 1987. *Bibliographie des textes médicaux latins: antiquité et haut moyen âge.* Saint-Étienne: Publications de l'Université de Saint-Étienne.

Savage-Smith, E. 2000. 'The Practice of Surgery in Islamic Lands: Myth and Reality', *Social History of Medicine* 13: 307–321.

Sigerist, H. 1934. 'The Medical Literature of the Early Middle Ages: A Program – and a Report of a Summer of Research in Italy', *Bulletin of the History of Medicine* 2: 26–50.

Siraisi, N. 1993. *Medieval and Early Renaissance Medicine: An Introduction to Knowledge and Practice.* Chicago: University of Chicago Press.

Stadler, H. (ed.) 1899. 'Dioscorides Langobardus (cod. lat. Monacensis 337)', *Romanische Forschungen* 10: 181–247 (first of four instalments of the edition).

Stoll, U. (ed.) 1992. *Das 'Lorscher Arzneibuch': ein medizinisches Kompendium des 8. Jahrhunderts (Codex Bambergensis Medicinalis 1)*, Sudhoffs Archiv Beihefte 28. Stuttgart: Franz Steiner.

Stürmer, J. 1982. 'Weitere Überlieferungen des mittelhochdeutschen "Geiertraktats" sowie eine althochdeutsche Übersetzung der "Epistula de vulture"', in G. Keil (ed.), *Gelêrter der arzenîe, ouch apotêker . . . Festschrift zum 70. Geburtstag von Willem F. Daems*, 443–478. Pattensen: H. Wellm.

Van Arsdall, A. 2005. 'Reading Medieval Medical Texts with an Open Mind', in E. Lane Furdell (ed.), *Textual Healing: Essays on Medieval and Early Modern Medicine*, 9–29. Leiden: Brill.

Van Arsdall, A. 2007. 'Challenging the "Eye of Newt" Image of Medieval Medicine', in B. Bowers (ed.), *The Medieval Hospital and Medical Practice*, 195–205. Aldershot: Ashgate.

Voigts, L. 1979. 'Anglo-Saxon Plant Remedies and the Anglo-Saxons', *Isis* 70: 250–268.

Voigts, L. 2008. 'Plants and Planets: Linking the Vegetable and the Celestial in Late Medieval Texts', in P. Dendle and A. Touwaide (eds), *Health and Healing from the Medieval Garden*, 29–46. Woodbridge: Boydell Press.

von Staden, H. 1992. 'Women and Dirt', *Helios* 19: 7–29.

Wallis, F. 1995a. 'Medicine in Medieval Calendar Manuscripts', in M. R. Schleiss-ner (ed.), *Manuscript Sources of Medieval Medicine*, 105–143. New York: Garland.

Wallis, F. 1995b. 'The Experience of the Book: Manuscripts, Texts, and the Role of Epistemology in Early Medieval Medicine', in D. Bates (ed.), *Knowledge and the Scholarly Medical Traditions*, 101–126. Cambridge: Cambridge University Press.

Wallis, F. 2000. 'Signs and Senses: Diagnosis and Prognosis in Early Medieval Pulse and Urine Texts', *Social History of Medicine* 13: 265–278.

Ward-Perkins, B. 2005. *The Fall of Rome and the End of Civilization*. Oxford: Oxford University Press.

Wickersheimer, E. 1966. *Les manuscrits latins de médecine du haut moyen âge dans les bibliothèques de France*. Paris: Centre National de la Recherche Scientifique.

Wlaschky, M. (ed.) 1928. '*Sapientia artis medicinae*: ein frühmittelalterliches Kompendium der Medizin', *Kyklos: Jahrbuch des Instituts für Geschichte der Medizin an der Universität Leipzig* 1: 103–113.

Wootton, D. 2006. *Bad Medicine: Doctors Doing Harm since Hippocrates*. Oxford: Oxford University Press.

Zipser B. (ed.) 2009. *John the Physician's 'Therapeutics': A Medical Handbook in Vernacular Greek*. Leiden: Brill.

POSTSCRIPT

I list here simply some of the references, either unpublished in 2010–11 when this article was in press or that I wish I had been aware of when writing.

I have been especially interested to come across some further evidence supporting my argument that apparently bizarre early medieval material continued to be transmitted through the later Middle Ages, the age of university learning. For example, the prognostication involving a dog and a lump of lard can be found in very similar form in Oxford, Bodley, MS Rawlinson C814, of the first half of the fourteenth century. See *Three Receptaria from Medieval England: The Languages of Medicine in the Fourteenth Century*, ed. Tony Hunt and Michael Benskin (Oxford, 2001), p. 51, kindly drawn to my attention by Joanne Edge. A version requiring yeast rather than lard appears in John Mirfield's (d. 1407) *Breviarium Bartholomei*, a medical anthology compiled for St Bartholomew's Hospital in London. It is most accessible, in translation, in Faith Wallis (ed.), *Medieval Medicine: A Reader* (Toronto, 2010), p. 484.

I should have noted a version of my very opening prognostication (which has the more plausible motion – turning towards you as a sign of future recovery) in the Old English Leechbook of Bald, book III, section 65, available (pending a modern scholarly edition) in Stephen Pollington, *Leechcraft: Early English Charms, Plant Lore, and Healing* (Hockwold-cum-Wilton, 2000), pp. 404–405.

On vultures, I should have risked a degree of naïve biological realism and mentioned the bird's widely attested capacity to digest, survive and neutralize anthrax in carrion. It really is a death-eater, and in that respect assists public health. I am grateful here to Emmett Sullivan.

On the vulture epistle and its transmission since antiquity, I should now want to cite María Teresa Santamaría Hernández, 'El capítulo *de vulture* del *Liber medicinae ex animalibus* de Sexto Placito: relacíon con la zooterapia Hermética y propuestas de enmienda al texto', *Traditio* 66 (2011), 1–26. I should already have read John A. C. Greppin, 'Birds in Armenian Medicine', *Medieval Encounters* 4.2 (1998), 93–114, which at pp. 98–99 takes us back to the *Cyranides* and forward to medieval medicine in Arabic. Citing some excellent work by Loren C. MacKinney, I should also have made space for his 'Animal Substances in Materia Medica: A Study in the Persistence of the Primitive', *Journal of the History of Medicine and Allied Sciences* 1.1 (1946), 149–170; one might phrase the subtitle differently today but the immense learning remains valuable.

The biological efficacy of medicine recorded in Old English, of which I was perhaps too dismissive, continues to be debated. See e.g. Frances Watkins, Barbara Pendry, Alberto Sanchez-Medina and Olivia Corcoran, 'Antimicrobial Assays of Three Native British Plants used in Anglo-Saxon Medicine for Wound Healing Formulations in 10th Century England', *Journal of Ethnopharmacology* 144 (2012), 408–415, with modest but positive results. For the headline-making 'Bald's eyesalve', reportedly effective against *Staphylococcus aureus*, see Freya Harrison, Aled E. L. Roberts, Rebecca Gabrilska, Kendra P. Rumbaugh, Christina Lee, and Stephen P. Diggle, 'A 1,000-Year-Old Antimicrobial Remedy with Antistaphylococcal Activity', *mBio* 6.4 (2015), e01129-15 [doi:10.1128/mBio.01129-15].

For onomancy see now Joanne T. Edge, '*Nomen omen*: The "Sphere of Life and Death" in England, c.1200–c.1500', unpublished PhD dissertation, Royal Holloway University of London, 2015, and her forthcoming monograph.

For Latin medical manuscripts in the early Salernitan period, see now Monica H. Green, 'Medical Books', in *The European Book in the Twelfth Century*, ed. Erik Kwakkel and Rodney Thomson (Cambridge, 2018), pp. 277–292.

A revised, partial version of Bennett 2003 has now been published, posthumously alas, as *Medicine and Pharmacy in Byzantine Hospitals: A Study of the Extant Formularies* (Abingdon, 2017). Alongside Fischer 1986 see now his 'Wenn kein Arzt erreichbar ist: medizinische Literatur für Laien in der Spätantike', *Medicina nei Secoli* 24.1 (2012) 379–401. Nutton 2004 should now be read in the revised edition of 2013.

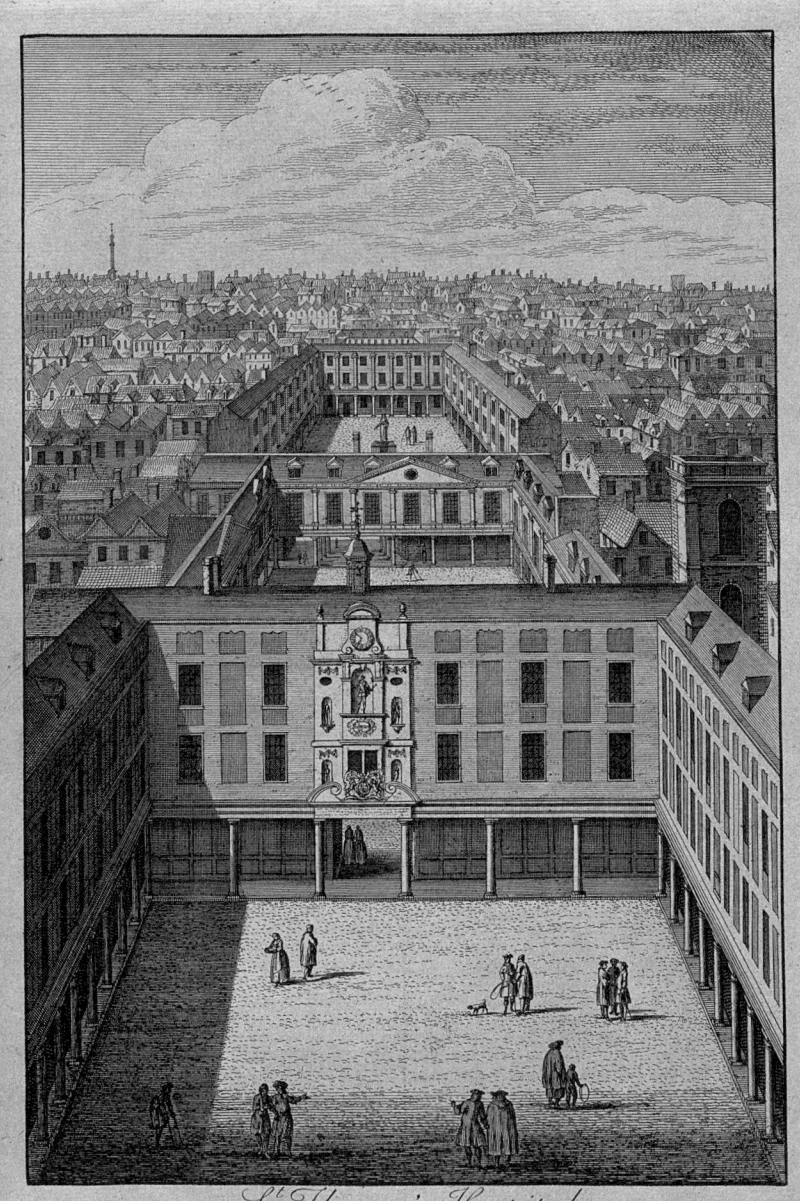

St Thomas's Hospital.

8

CITIES WITHIN CITIES

Early hospital foundations and urban space

1. Prospects

This prospect, or bird's-eye-view print, of St Thomas's Hospital, London, was engraved in the eighteenth century.[1] A medieval foundation, the hospital had survived the English Reformation and had escaped the Great Fire of London. Yet by the closing decade of the seventeenth century it had become dilapidated and was seen as unfit for purpose. Supported by voluntary subscription, its governors paid for it to be refurbished and enlarged, to consist of three quadrangles and a number of subordinate buildings. 'Prospect' prints of this sort were circulated in the eighteenth century to attract benefactions to public projects.[2] Some were notably successful. The greatest benefactor of St Thomas's was Sir Robert Clayton.[3] The governors acknowledged and proclaimed his outstanding generosity by erecting a statue to him inside the hospital. In the version of the prospect illustrated, published in 1756 in Maitland's *Survey of London*, the statue is visible in the quadrangle most distant from the viewer. The hospital, with its large connected courts, appears to drive a wedge through the capital's topography towards the distant horizon. No building round about seems to rival it in spaciousness. Its elegant architecture contrasts with the cramped zigzags of roofs everywhere else in view. And, in the middle distance on the central axis, stands the statue of its great benefactor, virtually its second founder. Did he hope for a statue or some such memorial when he transferred the funds that helped make all this possible? As Bernard Mandeville wrote in *The Fable of the Bees* in 1714, not long after Clayton would have earned his memorial, 'pride and vanity have built more hospitals than all the Virtues together'.[4] Clayton's wealth had refashioned not only the hospital but the entire landscape of this part of London (Southwark). Consider the likely number of patients housed around those three quadrangles, the staff needed to attend them, and the ramifications of an establishment on this apparent scale for the local movement of goods and people. Especially if we see St Thomas's through the eye of the engraver, who has magnified it, and heightened the contrast with its surrounding buildings, it is easy to envisage this hospital as a city within a city.

179

In the early modern period, that was an ambivalent position for a hospital – a presumed source of infection. To take an example from a different capital: the large, overcrowded, and reputedly highly insalubrious Hôtel-Dieu, the great hospital of Paris on the Île de la Cité opposite the façade of Notre Dame, was always seeking extra accommodation.[5] In 1548, though they acknowledged it to be 'like a heart in the middle of a man', the city governors rejected a request to expand onto two of the connecting bridges. They wanted to keep the hospital central yet – on account of its infectiousness – separate, literally insulated. In 1786, after the hospital had been gutted by fire, a similar request was rejected on similar grounds. A committee of the Académie des Sciences reminded the hospital authorities that, with its population of some 5,000, it was already like a city. Indeed, they added, it was bigger than three-quarters of the cities in France.

This paper takes seriously the idea that one kind of foundation, the hospital, can be city-like and, as such, can exercise a profound and potentially controversial influence on urban topography. It further raises the possibility that founders or benefactors of major hospitals foresaw this political dimension to their endeavours – political in both its literal (of the *polis*, the city) and its more usual, broader sense. And it does so by showing that that dimension is evident right at the beginning of hospital history, so far as Europe and the Mediterranean world is concerned: with some of the very early forerunners of St Thomas's and the Hôtel-Dieu.

2. The first hospital-city

Here is a verbal 'prospect' of a hospital thirteen hundred years older than St Thomas's:

> Go a little way from this city and gaze on the new city: the storehouse of piety, the common treasury of those with possessions, where the superfluities of wealth, as well as necessities, lie stored up because of his exhortation – shaking off the moths, giving no joy to the thieves, escaping the assaults of envy and the corruption of time – where disease is treated with philosophy, where misfortunes are called blessings, and compassion is held in real esteem.[6]

Gregory of Nazianzus in Cappadocia (modern Nenizi, Turkey), priest, rhetorician, and bishop, pronounced that injunction to visit a 'new city' in the course of his funeral oration for his friend, Basil, bishop of Caesarea (modern Kayseri, right in the middle of Turkey).[7] Basil had died in January 379. Gregory was prevented from attending Basil's funeral (he claims) by illness, and by what we might call religio-political preoccupation – combatting the so-called Arian heresy in Constantinople and trying to establish his leadership of the 'orthodox'. He probably did not speak about his departed friend and patron until the third anniversary of Basil's death, in early 382. By this time others had naturally orated, including Basil's brother, another bishop, Gregory of Nyssa, who may have delivered his own speech a year earlier.[8] The Nazianzen Gregory needed to make his mark. He wrote much more than Basil's brother did – more than could actually have been delivered; the text was either cut down for oral rendition or elaborated afterwards. And he went into much more detail of Basil's career and activities.

The 'new city' outside Caesarea, perhaps in its suburbs, was a complex of institutions that Basil had founded for the sick and needy. The description by Gregory of Nazianzus is allusive, even abstract. After all, his hearers – readers – could see for themselves. That is perhaps why, before him, Gregory of Nyssa did not mention these institutions at all. Gregory of Nazianzus, trying to go one better, needed to remind Caesareans of this achievement, but he did not need to describe. For a little more information we have to look to Basil himself. In a letter to the provincial governor, Elias, written when the complex was either very new or still under construction, Basil referred to a place for the reception of 'strangers', 'both for those on a journey, and for those needing therapies on account of sickness'.[9] He also seems to refer to the staff members who would tend them, people good at 'doctoring', and the workshops required by the support staff (or perhaps even for the temporary gainful employment of the transients). There was also a facility for housing or looking after lepers, the neediest of the sick. Some in the city had clearly found their presence, as beggars, offensive. In his oration Gregory of Nazianzus goes on to say that Basil's foundation had removed the 'terrible and piteous spectacle' of leprosy from civic gatherings, to a place where they could be objects of compassion rather than hatred. A later (sixth- or seventh-century) biography of Gregory of Nazianzus, by yet another Gregory, reports, plausibly, that Basil built several dwellings (plural) for the lepers, raised money for their maintenance from rich citizens, gathered all the sick into them (lepers presumably included), and called the buildings 'refuges [or secluded places, *phrontisteria*] for the poor'.[10]

The 'new city' was thus a centre for charity and healing. It offered lodging for needy transients, a medical facility for the sick, shelter for the poor. We should not worry about the different but overlapping target groups, and the varying terms used, any more than contemporaries did. The bigger point Gregory (of Nazianzus) makes in his eulogy is that 'because of Basil's persuasion', those with superfluous wealth had made pious benefactions to the philanthropic complex. Accumulated riches or goods are vulnerable to theft and depreciation. Wealth given to this hospital – as we can call it for brevity – stores up benefits which are there for the poor and sick when they require it. It also stores up future spiritual benefits for the wealthy, because they are addressing, however partially, the 'eye of the needle' problem set out for them by St Matthew.[11] They could gain those benefits not only from the act of charity itself, but also from the grateful prayers of the poor inmates of the institution. These had been offered compassion, and a 'philosophical' response to their ailments. This was philosophy of both a spiritual and a medical kind. Although the Christian way of life had long been promoted as 'the true philosophy', we also know that Basil himself had acquired some medical learning – medicine underpinned by Aristotelian philosophy – and he made sure that the poor people in his hospital received 'doctoring', if not from self-professed doctors then from those with some medical experience.[12] Thus was the hospital 'a stairway to heaven', as Gregory goes on to say, not in the sense that patients were all expected to die quickly, but because of the blessedness of the life lived there, and perhaps also because it enhanced the chances of salvation for the rich benefactors.

The philanthropic complex must have been quite sizeable. Gregory of Nazianzus continues his oration by likening it to the seven wonders of the (ancient) world. We should think, more realistically, of the hospital, or hospitals – presumably lepers were housed separately given the fear of infection at which Gregory hints in his discourse; of the church that would have been attached; of their outhouses and accommodation for support staff; of the rooms kept for the bishop, and for the provincial governor should he visit. We should think of all the comings and goings between old and new cities or between both and their common hinterland: that is, of families visiting inmates, of pious visitors, priests or monks, vendors or officials. Compare the new city to the old in size and prestige. In 1500, the earliest date for which any serious estimates are possible, the city could boast only 2,287 tax-paying adults.[13] A late antique population of only a few thousand citizens is entirely conceivable, indeed likely. On such a yardstick the population of the philanthropic complex was not infinitesimally small. And it was likely to grow. It may be that it formed the nucleus of modern Kayseri, which is not on the exact site of Caesarea. Just as new urban centres would crystallize round cathedrals in the early Middle Ages, a hospital and its associated community could also play some part in refocusing an urban population.

In Basil's time hospitals of this kind were beginning to change cities in many ways. It is essential to realize how very new such establishments were in the 370s and 380s – only two decades or so old as urban institutions, and scarcely much older as institutions in any setting, with virtually no precedents in classical antiquity. When Basil became a bishop in 370 they were still in many ways unusual. They had come about – to simplify – for two main reasons.[14] First, because the alms, the pious donations, of local Christian populations had long been channelled through the bishop (so much so that the laity were sometimes exhorted not to suppose themselves thereby off the hook, but to undertake direct giving to the poor). Second, because in the wake of the Constantinian revolution, the establishment of Christianity as the religion of empire, bishops and priests had benefited from considerable tax benefits and relief from public obligations – in return for the life of prayer *and charity* to which they could more effectively devote themselves.

To put it crudely, but not with undue cynicism, the Church needed a form of conspicuous expenditure to validate itself as a privileged institution. The hospital – as a permanent building, an architectural expression of charity more visible than say a distribution centre for food or money – answered this need admirably. And it was part of a revaluation of urban and suburban space by Christians of this period, the later fourth century, that also took in cemeteries for the poor as well as prisons where inmates might, in charitable spirit, be visited and supported.[15] All this, of course, along with church-building, an activity that reflected both some spectacular benefactions by the rich and smaller, but more numerous and perhaps in aggregate quite substantial, donations by those of modest means.

The framework within which such transfers of wealth were taking place – into churches, but also into hospitals – was changing, in ways that are far more clear-cut in retrospect than they will have seemed at the time. In the late antique Roman world, the long-established form of giving – the 'natural' transaction – was between citizens. Wealthy citizens paid for the erection or repair of public buildings (much as they would in eighteenth-century England) and also laid on games and distributions of food for the rest of their fellow citizens. The parameters of the gift were entirely civic: local non-citizen poor people and transients were not included. And it was a two-way process. Those who benefited would offer in return the adulation, fame, or political support that the rich expected. Such city-based philanthropy may have been in decline in volume in the Cappodocia of Basil's day. Nonetheless it retained its hold on the collective social 'imaginary', as it continues to do on that of modern historians, who have given it the label 'euergetism' and who associate it with the pagan classical world.[16] But there was a Christian euergetism too – so natural was it. Wealthy benefactors of churches, whose donations of silver bore their names, were inviting the gratitude of their fellow citizens in the churches in a way that would have been recognizable to their pagan forebears.[17]

Basil himself posed as a 'nourisher' of his city, an urban patron on the classical model. The hospital he founded came to bear his name – the Basileias – in a way that would remind future generations of his benevolence. One of the features of his achievement that marked him out as an ascetic monk-bishop rather than a pagan giver was the probability that he did not plan it this way. He did not seek to stamp his name on 'his' hospital.[18]

Of course there was more to it than a change of tone. Christian benefactors were making a down-payment on salvation, in a way the pagan ones were not. And however much the language of Christianity was accommodated to old civic patterns, there was a profoundly novel ingredient. The old transaction between rich citizens and the rest was being replaced by one between rich and poor. In the classical model the poor as poor had had no place. There were poor citizens, who counted, and poor non-citizens, who did not. The beggar was, in the strict sense, apolitical: outside the *polis*. The

Church's fastening on the case of the poor, as expressed most assertively in hospitals and institutional charity more generally, was meant to signal its concern for the very margins of society – destitute transients, beggars, the sick without means, above all lepers. And this care was offered to citizens and non-citizens alike. The old civic framework of giving was being dissolved.

Several 'new cities' were thus symbolized in Basil's suburban hospital. There was the city of God, to which the hospital was a stairway. In this life none had any continuing city; all were sojourners. Thus the strangers to which the hospital catered were such in a spiritual sense, even if they were not quite 'real' migrants (though some of them wold have been that too). There was the 'old city' that still made itself felt in the vocabulary of Christian benefactors. And the 'new' city that was – both symbolically and geographically – outside the old. In the name of God but under the name of Basil.

No wonder the whole early history of this hospital and its creator was politically fraught. Christians were still, in around 370, a minority in the population of Caesarea. It was only a few years since the death of the last pagan emperor, Julian, who may have admired and planned to imitate Christian charity but whose religious revival was still a chilling memory. Within Christian society itself, Basil's relations with his predecessor, with the local governor, and with the 'Arian' emperor Valens (d. 378, at the Battle of Adrianople) had all been strained. Even though Valens may at some point have provided for the hospital's endowment, there was clearly a sense that Basil's various philanthropic initiatives, in a time of severe food shortage, were damaging to state interests. It is hard for us now to credit how unsettling his help for the poor may have been, both before he became bishop and ran a soup kitchen and persuaded the rich not to hoard their grain, and after he was chosen bishop, and started on his 'new city'.[19] The Basileias shows us the politics of foundation and its effects on urban space. The reconfiguration of that space is indeed an essential aspect of the politics.

Every feature of organized charity is, or can become, a political matter. In Basil's time local churches were starting to keep lists of the poor they supported with their doles.[20] Those listed were, presumably, the vetted and approved poor, the demonstrably deserving. One of Basil's successors as bishop would fret that the Basileias might fill up with peasants escaping their obligations on the area's great estates.[21] Church leaders of different Christological persuasions would accuse each other of enrolling different groups of poor, those who were theologically sound more than genuinely deserving.[22] We do not know the details of any of the patients in Basil's hospital. We may guess they were as subject to 'ethical approval' as any pauper enrolled on the Church's list.

The question remains, however: what did Basil think he was doing? And how would he have articulated it if pressed? Out of undoubted piety, he wanted to help the poorest of the poor in a time of severe food stress, discharging to the full the responsibilities of his new position as bishop. Still, there were many ways of doing that. Charity ran in Basil's family, but mostly in the form of distributions. His soup kitchen was only the most recent in a line of such initiatives. Yet a hospital is more than a soup kitchen – in scale and in permanence. Basil's predecessor as bishop had undertaken no major new charitable works, so far as we know. He kept his head down. Basil, having somehow patched up a quarrel with him (the details are now obscure), acted, in that predecessor's last few years, virtually as coadjutant bishop. Once bishop in his own right – we may conjecture – he needed to consolidate his position: he needed a way of enhancing his reputation as a philanthropist and making his mark. Perhaps he thought he might impress the pagan population with his hospital complex. Julian after all had urged his co-religionists to build hospitals of their own.[23] But all this was obviously risky. We know how Basil justified himself when the governor took exception for some reason to the Basileias, probably while it was under construction. 'Who are we harming?' in setting up a hospital – and a suite for the governor – he asked with faux-naïveté.[24] Somehow, he involved the emperor. There is a later, yet credible report that Valens, the 'Arian', contributed to the endowment of the hospital of Basil, the adherent of Nicaea.[25] Basil would have been aware, as he assembled the financial resources for his project, of the politics that had to be played.

Quite how Basil's hospital was funded, and within what legal framework, we do not know. The evidence is altogether lacking. We cannot assume that what emerged as the law governing the establishment and endowment of pious foundations of this kind in later centuries was clear at the time the Basileias was being built. Churches had been able to own property since well before Constantine's conversion. Hospitals would be assimilated to them in their legal capacity. Yet did Basil put his own wealth into the hospital and if so how much, and in what form? Did Valens really support it with some grant of land, and if so by what mechanism of transfer, and as an individual or as the embodiment of the late Roman 'state'? Did the hospital benefit from hypothecated revenues from rural or urban property or from directly managed estates? Was it legally independent of the Church in Caesarea? How important were the continuing donations of local Christians to its economic survival? We can only speculate – and look forward, riskily, to the clearer legislation of the fourth and fifth centuries on the legal status of the *euageis oikoi*, the 'sacred houses' – a category that subsumed both philanthropic establishments and churches.[26] The one point we can make with reasonable confidence is the importance of knowing good accountants [*numerarioi*]. Basil corresponded with two of them, albeit about hospitals outside Caesarea.[27] Right from the start of its long history the endowment and financing of a hospital was never easy.

To attempt a summing up of Basil's endeavour. His foundation was not the first hospital we know of in fourth-century Asia Minor. But it still came very early on, belonging to the earliest wave of documented facilities. It was the first foundation of any scale, so far as we can tell, and the first in a major Byzantine city outside Constantinople. A political analysis of it would place it within the larger setting of the Church's attempts to legitimize or justify its newly growing wealth and its financial privileges. It would also place the hospital within the local setting of Basil's concern to secure his position as bishop and leader of the community. Basil and his hospital upset a lot of people: the emperor, the governor, other clerics, the non-Christian population. Not surprisingly: it changed Caesarea, both ideologically, through its novel representation of a Christian community, and topographically, through its reconfiguration of urban and suburban space. The first big hospital in the Mediterranean world, its effects are in some ways the clearest. The evidence for many other, later hospitals does not allow us to observe their effects with equal clarity. I suggest, nonetheless, that we envisage those later hospitals as *potentially* transformative in similar ways, sometimes to an even greater extent. The ambient details will be beyond recovery. A hospital may be built on virgin land, most likely on the edge of or outside a city. It may be on a 'brown-field' suburban site, or pre-existing houses or other buildings may be converted or demolished to make way for it. Each of these processes will have had subtly different effects on urban space, the local traffic of people and goods, and the way this part of the city, or indeed the city as a whole, is conceived. And yet the evidence is not detailed enough for us to differentiate these effects.

3. Capital spaces

Consider, as a second Byzantine example, the Sampson hospital of Constantinople.[28] Here was a late antique foundation that survived until the Latin conquest of the city, and, under Crusader control, spawned a new military order.[29] When the eponymous saint lived and how he came to set up a hospital are obscure. It is possible that Sampson lived in the fourth century, but the hospital first clearly enters the light of history in the sixth, when Justinian restored and enlarged it after it had been destroyed by fire in the Nika riot of 532. What is interesting in the present context is the way notions of urban space are built into how the hospital and its past were represented. The earliest biography of St Sampson, composed around 700, has him being born, not in Constantinople, but in Rome, to a senatorial family.[30] His parents were however related to the first Christian emperor, Constantine. In Rome he studied scripture and medicine. After his parents died he moved to Constantinople, where he combined those two strands in his education by opening his small house as a home for the charitable care of those who were destitute and seriously ill. Hospitals like Sampson's are being given a genealogy within the larger narrative of the establishment of Constantinople as the New Rome, and of the (entirely legendary) movement of philanthropic, hospital-founding senators from one capital, Rome, to the other, Constantinople.[31] The beginnings of the hospital are modest, a converted domicile – even though that does not sit with the orphaned future saint's presumed wealth.

Even before Justinian's re-foundation the hospital may already have grown quite sizeable. Its position was prime: in the symbolic heart of it the city, near to Hagia Sophia, between it and the Church of Hagia Eirene; and it may have begun as a dependent institution of Hagia Sophia since tradition, revealed in the early biography, has Sampson serving in the Great Church as a *skeuophylax* – sacristan, priest looking after the sacred treasures – which is in keeping with his supposed social background. Around 1300 one historian would claim that Justinian, in his re-foundation, won as much renown for the hospital as he did for Hagia Sophia – this at a time when the buildings were probably no longer functioning as a hospital.[32] Certainly Justinian worked on a considerable scale. His new, lavishly endowed Sampson hospital was a multi-storey affair, and it may be that the complex ground-plan, surrounding a central courtyard, which archaeologists have uncovered to the north-east of the Great Church really is that of the hospital. Justinian also established two further hospitals in the vicinity, as well as restoring the suburban church of St Mocius in which Sampson, thus present at both the centre and the periphery of the city, was buried. Under Latin occupation, and perhaps before 1204 too, the hospital had its own cemeteries and cistern.[33]

Unlike suburban Caesarea, this was of course no virgin site. But of the clearance of existing buildings on it, and the effects on local population and economy, we have no evidence. To understand anything of how the hospital interacted with the larger urban space and its various ecologies we have to change focus – to make the most of the evidence we do have.

For some light – highly refracted – on hospitals in Constantinople of the seventh century, the time when the first Life of Sampson was probably written, we can turn to a set of miracle stories. These are not the ones appended to later reworkings of Sampson's biography, but those of a saint whose shrine lay in the Church of St John Prodromos, in the Oxeia quarter of the city. The saint was Artemios, and his healing powers, at least as they were written up in around the 660s, seemed to concentrate on male genitals.[34]

> Stephen, deacon of the Great Church and a 'cheerleader' of the Blue Faction, related this tale: In my testicles I suffered a rupture . . . out of shame I concealed myself for a considerable time, watching for a chance to bathe alone in the small hours. At long last I disclosed my misfortune to my parents and after many treatments had been performed on me, finally, after taking counsel with them, I entrusted myself to the surgeons of the hospital of Sampson and I reclined in the hospital room near the entrance to the eye clinic.

After I had been treated all over for three nights and days with cold cauteries, surgery was performed on the fourth day. [Scar heals; apparent success; relapse; again shameful hiding.] I had a plan to approach the holy martyr [Artemios], as I had heard of his many great miracles. Still I was unwilling to wait in the venerable church, feeling ashamed before friends and acquaintances to be seen by them in such a condition. But I frequently used to pass by . . . and so I descended to the holy tomb of his precious relics and I cast some of his holy blessing, i.e. oil, on my testicles, hoping to procure a cure in this manner. And frequently I entreated him to deliver me from the troublesome condition. . . . one day because of some need I went out to the church, and . . . returned to my home at a late hour of the evening. But on the way the thought occurred to me to purchase candles and to approach the holy martyr . . . So taking the candles, I headed for the holy house and I lit them in the church, crying out to him from my soul. Next, after descending to the holy tomb, I found the doors in front open and I was astounded that they were open at such an hour. This was the doing of the martyr in his desire to pity me. Stretching out face down on the holy coffin, I straddled it and thus contrived to rub the corner of the same holy tomb on the spot where I was ailing. And with tears I spoke again to the martyr: 'St. Artemios, by God who has given you the gift of cures, no doctor on earth will ever touch me again. So if you please, cure me. But if not, to your everlasting shame I will live thus without a cure.' And after some days I went to the bath in the quarter of Anthemios, the one called Livanon, to bathe by myself at dawn in order not to be seen by anyone . . . upon exiting I had no injury.[35]

That passage, and a further one relating to yet another nearby hospital, the Christodotes, have normally been sifted for details of internal organization and medical personnel. What needs emphasis here is, rather, the different spaces involved, and the place of the hospital in the narrative, which is a narrative both of health-seeking and of the articulation of related yet contrasting spaces.

What spaces? Public ones, first. We have here the story of a deacon of the nearby Great Church, thereby reaffirming the long-standing link between it and the Sampson hospital: not a pauper in the strict sense but one of 'Christ's poor', a member of an enormous priestly and lay community. He has another public role, involving another great space. He is leader of one of the two circus factions that thronged the nearby Hippodrome, regularly focusing almost the whole population of the city on one central, agonistic space – a city at once united in its sporting addiction yet divided in its team loyalties. He must be a celibate too, and thus suffers the most shameful affliction of testicular rupture. He wants to go to the public baths – for hygiene, for recreation, perhaps in the hope of healing (in water that must in reality have been a soup of harmful bacteria). But he has to go when the baths are quiet – when the public space is empty. After retreating to the more private space of his home, he tells his parents, and is treated in the family house. His parents advise him to risk surgery (and the company of pauper patients) in the Sampson hospital. His bed is near the entrance to the eye clinic or ward, which presumably really was there since these miraculous stories had to seem realistic to a local audience. But its position is also symbolic of the discernment of whence his cure will ultimately be derived– the shrine of that patron saint (in effect) of afflictions such as his. There is a space beyond, a space of healing in which sight is restored, which he can glimpse but to which he does not quite yet have access. To cut the rest of the story short: only when he finds the crucial door unwontedly open, and straddles the martyr's tomb in quasi-sexual intimacy, rubbing his genitals against it, will he find relief. But not immediately: that happens only when he re-enters the public space of the bath, at dawn, symbolically the dawn of a new chapter in his life.

That is the spatial interpretation of the hospital and its place in the hierarchy of healing institutions – as seen by a hagiographer, for whom, of course, the saint's shrine rather than the hospital must be the setting of his story's triumphant conclusion. For a final Byzantine example, I could turn to the most discussed and most medicalized hospital, that of the Pantokrator Monastery and imperial mausoleum. But I have argued elsewhere that that hospital did not exist, at least as planned.[36] Instead let us look to a different kind of charitable institution, still in the heart of Constantinople, the great *Orphanotropheion* or orphanage.[37]

4. Eastern apogee

Whether or not established by a St Zotikos in the mid-fourth century – that is, just before the Basileias – the institution comes into the clear light of evidence only in the early twelfth century, by which time its patron saint seems to have been the Apostle Paul. It had long been lavishly endowed with estates and imperial revenues – and its successive directors, the *Orphanotrophoi*, could reasonably see their post as a stepping stone to a prominent career in the Church and at court. But by the time of Alexios I (from 1081) it was, however, clearly not functioning well. Alexios re-endowed it, including not only estates but (probably) tolls or customs dues levied on the city's commercial maritime traffic. Our most vivid, though not necessarily most reliable, information about what Alexios did for the orphanage itself comes from the celebrated memoir of his daughter Anna, the *Alexiad*. Like the Basileias, the restored philanthropic complex included a leprosarium (which may always have been the orphanage's twin institution). And it catered for the disabled as well as orphans. The residences of the disabled, two-storeyed to house both the needy and their designated attendants, formed a circle. That perhaps marked the perimeter of the complex. Within, built around the church of St Paul, were to be found the orphanage itself, a school for the orphans, and houses for deaconesses and female religious. On the Acropolis – the summit of the city – of Constantinople, the emperor 'built in this place another city within the imperial city'.[38] If this highly visible 'new city', set on a hill, was not all Alexios' doing, he certainly restored it and made it financially secure for a time.

This theme – of the hospital as a type of foundation at the heart of urban development, and attractive to funders and benefactors for precisely that reason – could be pursued in a number of directions. The examples so far given have concerned Byzantine history, the tradition of foundation that saw 'the birth of the hospital'.[39] If we look eastward to Baghdad in the ninth to tenth centuries, we can see the beginnings and early development of a distinct tradition of Islamic hospital foundation.[40] This owes much to Byzantine, as well as to Sasanian Persian, exemplars. It also reflects the translations, under court patronage, of medical texts, especially Galen's, from Greek into Arabic. That is relevant because the hospitals were founded by rulers, viziers, and courtiers in the major centres of power and their doctors came to be the hospital doctors too, shuttling between court and hospital in a way that had no precedent in Byzantium. The legal framework for such foundations, though again deriving much from Byzantine and Sasanian law, was also new. The *waqf*, or perpetual pious endowment, did not initially develop to support hospitals but rather seems to have functioned as a family trust.[41] Yet though its main objects came to be the *madrasa* and the mosque, hospitals certainly fell within its scope. And by the twelfth century, royal or elite foundations could be massive complexes, including mosques, mausoleums, and hospitals – as with that of Nur al-Din in Damascus.[42]

The apogee of this development came in the Ottoman empire. Waqfs in general seemed to underlie a considerable proportion of all urban space in the major centres and to determine its very fabric.[43] Complexes including mosques and hospitals became bigger than ever before. The Süleymaniye, of Süleyman I, in Istanbul, comprised (besides a hospital) a mosque big enough to hold several thousand, four colleges (*medrese*), a primary school, a soup kitchen, an insane asylum, a *hamam* (bathhouse), a *caravanserai*, a guest house offering food and lodging to travellers for three nights, and a large public courtyard.[44] Writing of such complexes Singer notes that 'it is easy to understand how a neighbourhood of the city grew up around them, taking advantage of the public and commercial spaces, and the social services that they offered, as well as opportunities for employment. Seen from this perspective, the Süleymaniye and other complexes were high-profile urban development projects and answered the obvious needs of a growing metropolis.[45] Where such foundations were initially extra-mural, as at another

Ottoman capital, Bursa, the city can be seen to have expanded its suburbs to embrace them.[46]

Nothing on this scale could have been found in Byzantium, or in medieval western Europe, although the Hôtel-Dieu in early modern Paris might have approached it. As 'the hospital idea' had, in the earlier Middle Ages, spread slowly from Constantinople and Asia Minor round the Mediterranean and north into the Frankish world, we can discern charitable foundations enhancing the complex of cathedral and bishop's house in the centre of some cities, but not having the obvious effects that a Basil or a Süleyman would have witnessed in their own life times.[47] Later in the Middle Ages, when the evidence of urban topography and its evolution becomes much more plentiful, many hospitals can be seen to have been founded on extra-mural sites, but not because of fear of infection or a precocious predilection for the liminal – that nebulous state once beloved of historians as of anthropologists. Rather, they were taking advantage of the greater availability of building space, and they lay on major thoroughfares, well placed to attract benefactions. They also marked the foci or the boundaries of lay lordships or communal jurisdictions. In idealized views of Renaissance cities, the forerunners of those prospects with which we began, hospitals configured urban topography along with other monuments of civic pride.[48] Even small hospitals in minor conurbations – along with their other functions of helping the poor and redeeming their founders' souls – had a political point to make about urban topography. 'Whether directed towards those visiting or living within the town, these public displays of charity aimed to shape both a day-to-day experience of government and the perception of its reach.'[49] That was written of English towns of the twelfth to thirteenth centuries. But it applies also, for example, to the little hospital that nestled beside, and connected with, the imposing central tower erected by a consul in the French city of Montauban in the early fourteenth century; possibly the best-defended hospital of its age.[50] Abstracted from its particular economic and social context, the view of a hospital's role in urban politics implied by its proximity to that tower is one that Basil of Caesarea could have recognized and endorsed.

Notes

1 Image reproduced by permission of the Wellcome Library, London. For what follows see Christine Stevenson, *Medicine and Magnificence: British Hospital and Asylum Architecture, 1660–1815* (New Haven, CT, 2000), 128.

2 Christine Stevenson, 'Prints "Proper to Shew to Gentlemen": Representing the British Hospital', in John Henderson, Peregrine Horden, and Alessandro Pastore (eds), *The Impact of Hospitals 300–2000* (Oxford, 2007), 195–218.

3 William Maitland, *The History and Survey of London from its Foundation to the Present Time*, vol. 2 (London, 1756), 1322.

4 Frederick Benjamin Kaye (ed.), *Bernard Mandeville, The Fable of the Bees, or, Private Vices, Publick Benefits* (Oxford, 1924), vol. 1, 261.

5 Stevenson, *Medicine and Magnificence*, 184, citing Michel Foucault et al., *Les machines à guérir* (Brussels, 1979), 94. For context see Tim McHugh, *Hospital Politics in Seventeenth-Century France: The Crown, Urban Elites and the Poor* (Aldershot, 2007).

6 Gregory of Nazianzus, Oration 43.63, 1–7, ed. and trans. Jean Bernardi, *Grégoire de Nazianze, Discours* 42, 43 (Sources chrétiennes, vol. 384) (Paris, 1992), 260–262. My translation differs slightly from Bernardi's French version.

7 For full detail and references on what follows, see Peregrine Horden, 'Poverty, Charity and the Invention of the Hospital', in Scott Fitzgerald Johnson (ed.), *The Oxford Companion to Late Antiquity* (Oxford, 2012), 715–743, esp. 715–718. See also Brian Daley, 'Building a New City. The Cappadocian Fathers and the Rhetoric of Philanthropy', *Journal of Early Christian Studies* 7 (1999), 431–461. For the genre of funerary oration, see David Konstan, 'How to Praise a Friend: St. Gregory of Nazianzus's Funeral Oration for St. Basil the Great', in Tomas Hägg, Philip Rousseau, and Christian Høgel (eds), *Greek Biography and Panegyric in Late Antiquity* (Berkeley, CA, 2000), 160–179.

8 Gregory of Nyssa, *Opera Omnia*, vol. X/1, ed. Otto Lendle (Leiden, 1990), 109–134.

9 Basil of Caesarea, Letter 94, ed. Yves Courtonne, *Saint Basile, Lettres*, 3 vols (Paris, 1957–1966), vol. I, 204–208.

10 *Gregorii presbyteri vita sancti Gregorii theologi*, 11, ed. and trans. Xavier Lequeux (Corpus Christianorum series graeca, vol. 44) (Leuven, 2001), 156–159.

11 See now Peter Brown, *Through the Eye of a Needle: Wealth, the Fall of Rome, and the Making of Christianity in the West, 350–550 AD* (Princeton, NJ: 2012).

12 Owsei Temkin, *Hippocrates in a World of Pagans and Christians* (Princeton, NJ, 1991), 172–177.

13 Suraiya Faroqhi, *Men of Modest Substance: House Owners and House Property in Seventeenth-Century Ankara and Kayseri* (Cambridge, 1987), 43.

14 Peter Brown, *Poverty and Leadership in the Later Roman Empire* (Hanover, 2002), 29–35. Brown, *Eye of a Needle*, 35–36.

15 Horden, 'Poverty', 719–720.

16 Paul Veyne, *Le pain et le cirque. Sociologie historique d'un pluralisme politique* (Paris 1976) remains the classic account.

17 Brown, *Poverty and Leadership*, 29.

18 For hospital naming see Peregrine Horden, 'Alms and the Man: Hospital Founders in Byzantium', in Henderson et al., *The Impact of Hospitals 300–2000*, 59–76 [reprinted as Ch. 9 in the present volume].

19 For more detail on what follows see Horden, 'Poverty', 719–720. Also, for a different approach, Richard Finn, *Almsgiving in the Later Roman Empire* (Oxford, 2006), 228–231.

20 Finn, *Almsgiving*, 74–76.

21 Firmus of Caesarea, Letter 43, ed. Marie-Ange Calvet-Sebasti and Pierre-Louis Gatier, *Firmus de Césarée, Lettres* (Sources chrétiennes, vol. 350) (Paris, 1989), 166–167.

22 For some context see David Gwynn, *Athanasius of Alexandria: Bishop, Theologian, Ascetic, Father* (Oxford, 2012), 39–40, 137–138.

23 Jean Bouffartigue, 'L'authenticité de la Lettre 84 de l'empereur Julien', *Revue de philologie* 79 (2005), 231–242, defends the authenticity of the document in question.

24 Basil, *Letter* 94.
25 Theodoret of Cyr, *Ecclesiastical History*, 4.19, ed. Léon Parmentier and Günther Christian Hansen, *Theodoret Kirchengeschichte*, 3rd edn (Berlin, 1998), 245. I am much indebted to the dossier of texts on hospitals as well as the discussion of them in Mark Anderson, 'Hospitals, Hospices and Shelters for the Poor in Late Antiquity' (PhD dissertation, Yale University, 2012), esp. 232–238, and to the author for permission to cite his work here.
26 Aleksandr Petrovich Kazhdan, Alice-Mary Talbot, and Anthony Cutler (eds), *The Oxford Dictionary of Byzantium*, 3 vols (Oxford, 1991), s.v. 'euageis oikoi'.
27 Basil, *Letters* 142, 143; Anderson, 'Hospitals', 231–232.
28 See Timothy Miller, 'The Sampson Hospital of Constantinople', *Byzantinische Forschungen* 15 (1990), 101–135. I am greatly indebted to this paper for details of the various biographies of Sampson, set out in n. 1, while differing from several of its interpretations. See also Anderson, 'Hospitals', 209–212.
29 Dionysios Stathakopoulos, 'Discovering a Military Order of the Crusades: The Hospital of St. Sampson of Constantinople', *Viator* 37 (2006), 255–268.
30 Miller, 'Sampson Hospital', 104–105.
31 Gilbert Dagron, *Naissance d'une capitale. Constantinople et ses institutions de 330 à 451* (Paris, 1974).
32 Miller, 'Sampson Hospital', 101–102.
33 Anderson, 'Hospitals', 213, nos 25, 26; Stathakopoulos, 'Military Order', 259.
34 Miller, 'Sampson Hospital', 116–117, 120–122. The miracles of Artemios were edited in Athanasios Papadopoulos-Kerameus, *Varia graeca sacra* (St Petersburg, 1909). This edition was reprinted, with translation, in Virgil Crisafulli and John Nesbitt, *The Miracles of St. Artemios* (Leiden, 1997).
35 Ibid. 127–129, Miracle 21.
36 Peregrine Horden, 'How Medicalized Were Byzantine Hospitals?' in Neithard Bulst and Karl-Heinz Spiess (eds), *Sozialgeschichte Mittelalterlicher Hospitäler* (Vorträge und Forschungen, vol. 65) (Ostfildern, 2007), 213–235.
37 For what follows see esp. Timothy Miller, *The Orphans of Byzantium: Child Welfare in the Christian Empire* (Washington, DC, 2003), 176–246.
38 Alexiad, 15.7.4, ed. Bernard Leib, *Anne Comnène, Alexiade*, vol. 3 (Paris, 1945), 215.
39 Timothy Miller, *The Birth of the Hospital in the Byzantine Empire*, 2nd edn (Baltimore, MD, 1997).
40 For what follows see Peter E. Pormann, 'Islamic Hospitals in the Time of Al-Muqtadir', in John Nawas (ed.), *'Abbasid Studies* II (Orientalia Lovanensia Analecta, vol. 177) (Leuven, 2010), 337–381. I return to the topic in more detail in a forthcoming monograph.
41 Adam Sabra, 'Public Policy or Private Charity? The Ambivalent Character of Islamic Charitable Endowments', in Michael Borgolte (ed.), *Stiftungen in Christentum, Judentum und Islam vor der Moderne. Auf der Suche nach ihren Gemeinsamkeiten und Unterschieden in religiösen Grundlagen, praktischen Zwecken und historischen Transformationen* (Berlin, 2005), 95–108.
42 Peter E. Pormann and Emilie Savage-Smith, *Medieval Islamic Medicine* (Edinburgh, 2007), 98–99.
43 Richard van Leeuwen, *Waqfs and Urban Structure: The Case of Ottoman Damascus* (Leiden, 1999. [See also Ethel Sara Wolper, *Cities and Saints: Sufism and the Transformation of Urban Space in Medieval Anatolia* (University Park, PA, 2003), for the transformative effect of powerful dervish lodges on urban space in thirteenth-century Anatolia.]

44 Godfrey Goodwin, *A History of Ottoman Architecture* (London, 1987), 215–217.
45 Amy Singer, *Charity in Islamic Societies* (Cambridge, 2008), 104. I am indebted to Professor Singer for further advice here.
46 Miri Shefer-Mossensohn, *Ottoman Medicine. Healing and Medical Institutions, 1500–1700* (Albany, NY, 2009), 154–155; Aptullah Kuran, 'A Spatial Study of Three Ottoman Capitals. Bursa, Edirne, and Istanbul', *Muqarnas* 13 (1996), 117.
47 Peregrine Horden, 'The Earliest Hospitals in Byzantium, Western Europe, and Islam', in Mark Cohen (ed.), *Journal of Interdisciplinary History* 35 (2005), 361–389 (special issue, 'Poverty and Charity: Judaism, Christianity, Islam') [reprinted as Ch. 2 in the present volume]; Thomas Sternberg, *Orientalium more secutus. Räume und Institutionen der Caritas des 5. bis 7. Jahrhunderts in Gallien* (Münster, 1991).
48 John Henderson, *The Renaissance Hospital: Healing the Body and Healing the Soul* (New Haven, CT, 2006), 3–12. I am grateful to Professor Henderson for discussion.
49 Sethina Watson, 'City as Charter: Charity and the Lordship of English Towns, 1170–1250', in Caroline Goodson, Anne E. Lester, and Carol Symes (eds), *Cities, Texts, and Social Networks. Experiences and Perceptions of Medieval Urban Space* (Farnham, 2010), 235–62 (quotation from p. 262).
50 Claude Collu, 'Urbanisme et cadres d'assistance à Montauban (XIIIe–XVI siècles)', in François-Olivier Touati (ed.), *Archéologie et architecture hospitalières de l'antiquité tardive à l'aube des temps modernes* (Paris, 2004), 305–324.

9

ALMS AND THE MAN
Hospital founders in Byzantium

'Pride and vanity have built more hospitals than all the Virtues together.'[1] So wrote the Dutch physician Bernard de Mandeville in *The Fable of the Bees* (1714). He added:

> Men are so tenacious of their Possessions, and Selfishness is so rivited in our nature, that whoever in any ways can conquer it shall have the Applause of the Publick.[2]

Mandeville was composing his satire on the eve of the 'voluntary hospital' movement in his adopted England. Georgian propertied classes found in the voluntary hospital a way of dignifying their pride and vanity and mitigating their possessiveness. Their subscriptions to hospitals purchased not only the esteem of their peers but the right to nominate suitable deserving patients. It was seen as prudent to help such people get back to work.[3] It was a social obligation, a Christian duty, a loan to God – Proverbs 19.17, but with extra resonance in the early Georgian economy – a loan that would be repaid at Judgement Day. Not least, it was a pleasure. As the *Gentleman's Magazine* put it in 1732, one year before Mandeville's death, charity was 'the most lasting, valuable and exquisite pleasure'.[4]

I

What would Mandeville have made of Byzantine hospitals and their founders? The *philanthropia* of the empire's inhabitants in general, and its particular expression in charitable institutions, has been lauded from early Byzantine times onwards. Most recently and influentially, some of those charitable institutions have been the subject of an 'upbeat', optimistic monograph by Tim Miller, *The Birth of the Hospital in the Byzantine Empire*. Yet, in all the literature, there has been surprisingly little discussion of founder's motives. It is as if it were enough to rehearse the biblical and patristic proof texts on almsgiving, and then invoke economic circumstances – that is, clear need – as the demand that straightforwardly

195

induced the charitable supply – compassion for the poor.[5] This confidence that the answer is obvious is one possible reason for lack of interest in the subject of motivation. Another, equally powerful, is paucity of evidence. The period of Byzantine history that concerns me runs from the fourth century to the twelfth, though with some excursion into the later, Palaiologan period (after the end of Latin rule in 1261).[6] Throughout that period, we mostly lack the kinds of personal detail that would give some glimpse of what really motivated founders. With a few exceptions, to which I shall return, we also lack even the more formulaic statements of founders' aspirations: what they wanted people to think were their motives. Yet it is, I think, still possible to recover something of the Byzantine founder's mind-set.

The foundations to be considered here have been arbitrarily excerpted from the wider subject of charity in Byzantium. They were for the overnight accommodation of the poor, transients, the sick, lepers, the old, the orphaned, occasionally the blind, and others. I shall refer to all these for convenience as hospitals, generalizing about them somewhat as Roman law did in its category of *piae causae* (literally pious causes) or *euageis oikoi* (holy houses) – a category that could, however, also include, as I shall not, churches and monasteries.[7] Such foundations were above all religious establishments. This was so not only in a basic legal sense: whatever their origin in the foundations of private individuals (clerical or lay), of churches, of monks, or of members of imperial families, hospitals tended to fall under ecclesiastical jurisdiction. More importantly, even in the most 'medicalized' hospital – the one with the most doctors – the Divine Liturgy was far more central to daily life than the ward round.[8] Yet it remains hard to pin down the particular way in which that religious aspect, and the theology underpinning it, affected, or reflected, Byzantine hospital founders' motivation.

Contrast for the moment the (as I see it) difficult topic of Byzantine foundations with the clearer picture that presents itself to a *later* medievalist studying, say, England.[9] In a typical later medieval hospital – a hospital that housed a few paupers and pensioners – the chief beneficiary was not the inmates but the founder. The secular gratitude and recognition of the poor and all those (such as nurses, servants, and priests) who benefited from the hospital's existence could be expressed in prayer for the founder's soul. That gratitude was constantly renewed in the recitation of foundation statutes and rolls of benefactors, as well as in masses for the dead. The founder's name rang in the ears of the grateful poor, and his or her image assailed them on every side. Such was *memoria*, that (primarily liturgical) commemoration of the dead on which scholars, especially in Germany, have lavished such attention.[10] In these circumstances it was, perhaps, much harder to forget than to remember. And the purpose of remembering was theologically explicit; it was either to assure the founder's place in heaven or to abbreviate his or her passage through purgatory. The connection between one's own salvation and the almsgiving, prayers, fasting, and (particularly) masses of other people was clear – even quantifiable. With its 'treasury of merits', its complex transactions between living and dead, this really was a 'spiritual economy' – aspects of which might have appealed to the Georgians if they could have overcome their Protestant aversion.[11]

Many facets of this western hospital scene are familiar to Byzantinists. How could they not be, given the common patristic roots of both eastern and western doctrinal traditions? But there is a temptation to see the less tightly coherent Byzantine scene either as a somehow incomplete version of Europe or as a completely alien religious culture. In this as in so many respects, however, Byzantium is both similar to and different from the West. The hard task is to disentangle those similarities and differences.

Pursuing them in what follows, I shall look first, for background, at the theology of almsgiving in late antiquity (section II). Then (section III), with reference to two of the most significant Byzantine hospitals, I shall explore the methodological problem of inferring founders' intentions from the various explanations that historians have been tempted to give of their foundations. Next (in section IV), I shall review some Byzantine evidence for the mixed motives of hospitals patrons – especially concern for reputation in this world as evidenced in the little-considered topic of the naming of hospitals. After that (section V), I shall give some examples of the most elaborate accounts of founders' aspirations that survive from Byzantium: those found in *typika* (foundation documents), with all their liturgical and commemorative specifications and their hopes of everlasting benefit to be derived from acts of philanthropy. Finally (in section VI), I shall ask what these benefits were thought to be in a religious culture which had no formal doctrine of purgatory. Why should hospital patients pray for a deceased founder?

II

First, the theology. The basic doctrine concerning almsgiving and its link with salvation, fortunately, is clear enough. The need for charity to the poor is emphasized again and again in the Judaeo-early Christian material from the Deuteronomic code onwards.[12] He who sows in almsgiving shall reap the fruit of life (Hosea 10:12). Almsgiving atones for sins (Sirach 3:30). This tradition Matthew especially, among the gospel writers, glosses with the familiar injunction to lay up treasures in heaven, not on earth. And he adds (at 25:31f.) the parable of the sheep and the goats, according to which, of course, the basis for the Last Judgement will be the treatment of Christ present in anyone who is hungry, thirsty, naked, and so on.

If anything, the emphasis on the salvific value of charity only increases in early Christian literature. 'Almsgiving is as good as repentance from sin, fasting is better than prayer; almsgiving is better than either.'[13]

> When the rich man rests upon the poor [...] he believes that what he does for the poor can find a reward with God, for the poor man is rich in intercession.[14]

This is developed at great length in well-known homilies by, above all, John Chrysostom among the fourth-century Fathers. For him, alms erase post-baptismal sins, preserve from damnation, procure God's mercy; they are essential to salvation. These effects can be obtained for others: alms can be given vicariously – on behalf of the dead.[15] Commemoration of almsgivers came chiefly in prayers and in petitions in the liturgies of Chrysostom and Basil. 'Remember Lord those who are mindful of the poor. Give them your rich and heavenly gifts.'[16]

Such is the theological context for the emergence of Christian hospitals. Doubtless it is also a considerable part of the explanation for that emergence. In what follows I do not mean to cast aspersions on founders. Most, if not all, will have been deeply aware of the Bible's charitable imperative, will have felt some compassion for the poor, and will, especially, have been anxious about their prospects in the afterlife. A saint in the making will have been acutely – to us, perhaps disproportionately – aware of the tiniest spiritual blemish. For such a blemish might put the 'bosom of Abraham' beyond reach. A bishop or priest, answerable for his conduct towards the souls entrusted to his care, will have been hypersensitive to any pastoral failing on which divine judgement might focus. An 'ordinary' lay sinner, and still more an emperor with blood on his hands, will have wondered if hell could be avoided. Take for example the story recorded by John Moschus in the early seventh century, about how the Emperor Zeno was saved from the retribution of the Mother of God on behalf of a woman he had wronged. 'Believe me, woman,' says the Virgin appearing in a vision to the wronged woman's mother, 'I frequently tried to get satisfaction for you, but his [God's] right hand prevents me' – because, Moschus adds, the emperor was a very good almsgiver.[17] All – emperors, saints, others – in their different ways could seek spiritual merit, as well as earthly acclaim, through the founding of a hospital.

There must, however, be more to be said. Let us take two examples from opposite ends of my chosen period. First, some of the first hospitals we know about; second, the best-documented, and most impressive, Byzantine hospital, from the early twelfth century.

III

To begin at the beginning, with the earliest Christian hospitals. It is not enough to see hospitals as an inevitable outgrowth of the early Christian charitable impulse, a natural development from doorstep distributions to overnight shelter, and therefore needing no particular explanation beyond the religious motives that I have just outlined. The early Christian hospital was an invention. It was, apparently, invented quite suddenly – not in Jewish communities of the first three centuries CE, not in *pre*-Constantinian Christian communities, not even in the reign of Constantine himself, for all his lavish patronage of the Church. It was an invention of (roughly) the 350s, in the reign of Constantius II, and in the heart of Anatolia, not just in Constantinople.[18]

Why? Many explanations have been offered. They have been couched in terms of the demography of the poor; of competition for support between Arian and Catholic; of the self-expression of an extremely ascetic form of urban monasticism; and, most recently, by Peter Brown, as an aspect of the fourth-century bishops' 'pitch' for urban leadership, and a visible 'quid pro quo' for imperial patronage.[19] 'Whom do we harm', wrote St Basil, founder of the first big philanthropic 'multiplex' at Caesarea around 370, 'if we build shelters for passers-by who need someone's attention because of ill health [...]?'[20] The answer is that quite a few will have been disturbed by his hospital's affront to traditional civic values, even to civic topography. And this despite the fact that hospitals can also be seen as traditional euergetism (civic beneficence) continued by non-traditional means. The bishop, according to Brown, was in a sense inventing the poor – and 'a fortiori' the hospital for the poor. He was seeing them as 'good to think with'. The hospital was not just a new type of building (it had precedents but few close analogues in the classical world). It was a conceptual tool in an urban revolution.

My purpose in reviewing these various explanations of what has rightly been called 'the birth of the hospital in the Byzantine empire'[21] is not to adjudicate among them. (We do not have to choose; several explanations will have applied; the hospital is always an 'overdetermined' phenomenon.) My purpose is, rather, to draw attention to a methodological problem. All these explanations offered by historians – essentially functional explanations – can, *mutatis mutandis*, be converted into guesses about founder's explicit or half-formed aspirations or motives. How we establish the criteria for a plausible guess is the methodological problem to which I have referred – and to which I am not sure that we yet have a solution.

A second illustration of the problem, as substitute for a solution. If Basil's is the first of the big foundations, the last, and in any ways the most impressive of them before the Latin conquest, is that of the Pantocrator founded, in effect jointly, by the emperor John II Comnenos and his wife, Irene, in 1126. This monastery and its hospital is famed for its *typikon* or foundation charter (to which I return below), and for the number of doctors and support staff that the imperial couple planned for the hospital's patients – an almost 1:1 ratio.[22]

Some historians have seen this hospital as a fantasy that existed only on parchment; some as a short-lived experiment in intensive medical care; some as a symbol of the modernity of Byzantine community medicine and as a guide to the standard facilities of other, less well-documented establishments.[23] I align myself with those who see the hospital as highly unusual, at least in its medical aspect. I think that the medical presence planned for it can be analysed in terms of an imperial extension, to the medical profession, of what Paul Magdalino has called 'lordship over the professional classes'.[24] Indeed, through his patronage of hospital doctors, who were clearly not to be workaday quacks but 'consultants', the emperor can be seen as beginning to consolidate, even to create, the upper echelons of that profession.

I am encouraged in this interpretation by a comparison with a later hospital. The value of associating a major imperial foundation (and, as we shall see, family mausoleum) with a heavy medical presence in the monastery's hospital seems to have been as evident to the Palaiologans as it was to the Comneni. Despite the eulogies of Michael VIII's *philanthropia* to have come down to us, the first clearly documented hospital foundation after 1261 was undertaken by Michael's widow, Theodora, towards the end of the century. She restored the tenth-century monastery established, it seems, by Constantine Lips, turning it into a large monastic multiplex with fifty nuns and a hospital for twelve female patients clearly modelled on the women's section of the Pantocrator hospital. Twelve patients were to be looked after by three male doctors and one assistant, one nurse, one head pharmacist and two others, six attendants, a phlebotomist, three servants, a cook, and a laundress.[25]

It is one thing, though, for me to analyse all this in terms of imperial patronage of medicine; quite another to suggest that this was how the founders' thoughts ran as they drafted their *typika*. The methodological problem remains, ultimately, because of a lack of sufficiently intimate evidence about founders' ideas. In her splendid study of benefactors' motives in Turin, *Charity and Power in Early Modern Italy*, Sandra Cavallo takes religious motives as a standard lowest common denominator among benefactors.[26] She could thus leave religion virtually on one side and look at how changing expressions of institutional charity reflected changing political structures and concomitantly changing aspirations among elite benefactors. None of this subtlety is possible for a Byzantinist concerned with the early and middle phases of the empire's history.

IV

Of course, Byzantine writers were as aware as any modern scholar that founders' motives were mixed. They also knew that those motives were not always commendable. In one of his sermons on loving the poor, Gregory of Nyssa, in the fourth century, for example, seemingly castigated those who saw hospitals as a means of getting beggars off the streets and out of sight.[27] The most emphatic identification of inappropriate motives for philanthropy

comes in the well-known novel (new law) of the Emperor Nicephorus
Phocas, perhaps drafted by Symeon Metaphrastes, and issued in 964 in a
vain attempt to protect the empire's financial and military base from erosion
by the tax dodges of 'the powerful'.[28]

> What is then the matter with the people who, moved by the wish to
> do something to please the Lord and to have their sins pardoned,
> neglect thus the easy commandment of Christ which enjoins them
> to be free of care and, selling their property, to distribute its pro-
> ceeds among the poor? But instead of following this commandment
> they [...] subject themselves to more worries by seeking to establish
> [private] monasteries, hospitals and houses for the old. In times gone
> by when such institutions were not sufficient, the establishment of
> them was praiseworthy and very useful [...] But when their num-
> ber has increased greatly and has become disproportionate to the
> need and people still turn to the founding of monasteries, how is
> it possible to think that this good is not mixed with evil [...]? And
> moreover, who will not say that piety has become a screen for vanity
> [Mandeville would have enjoyed this] when those who do good, do so
> in order that they may be seen by all the others? They are not satisfied
> that their virtuous deeds be witnessed by their contemporaries only,
> but wish also that future generations be not ignorant of them.

The emperor had his own reasons for exaggerating hospital founders'
pursuit of worldly renown. When he asserted that the empire already had
enough hospitals, he was not offering a considered estimate of the needs of
the poor. Still, he raises for us the question of how easy it was in Byzantium
to be remembered for having founded a hospital.

One way in which we can pursue this question is through the topic of
hospital names. A late antique commentator on Aristotle's *Art of Rhetoric*
puts hospitals first in a list – before churches – of things that perpetuate the
memory of an individual after death.[29] Was the philosopher's advice heeded?
St Basil's suburban philanthropic centre at Caesarea came to be called the
Basileias, but not (one guesses) at his instigation. So far as we can tell from
Procopius in his panegyric, *De Aedificiis*, the emperor Justinian, one of the
great founders and restorers of Byzantine hospitals, does not seem to have
named any of them after himself: uncharacteristic modesty. The Pantocrator
hospital, to which I have also already referred, was named for its monastery,
not its imperial founder. As for other major establishments in Constantinople: the premier orphanage was St Paul's;[30] St Sampson did found the Sampson hospital, but exactly when is obscure, and the name probably derived
from popular association rather than the holy man's choosing.[31]

How many known hospitals in the early Byzantine empire are in fact
securely named after their founders as a way of preserving those founders'

memoria? The apparent answer is: surprisingly few.[32] And this is not, as it would be in the West, because most hospitals are named for saints such as John the Baptist, although Theodore and George do have a few Byzantine adherents. Some 150 hospitals and similar establishments are known from the provinces of the empire from the fourth to the eighth centuries. Only about twenty of these are apparently named after their founders. Where a name is preserved at all, it usually identifies the hospital by its location or its mother religious house.

Now the figures that I have given are no more than rough estimates. There will have been many more hospitals founded than we know about. Of those that are known to us, only a few (about eight) are recorded in surviving inscriptions. But there must once have been many more of those inscriptions, each of which would presumably have announced the founder to all visitors and inmates. Even in the minority of cases in which the identity of a founder is recorded, that is not necessarily the same as the hospital's being named after him or her. The transmission of such information was not necessarily subject to the founder's control. Only in the Egyptian papyri do founders' names occur with any frequency, though still in a minority of the seventy-five references to hospitals now recovered.[33]

These crude statistics concern the provinces. In the capital, the picture is a little different. I think that twenty-three out of some fifty-eight establishments were known by the founder's name (or the founder's status, as with the 'Hospital of the King' (*tou Krale*), founded *c*.1300 by the Serbian Stephan Milutin).[34] But in so many cases the evidence is ambiguous, and a fair number of these names are found in the strange writings of those not wholly reliable historians of urban folklore known as the patriographers.[35]

V

Ultimately, the renown that came from founding a hospital, whether it was transmitted orally, in the name of the establishment, or in an inscription over the door, was only a means to an end. Secular commemoration was principally valuable as an incitement to liturgical commemoration. I come back to the religious aspect of hospitals, shifting from the earlier to the later part of my period because that is where the evidence is. As John Thomas has commented,[36] after the papyri the most vivid evidence for Byzantine religious foundations comes from monastic *typika* or foundation documents. Here, in *typika* drawn up for houses with philanthropic establishments attached, we read founders' own characterisation of their religious motives. Naturally they write in acceptable and predictable formulae: these are not 'confessions'. But they are the nearest that we can come to the mentality of a hospital founder of the eleventh and twelfth centuries.

Thus in 1077 the senator and judge Michael Attaliates founds an almshouse and a monastery with two dependent poorhouses.[37] He owes thanks to God for allowing him to rise from a humble and foreign background to the rank of senator, although he is a great sinner. He thinks daily about the account that he will have to render in the world to come, and wants to grant the Almighty some small pleasure. The poorhouses will, he hopes, propitiate his sins. (They would also effectively protect his family property.)[38]

A second example: in 1083 Gregory Pakourianos establishes a monastery in Bačkovo with three hospitals and with outdoor distributions.[39] He gives to God the ransom for his soul (Matthew 20.28), hoping to gain release from sins and from the threat of hellfire. On the anniversaries of his death and his relatives' deaths there are, for the salvation of their souls, to be offerings of the divine mysteries, memorial feasts, and distributions to the poor.

As we should expect from what can be learned about the Pantocrator hospital, the most elaborate provisions of this kind are to be found in that monastery's *typkon*.[40] In this mausoleum, monks, clerics, patients, and doctors are all intercessors:

> Yet though I am not able to fathom the depths of thine incomprehensible wisdom which beneficially manages our lives, I [the emperor, somewhat suppressing the role of his wife, Irene] give thanks for thy patience and at last according to my capabilities I unveil my enterprise, bringing thee a band of ascetics, a precious gathering of monks, whose duty it is to devote themselves to the monastery and propitiate thy goodness for our sins [...] Along with these I bring thee, the Lover of goodness, some fellow-servants, whom thou in thy compassion called brothers [Matthew 25.40], worn out by old age and toil, oppressed by poverty and suffering from diseases of many kinds [...] We bring thee these people as ambassadors to intercede for our sins; by them we attract thy favor and through them we plead for thy compassion.

The emperor's memory (*mnemosyne*), and that of his immediate family buried in the mausoleum, were to be lastingly preserved in several ways: (1) by regular mention in the daily services of the monastery and four times a week at services attended by hospital patients; (2) in two candles burning at the emperor's tomb; (3) by the offering of a daily communion loaf; (4) in weekly prayers for the dead at his tomb; (5) through annual commemorations associated with a visit to the monastery by a great icon of the Virgin.[41] And this was not all, because the *typikon* refers to other commemorations outlined in a separate confidential document, which does not survive.

It should not be thought that this kind of arrangement was at all new to the eleventh or twelfth century. The *typika* are bringing older practices into the light of our evidence. For instance, an edifying tale that is the sole survivor from the biography of a ninth-century recluse, Isaiah of Nicomedia, shows the extreme spiritual danger risked by a high-ranking official on the point of death. He had instructed his wife to distribute his fortune to the poor, but had oddly refused to pay fees to priests to celebrate the Divine Liturgy on the fortieth day after his demise.[42] A law of Leo VI (c.900) expresses concern about private foundations that cannot support their complement of priests so that the divine mysteries are not celebrated. The 'memorial' consequences of that failing are clear: anniversaries of the dead pass unhallowed for lack of priests, to the detriment of both those who live here below and those 'who possess the life thereafter'.[43]

Founders rightly feared that their provisions would not meet the expenses of the commemorations that they planned. Some of John II's arrangements had apparently broken down within less than a decade after his death. As a monk wrote to the emperor's daughter-in-law, he

> desired very strongly [...] that his memory should not disappear into oblivion, and left no stone unturned in planning it and tried very hard in this connection, but failed.[44]

VI

If founders rightly feared such failures, they also feared that their foundations, however well-intentioned and piously managed, would be insufficient to expiate their sins. What would happen to them? If they did not reach 'the bosom of Abraham', could they yet avoid the fires of hell? Orthodox thought, as I understand it, has always discouraged questioning what happens to the soul after death, or formulating any precise or mechanistic connection between the fate of the dead and the prayers and memorial liturgies of the living. God is not to be bribed or bargained with in prayer.

Despite the endorsement of prayers for the dead by such figures as John the Almsgiver onwards,[45] and the clear evidence of liturgical commemoration, some monastic moralists and church authorities discouraged the idea that the prayers of others can have any effect on one's soul in the afterlife. Paul of Evergetis (d. 1054) in his *Synagoge* offers a stern warning: repent now, because there is nothing you or anyone else can do after death to change your fate in the other world. The second *hypostasis* of the first book of the *Synagoge*, which became the chief manual for the monastic and spiritual life, states categorically that, 'as long as we are in the present life, we must do good here, and not delay until the future. For after death, we cannot set things aright.'[46]

Within Orthodoxy there was thus room for a spectrum of opinion. The gaps that official pronouncements left were, for the ordinary believer, filled in by a variety of written 'questions and answers', hagiographical anecdotes, edifying tales, apocryphal revelations, and visions that circulated throughout Byzantine history in the penumbra of orthodoxy.[47] Some of the material was cautious. A question addressed to Anastasius of Sinai in the seventh century produced an answer to the effect that suffrages for the dead are of some use for light sins, but it is better to rely on one's own actions.[48] Other tales showed in more detail why the dead were worth remembering.[49] I give two visionary examples. The first concerns Philentolos. He was renowned both for his charity (he built a hospital) and for his sexual conquests. After his death an archbishop was consulted about the fate of his soul but, with true orthodoxy, claimed not to know. Instead a hermit was granted a vision of Philentolos suspended between Paradise and Hell.

The second example is a vision attributed to a nun, Anastasia, in an apocalypse of *c*.1000. This shows how the charity and good behaviour of the living does actually determine the condition of the dead – the dead in a zone of interim punishment that is not hell, but is not some hitherto undetected Byzantine purgatory either.[50]

> And again the angel turned back to where the sinners were being punished, and said to them, 'Behold! Here is a person from this life [Anastasia], and I am about to return her again to there, by the command of God.' And all [the sinners] raised a great voice to me, saying, 'We have left behind parents and children and wives. Passing over, send a message to them, so that they might be vigilant, lest they also come into these fearsome places of punishment – but truly, also, *so that they might make supplication to God on our behalf, and [do] almsgiving, namely that very money that we designated for the salvation of our souls. They have not given it, and we do not find any respite.* [Tell them]: you will come here too, where we are being punished. Look – do not be condemned by the righteous judge, because of our designations!'
>
> Then I saw someone else, and they threw him into the pitch, which boiled over a thousand fathoms deep. And the angel said to him, 'She is from the vain world, and I am about to return her back there again, so send a message, if you wish.' And [the sinner] cried out with weeping and lamentation and gnashing, saying, 'I am from the west, Peter by name, from the *kastron* of Corinth, by rank, *protospatharios*. And in my presence a person neither rejoiced nor obtained anything, but I wronged many in the vain life, and snatched away estates, wronged widows and orphans, arranged murders and did not judge justly because of money. *I never practised almsgiving, and the earth did not accept my body*, but God did not conceal my soul. I left behind wealth and much treasure. Report these things to my wife and to my children: be vigilant, lest you enter these fearsome places of punishment! *Be zealous through almsgiving, and supplicate God, and give these things on my behalf, that I might have rest from this bitter torment!*'

In his message from the place of punishment, the sinner did not mention hospitals as a form of almsgiving. But clearly if he had founded a hospital, or if his family at once proceeded to found one, his punishments would not be so severe. That was a message indeed worth remembering. It reveals to us a Byzantium that we do not find in the usual kinds of evidence. It is a Byzantium that is closer to the West in its theology of prudential hospital foundation than we might have expected – the West in the earlier Middle Ages, before the 'birth of Purgatory'.[51]

Notes

1 With the permission of the publishers, Akademie Verlag, this paper draws on material first presented in my 'Memoria, Salvation, and Other Motives of Byzantine Philanthropists', in M. Borgolte (ed.), *Stiftungen in Christentum, Judentum und Islam vor der Moderne* (Berlin, 2005), pp. 137–146.

2 *The Fable of the Bees, or, Private Vices, Publick Benefits*, ed. F. B. Kaye (Oxford, 1924), I, p. 261.

3 R. Porter, 'The Gift Relation: Philanthropy and Provincial Hospitals in Eighteenth-Century England', in L. Granshaw and R. Porter (eds), *The Hospital in History* (London, 1989), pp. 162–163.

4 Quoted ibid. p. 162.

5 T. S. Miller, *The Birth of the Hospital in the Byzantine Empire*, 2nd edn (Baltimore, MD, 1997). See also D. J. Constantelos, *Byzantine Philanthropy and Social Welfare*, 2nd edn (New Rochelle, NY, 1991), esp. pp. 15–21 on founders' motives, and E. Patlagean, *Pauvreté économique et pauvreté sociale à Byzance 4e–7e siècle* (Paris, 1977), pp. 185–188, 231–235, for the initial demographic and political setting. For more recent work, see P. Horden, 'The Earliest Hospitals in Byzantium, Western Europe, and Islam', *Journal of Interdisciplinary History* 35 (2005), pp. 361–389 [reprinted as Ch. 2 in this volume]

6 On which see D. Stathakopoulos, 'Stiftungen von Spitälern in spätbyzantinischer Zeit (1261–1453)', in Borgolte, *Stiftungen*, pp. 147–157.

7 A. P. Kazhdan et al. (eds), *The Oxford Dictionary of Byzantium*, 3 vols (New York, 1991), s.v. 'euageis oikoi'.

8 P. Horden, 'Religion as Medicine: Music in Medieval Hospitals', in P. Biller and J. Ziegler (eds), *Religion and Medicine in the Middle Ages* (Woodbridge, 2001), pp. 135–153.

9 C. Rawcliffe, *Medicine for the Soul: The Life, Death and Resurrection of an English Medieval Hospital* (Stroud, 1999), pp. 103–132. See also S. Sweetinburgh, *The Role of the Hospital in Medieval England: Gift Giving and the Spiritual Economy* (Dublin, 2004).

10 K. Schmid and J. Wollasch (eds), *Memoria: der geschichtliche Zeugniswert des liturgischen Gedenkens im Mittelalter* (Munich, 1984); O. G. Oexle, 'Memoria und Memorialüberlieferung im früheren Mittelalter', *Frühmittelalterliche Studien* 10 (1976), pp. 70–95.

11 J. Chiffoleau, *La comptabilité de l'au-delà: les hommes, la mort et la religion dans la région d'Avignon à la fin du moyen âge (vers 1320–vers 1480)* (Rome, 1980), remains classic.

12 R. M. Grant, *Early Christianity and Society* (London, 1978), pp. 124–145. For what follows see now also R. Finn, *Almsgiving in the Later Roman Empire: Christian Promotion and Practice (313–450)* (Oxford, 2006), esp. pp. 29–30,

177–182. [Also G. A. Anderson, *Charity: The Place of the Poor in the Biblical Tradition* (New Haven, CT, 2015); D. J. Downs, *Alms: Charity, Reward, and Atonement in Early Christianity* (Waco, TX, 2016).]

13 *II Clement* 16.4, ed. and trans. B. D. Ehrman, *The Apostolic Fathers*, 2 vols, Loeb Classical Library (Cambridge, MA, 2003), I, p. 122. Trans. quoted is from Grant, *Early Christianity*, p. 128.

14 Hermas, *The Shepherd* 51 (Parable 2), 5–7, ed. Ehrman, *Apostolic Fathers*, II, pp. 310–312; Grant, *Early Christianity*, p. 130.

15 Finn, *Almsgiving*, pp. 150–155; more generally O. Plassmann, *Das Almosen bei Johannes Chrysostomus* (Münster in Westfalen, 1961).

16 Constantelos, *Byzantine Philanthropy*, p. 49.

17 John Moschus, *The Spiritual Meadow* (*Pratum spirituale*), p. 175, in J.-P. Migne (ed.), *Patrologia cursus completus, series graeca* (hereafter *PG*), 161 vols (Paris, 1857–66), LXXXVII, col. 3044B, trans. J. Wortley, *The Spiritual Meadow of John Mochos* (Kalamazoo, MI, 1992), p. 144.

18 For what follows, see P. Horden, 'The Christian Hospital in Late Antiquity: Break or Bridge?' in F. Steger and K. P. Jankrift (eds), *Gesundheit-Krankheit: Kulturtransfer medizinischen Wissens von der Spätantike bis in die Frühe Neuzeit*, Beihefte zum Archiv für Kulturgeschichte 55 (Cologne, 2004), pp. 77–99.

19 P. Brown, *Poverty and Leadership in the Later Roman Empire* (Hanover, 2002), pp. 26–35.

20 Letter 94, *Saint Basile, Lettres*, ed. Y. Courtonne, 3 vols (Paris, 1957–66), I, p. 206.

21 Miller, *Birth*.

22 P. Horden, 'How Medicalised Were Byzantine Hospitals?', *Medicina e storia* 5 (2005, published 2006), pp. 45–74; Miller, *Birth*, pp. 14–21, with further bibliography.

23 Contrast E. Kislinger, 'Der Pantokrator-Xenon, ein trügerisches Ideal?' *Jahrbuch der Österreichischen Byzantinistik* 37 (1987), pp. 173–179; Miller, *Birth*.

24 P. Magdalino, *The Empire of Manuel I Komnenus 1143–1180* (Cambridge, 1993), p. 220.

25 J. P. Thomas and A. Constantinides Hero (eds), *Byzantine Monastic Foundation Documents: A Complete Translation of the Surviving Founders' Typika and Testaments* (hereafter *Typika*), 5 vols (Washington, DC, 2000), no. 39, vol. V, pp. 1254–1286, at 1281; Stathakopoulos, 'Stiftungen', pp. 152–153.

26 S. Cavallo, *Charity and Power in Early Modern Italy: Benefactors and their Motives in Turin, 1541–1789* (Cambridge, 1995).

27 S. R. Holman, *The Hungry Are Dying: Beggars and Bishops in Roman Cappadocia* (Oxford, 2001), pp. 147, 203.

28 J. Zepos and P. Zepos, *Jus graecoromanum*, 8 vols (Athens: Phexe, 1931), I, pp. 251–252, trans. P. Charanis, 'Monastic Properties and the State in the Byzantine Empire', *Dumbarton Oaks Papers* 4 (1948), pp. 56–57. The text is also translated in E. McGeer, *The Land Legislation of the Macedonian Emperors* (Toronto, 2000), p. 95.

29 H. Rabe (ed.), *Anonymi et Stephani in Artem Rhetoricam commentaria* (Berlin, 1896), p. 52, cited by P. van Minnen, 'Medical Care in Late Antiquity', in P. J. van der Eijk, H. F. J. Horstmanshoff, and P. H. Schrijvers (eds), *Ancient Medicine in its Socio-Cultural Context*, 2 vols (Amsterdam, 1995), I, pp. 153–169, at 163 n. 39.

30 T. S. Miller, *The Orphans of Byzantium* (Washington, DC, 2003), pp. 176–246.

31 T. S. Miller, 'The Sampson Hospital of Constantinople', *Byzantinische Forschungen* 15 (1990), pp. 101–135.

32 What followers derives from my reading of the often-ambiguous evidence usefully collected by K. Mentzou-Meimare, 'Eparchiaka evage hidrymata mechri tou telous tes eikonomachias', *Byzantina* 11 (1982), pp. 243–308.

33 Van Minnen, 'Medical Care'.

34 R. Janin, *Les églises et les monastères*, La geographie ecclésiastique de l'empire byzantin I.3, 2nd edn (Paris, 1969), pp. 552–569; M. Živojinović, 'Bolnica Kralja Milutina u Carigradu', *Zbornik Radova Vizantoloshkog Instituta* 16 (1975), pp. 105–117; Stathakopoulos, 'Stiftungen', pp. 156–157.

35 On whom see G. Dagron, *Constantinople imaginaire* (Paris, 1984).

36 J. P. Thomas, *Private Religious Foundations in the Byzantine Empire* (Washington, DC, 1987), p. 171.

37 Thomas and Hero, *Typika*, no. 19, vol. I, pp. 326–376, at 333–334, 336–337, 349.

38 Thomas, *Private Religious Foundations*, pp. 179–185.

39 Thomas and Hero, *Typika*, no. 23, vol. II, pp. 507–563, at 522, 544–556, 549–550. See also E. Patlagean, 'Les donateurs, les moines et les pauvres dans quelques documents byzantins des XIe et XIIe siècles', in H. Dubois, J.-C. Hocquet, and André Vauchez (eds), *Horizons marins, itinéraires spirituels (Ve–XVIIIe siècles)*, 2 vols (Paris, 1987), I, pp. 223–231.

40 Thomas and Hero, *Typika*, no. 28, vol. II, pp. 725–781. For the hospital, see pp. 757–766.

41 See also A. W. Epstein, 'Formulas for Salvation: A Comparison of Two Byzantine Monasteries and their Founders', *Church History* 50 (1981), pp. 385–400; E. A. Congdon, 'Imperial Commemoration and Ritual in the *Typikon* of the Monastery of Christ Pantocrator', *Revue des études byzantines* 54 (1996), pp. 161–199.

42 D. Sternon, 'La vision d'Isaïe de Nicomédie', *Revue des études byzantines* 35 (1977), pp. 5–42 at 25.

43 P.-B. Noailles and A. Dain (eds), *Les novelles de Léon VI le sage* (Paris, 1944), p. 25, no. 4.

44 M. Jeffreys and E. Jeffreys, 'Immortality in the Pantokrator?' *Byzantion* 64 (1994), pp. 195–196. For wider context, see J. Thomas, '*In perpetuum*: Social and Political Consequences of Byzantine Patrons' Aspirations for Permanence for their Foundations', in Borgolte, *Stiftungen*, pp. 129–132.

45 *Life of John the Almsgiver* 24, in A.-J. Festugière (ed.), *Léontios de Néapolis, Vie de Syméon le Fou et Vie de Jean de Chypre* (Paris, 1974), pp. 375–376. See also the 'Oration on those who have fallen asleep in the faith' and on the value of alms for the salvation of their souls, once (wrongly) attributed to John of Damascus, *PG* XCV, cols 247–278.

46 V. Matthaios (ed), *Evergetinos etoi Synagoge [...] tomos protos* (Athens, 1957), p. 42; Bishop Chrysostomos et al. (ed. and trans.), *The Evergetinos: A Complete Text. Volume I of the First Book* (Etna, CA, 1988), p. 57.

47 J. Wortley, 'Death, Judgement, Heaven, and Hell in Byzantine "Beneficial Tales"', *Dumbarton Oaks Papers* 55 (2001), pp. 53–69, at 55, and N. Constas, '"To Sleep, Perchance to Dream": The Middle State of Souls in Patristic and Byzantine Literature', ibid. pp. 91–124.

48 (Pseudo-)Anastasius of Sinai, *Questions and Answers* 22, in *PG* LXXXIX, col. 536C.

49 F. Halkin, 'La vision de Kaioumos et le sort éternel de Philentolos Olympiou', *Analecta Bollandiana* 63 (1945), pp. 56–64.

50 R. Homburg (ed.), *Apocalypsis Anastasiae* (Leipzig, 1903), pp. 27–30, trans. J. Baun, *Tales from Another Byzantium: Celestial Journey and Local Community in the Medieval Greek Apocrypha* (Cambridge, 2007), p. 41, adapted, and with

italics added. [For wider context see now V. Marinis, *Death and the Afterlife in Byzantium* (Cambridge, 2017). Some late Byzantine texts linking good works for the poor and the remission of sins are translated, in convenient excerpts, in D. J. Geanakoplos, *Byzantium: Church, Society, and Civilization Seen Through Contemporary Eyes* (Chicago, 1984).]

51 J. Le Goff, *The Birth of Purgatory* (Aldershot, 1984); M. McLaughlin, *Consorting with Saints: Prayer for the Dead in Early Medieval France* (Ithaca, NY, 1994).

10

THE USES OF MEDICAL
MANUSCRIPTS

Much of this collection of articles [on Byzantine medical books] concerns medical texts that seem eminently 'practical' or 'useful'.[1] But what does either of those adjectives mean? How can historians of medieval Greek medicine, usually working on writings that now lack contextual evidence of origins and application, establish criteria of usefulness or practicality? Those who study medical remedies of the pre-modern period are often asked – by 'lay', non-specialist audiences in particular – 'Did they work?' The question usually presupposes a certain kind of effectiveness as the yardstick: that of modern, laboratory-based biomedicine with its high levels of pain relief – on which yardstick medieval remedies generally fall short, proving neutral at best.[2] In the same way, the question put (in effect) to scholars of medieval medical manuscripts – 'Were they used?' – presupposes a certain vision of the texts' *Sitz im Leben* as providing the sole criterion.[3] In effect, if the text did not sit in the consulting room, and if it was not frequently in the doctor's hand, at least between patients and perhaps during a consultation, it was not or useful. What follows is a short statement of the obvious contrary position. Just as there are many kinds of effect and effectiveness that can be ascribed to remedies,[4] so there are many kinds of usefulness with respect to medical texts. In each case we need to separate out the different kinds to arrive at a suitable typology, and we need to try to arrive at criteria for each kind – ideally, in the case of texts, related to aspects of the manuscripts in which we find them.

The starting point must be that the production of a manuscript – either to create a text or texts for the first time or to copy an existing exemplar – had some perceived value in the Byzantine world. Nigel Wilson has shown that, in the middle Byzantine period, the cost of a manuscript of some 400 folios was the equivalent of several months' salary for a low-ranking civil servant. That cost included the production of the writing materials as well as the copyist's skill and time.[5] We need not worry here about the exact period or the exact salary. The point is the order of magnitude. In simple terms of price, the modern equivalent to producing or commissioning a manuscript was, shall we say, buying a small car. It was not the equivalent of buying a modern hardback volume. The best evidence of the preciousness of parchment or vellum is its re-use – the palimpsest. Witness, most strikingly for us today, the codex containing three 'new' texts of Archimedes.[6] Thus, a medical manual such as that of John the Physician, 90 folios including *pinax* in one quarto manuscript, might have cost our civil servant one month's salary.[7] Even such a *iatrosophion*, when copied on vellum, required a number of hides from sheep or goats (hardly more than four folia per animal)[8] and would have taken several months to write out. And when various types of paper became generally available as a substitute writing material from the eleventh to twelfth century onwards, it was not, at least to begin with, very much cheaper in the Byzantine empire.[9] So it can be taken as axiomatic in this context that no text was written out, no copy made, automatically – without some calculation, however rapid, however subconscious, of costs and benefits: the cost of the material, the benefit of the text or texts that it might already bear (in the case of a palimpsest), the benefit of the text or texts that might be written on it. With the Archimedes manuscript, the value of the writing material, the lack of alternative sources of parchment, and the Palestinian scribe-priest's need for a copy of a prayer book clearly trumped any need felt to preserve mathematics or philosophy from pagan antiquity. That is why, more generally, we find the filling up of blank pages or half-pages in manuscripts: such spaces were a waste of a rare and costly medium.

Of course, we always have to bear in mind that we are generalizing about what survives, not what once existed – about which we can only conjecture.[10] Crossings-out, or other signs of editing, are unusual in the codices that have come down to us because for the most part only 'fair copies', finished products and their derivatives have been preserved.[11] (At least in the medical sphere, not even the ancient and late antique papyri have revealed anything much that could be identified as rough draft or working copy.[12]) We presume that authors or compilers, or those reworking some earlier material, roughed out their texts on papyrus off-cuts, slates, ostraca, or individual palimpsest sheets of parchment. These were ephemeral: they have not come down to us. Nor, we may guess, have the large majority of the more polished manuscripts that existed in the Byzantine period. (Think, for a non-literary parallel, of the 50,000 or so lead seals that have survived – without the documents they once authenticated.) That attrition strengthens the point that what was deliberately kept, as distinct from what was accidentally lost, or censored, or destroyed in violent circumstances (what one might call the *Name of the Rose* scenario) was what had some perceived value. We should take it as a working hypothesis that no writing was kept unthinkingly. If for example Byzantine scribes stopped copying Galen's longer and more theoretical works in the ninth to tenth centuries, so that they survive if at all only in Arabic, that was because these substantial treatises were no longer thought worth keeping, given the expense of the parchment and of the copyist's time that such works would require, their unwieldy size, the perceived redundancy of some of their information, or the novel availability of more compact alternatives.[13]

Therefore, if we are trying to set out the possible reasons for creating or keeping a manuscript of medical writings in Byzantium, the simple preservation of the text for its own sake, or merely out of respect for the standing of its presumed author, is perhaps the least likely – even if that author was Galen. Pure antiquarianism as an explanation should be automatically suspect.

After respect – in ascending order of usefulness – might come luxury or display. Under this heading we could group those manuscripts commissioned by a patron to show off his (nearly always 'his') learning, or prepared by an author, compiler, or scribe to attract or retain the interest of a patron. The copies of Galen in Greek that end up in Italy after the fall of Constantinople exemplify this category.[14] The 'usefulness' here is symbolic – of wealth, of taste, of learning. We should not underestimate the role of display copies in the Greek medical manuscript tradition.

Then, scholarship. Medical manuscripts had their uses for scholars living in the Middle Ages that had nothing to do with medicine. These range from the literary – the text in the manuscript as a model of good style – to what in modern terms would be science, that is, information about the world: about the environment and the ways humanity is made up (reproduction, generation, anatomy, physiology). Perhaps a common mistake in hoping to establish the *Sitz im Leben* of many medical manuscripts has been to confuse the 'scientific' and the medical; to assume that the usefulness of medical texts lay only in therapy.

This is not of course to diminish some therapeutic application as a substantial category. But the place of a manuscript – a text or a collection of texts – in a doctor's practice can be just as variable as its non-medical uses. We must remain alert to the whole range of possibilities, rather than draw conclusions too hastily.

What are these possibilities? The first is broadly educational – to do with medical training, the making of a medical career (if only part-time). Does the codex in question suggest a school, an individual teacher, self-instruction? Does it suggest display here too – self-validation, image-making? What does its size tell us about where it might have been kept and opened? Could it literally have been a *vade mecum* or would it have stayed on the shelf for only occasional reference? What can we infer from its contents about the possible circumstances of its application? Or from the way the text is laid out, and the ease with which it would have been possible to find one's way about it?

If that is the range of possibilities, then the task becomes one of trying to map features of surviving manuscripts onto it – not in any hope of precision but simply to establish a working framework that can be constantly revised as new evidence is considered. How much theory, of humours or complexions, do we take to be more redolent of medical training than of clinical practice? Are commentaries on standard texts a sign of an educational syllabus?[15]

What can we infer from the apparent absence of such commentaries? What size of manuscript is portable – on foot, by pack animal? Quarto size or smaller is genuinely portable; but how would one preserve the precious book from water damage? How many such small volumes could one easily transport? What signs of discolouration from handling, even what density of fingerprinting, do particular folia display?[16] What, if anything, *a priori* (simply as starting point for investigation) might we infer from the presence of non-medical texts in a medical manuscript? Are there prefaces that yield any clues about intended use? What kind of anthology of abbreviated or excerpted material do we find in the manuscripts, and are there any criteria by which we might distinguish their compilers' purposes? What is the significance of linguistic reworking – from 'classical' to 'demotic'?[17] What 'finding aids' are there (indexes, headings, spacing out, marginal marks of significant passages), and how comprehensive and how effective would they have been in facilitating ready reference in the 'consulting room', the *iatreion*, or at the bedside? Serious comparative work has begun on a number of the fronts bound up in that agenda; some of it is to be found in the chapters below. Yet much remains to be done before we can pronounce with any confidence about when, in what circumstances, a text was 'useful'.[18]

Notes

1 The conference from which it derives was indeed conceived as a collective study of Byzantine medieval manuals, or *iatrosophia* (for the definition of which see V. Nutton, 'Byzantine Medicine, Genres, and the Ravages of Time', in B. Zipser (ed.), *Medical Books in the Byzantine World* (*Eikasmós: Quaderni bolognesi di filologia classica*, Studi Online 2, Bologna 2013), 7–18. In what follows I am grateful throughout for advice from Barbara Zipser and Nigel Wilson.

2 See e.g. B. Brennessel, M. D. C. Drout, and R. Gravel, 'A Reassessment of the Efficacy of Anglo-Saxon Medicine', *Anglo-Saxon England* 34 (2005): 183–195. [See further Postscript to Ch. 7, this volume.]

3 To borrow a term from biblical form criticism.

4 E. Hsu, 'Medical Anthropology, Material Culture, and New Directions in Medical Archaeology', in P. A. Baker and G. Carr (eds), *Practitioners, Practices and Patients: New Approaches to Medical Archaeology and Anthropology* (Oxford, 2002), 1–15, suggests that we substitute 'Was it successful?' (in meeting patients' expectations) for 'Did it work?' (in relieving symptoms or pain) as our main question.

5 N. Wilson, 'Books and Readers in Byzantium', in *Byzantine Books and Book-Men* (Washington, DC, 1975), 3f., with C. Mango, 'The Availability of Books in the Byzantine Empire, A.D. 750–850', ibid. 38f.

6 *The Archimedes Palimpsest*, ed. R. Netz et al., 2 vols (Cambridge, 2011).

7 B. Zipser, *John the Physician's Therapeutics: A Medical Handbook in Vernacular Greek* (Leiden, 2009), 18. This estimate is based on manuscript M, the only complete witness of the text.

8 Wilson, *Books and Readers*, 2.

9 R. S. Bagnall, *Early Christian Books in Egypt* (Princeton, NJ, 2009), ch. 3, for the costs of papyrus rolls and codices; J. Bloom, *Paper Before Print: The History and Impact of Paper in the Islamic World* (New Haven, CT, 2001).

10 See V. Nutton, *Ancient Medicine* (Abingdon, 2004), ch. 1.

11 For a rare example of crossing-out, see B. Zipser, 'Deleted Text in a Manuscript: Galen On the Eye and the Marc. gr. 276', *Galenos* 3 (2009): 107–112.

12 R. S. Bagnall, *Everyday Writing in the Graeco-Roman East* (Berkeley, CA, 2011).

13 V. Nutton, 'Galen in Byzantium', in M. Grünbart, E. Kislinger, A. Muthesius, and D. Stathakopoulos (eds), *Material Culture and Well-Being in Byzantium* (Vienna, 2007), 174; see also N. Wilson, 'Aspects of the Transmission of Galen', in G. Cavallo (ed.), *Le strade del testo* (Bari, 1987), 47–64 [and now P. Bouras-Vallianatos, 'Reading Galen in Byzantium: The Fate of "Therapeutics to Glaucon"', in P. Bouras-Vallianatos and S. Xenophontos (eds), *Greek Medical Literature and its Readers* (Abingdon, 2018), 180–221.]

14 Nutton, 'Galen in Byzantium', 175.

15 The second version of *John the Physician* is in effect a commentary on the earlier one (Zipser, *John the Physician*, 38–41), made as an aid to translation, not education. Contrast the material mentioned by Nutton, 'Byzantine Medicine, Genres, and the Ravages of Time', at nn. 6–8.

16 See e.g. the [still] classic K. M. Rudy, 'Dirty Books: Quantifying Patterns of Use in Medieval Manuscripts Using a Densitometer', *Journal of Historians of Netherlandish Art* 2 (2010): 1–2, DOI: 10.5092/jhna.2010.2.1.1, available at https://jhna.org/articles/dirty-books-quantifying-patterns-of-use-medieval-manuscripts-using-a-densitometer/ (accessed 27 July 2018). [Also M. D. Teasdale et al., 'The York Gospels: A 1000-Year Biological Palimpsest', *Royal Society Open Science* 4 (2017): 170988, 1–11, DOI: 10.1098/rsos.170988, available at http://rsos.royalsocietypublishing.org/content/4/10/170988/ (accessed 27 July 2018).]

17 Zipser, *John the Physician*, 28–30.

18 G. Cavallo, 'Il libro come oggetto d'uso nel mondo Bizantino', *Jahrbuch der österreichischen Byzantinistik* 31.2 (1981): 395–423, has only brief comments on medical texts, at p. 409.

11

MEDIEVAL HOSPITAL
FORMULARIES

Byzantium and Islam compared

I

The novel availability of editions or transcriptions of medical writings associated with hospitals in the medieval Middle East makes possible something that has not been attempted before: comparison of Byzantine and Islamic examples of such material.[1]

This comparison – of what we can label hospital *iatrosophia*[2] – is important for two reasons. First, it makes good long neglect. If *iatrosophia* in general have largely been ignored, those relating to hospital practice have, until quite recently, remained wholly unknown. Second, the comparison adds a fresh dimension to the debate about hospital medicalization in the Middle Ages. This is a more intricate task.

Great claims have by turns been made for the quasi-modernity of both Byzantine and medieval Islamic hospitals. 'Philanthropic social welfare and medical assistance institutions [in Byzantium] [. . .] were in every respect perfect and nearly similar to present day institutions of this kind [. . .] they were the first fully equipped European hospitals.'[3] No serious historian would write in such terms now. Yet the medical superiority of Byzantine hospitals, at least over those to be found in contemporary western Europe, has been stoutly maintained by Timothy Miller in a number of publications. '*Xenones* [or *nosokomeia* – hospitals] evolved [he writes, in 2008] as the principal centres of Byzantine medicine because of their link to the *archiatroi*, the ancient chief physicians of the polis.' And he adds: 'that members of the ruling elite sought treatment at Byzantine hospitals demonstrates how different these institutions were from the Hôtel-Dieu in Paris or Saint Bartholomew in London.'[4] Even such modified eulogy of Byzantine charitable establishments has been questioned. Yet this way of describing medieval hospitals lives on – in effect asserting the superiority of one culture over another by reference to the degree to which its hospitals were in some sense medicalized.

It lives on, indeed has long flourished, in the realm of scholarship about early Islamic hospitals. 'The emergence of the prototype of the modern hospital in medieval Islam': the title says it all.[5] That is from 1980. The latest, and also the most learned and authoritative, exponent of such a view has been Peter E. Pormann. With him, the *comparandum* is Byzantium, not western Europe: it is always the poorer neighbour. And the contrast drawn is between (implicitly) backward Christian health care in Byzantium and forward-looking, secular, or at least multi-faith, establishments in Islam. In these hospitals, as in Miller's version of Byzantium, elite patients were treated by elite physicians. And the density of hospital provision in tenth-century Baghdad is ultimately validated by estimating its statistical superiority to that of modern Pakistan:[6]

> It is therefore evident that the medieval Islamic hospital was a more elaborate institution with a wider range of functions than the earlier poor and sick relief facilities offered by some Christian monasteries and hospices. The care for the insane in hospitals was unprecedented and an important part of even the earliest Islamic hospitals. Although early Islamic hospitals drew on Christian models, there are some things which make them unique. First, unlike their Christian counterparts, the medicine practised there was secular in character, insofar as it was based on the principles of humoral pathology rather than religion. Treatment in Christian institutions before the eighth century would customarily begin with a confession, and be carried out by monks or priests – that is to say, by Christians for Christians through Christian ritual (although of course not limited to it). In contrast, there were no mosques or places for religious ritual associated with Islamic hospitals, though in a few instances mosques were attached at a later date. In Islamic hospitals from the tenth century onwards (as far as we know), Muslim, Jewish, Christian, and even pagan doctors worked together, treating not only patients of their own community, but also those of other communities. Secondly, *elite medical theory and practice came together* in Islamic hospitals in a way that they had not done so before. This is illustrated by the fact that some of the best physicians of the time worked in hospitals and produced there some of their most advanced and innovative research. Thirdly, over time hospitals became *centres for the teaching of medicine*, in which students were encouraged to obtain their medical education. Finally, hospitals were *part of wider public health efforts* promoted by the ruling elite.

Again, therefore, the hospital is presented as a centre of medical excellence – of research, teaching, and practice informed by theory. It is a medical-history equivalent of the *translatio imperii*: from Constantinople to Baghdad. The *translatio* may turn out to be entirely justified, but its basis needs testing – and on as many fronts as the evidence permits.

There are various ways in which the accuracy of the Byzantine–Islamic comparison could be appraised. But some obvious methodological caveats must be heeded first. Is like being compared with like – or does the starkness of the presumed contrast between a Christian and a secular ethos vitiate further discussion? Is what is being compared the generality of hospitals in each culture, which is what the rhetoric of both Miller and Pormann implies? Or are really only a few metropolitan hospitals in question, as the specific supporting examples (such as Baghdad) suggest? Still more to the point, on what yardstick is medicalization being measured – the mere presence or absence of doctors; the degree of authority they wielded; whether they were courtiers; the number of beds at their disposal; what sort of medicine they were therefore likely to have dispensed; or how that medicine's efficacy would have been assessed in the modern laboratory?[7]

On a practical level, answers to these methodological questions must be sought using contemporary evidence, or as near to contemporary as possible. This is not the place to review that evidence, which (very much in Pormann's favour, let it be stressed) does include some first-hand, contemporary descriptive texts of elite physicians active in hospitals, as well as later, retrospective narratives in the same vein; prescriptive (deontological) exhortations to learn medicine in hospitals; and medical casebooks that record experiments with treatments that in some ways might be seen to anticipate modern clinical trials.[8]

What should be mentioned here is a wider trend within the scholarship of early Islamic medicine, that is, medicine from the ninth century onwards. This trend is to point up the contrast, not between Islam and some other culture, but within Islamic medicine itself – a contrast between the sophisticated procedures and treatments advocated on the theoretical and technical medical literature of the period and the much simpler responses to the same medical problems recorded in the case histories.[9] The contrast is more than a matter of the doctors' selecting a narrow range of treatments from the large arsenal in principle available to them.[10] It suggests a deliberate avoidance of the sophistication paraded in those writings intended to attract and hold the attention of potential patrons. It seems almost to concede that these writings were only (to recall the gloomy tones of Manfred Ullmann) 'lifeless theory [...] mere book knowledge'.[11] Perhaps the practice of elite medicine in hospitals was different from the theory.

The possible implications of that for the comparison of Byzantine and Islamic medical literature deserve further exploration – elsewhere. For the moment it is simply worth bearing them in mind as we come to the one type of evidence that has not so far been pressed into service when juxtaposing the hospitals of the two empires: the Greek hospital *iatrosophia* and their Arabic equivalents, the hospital *aqrabadhinat*.[12]

II

The first task is to establish the corpora involved. On the Byzantine side, David Bennett has surveyed the relevant manuscripts, in a discussion that supersedes all others in both scope and thoroughness.[13] I am indebted to him for permission to summarize and continue disseminating his main findings.

There are five or six texts in question – depending on how one counts a text that has at some point been divided into two by its copyists.

1. 'Prescriptions and classifications [of fever?] of the great hospitals, of the kind that doctors prescribe from experience for healing, especially for patients in the hospitals.' That is the translated title of one version of a compilation of treatments (parts of which, including the title, variously appear in at least four other manuscripts). The compilation is divided under sixteen very miscellaneous headings and dates from approximately 1050. It is found in the fourteenth-century *Vat.* gr. 292. Three other manuscripts (nos 2, 4, and 5 below) also preserve these 'prescriptions and classifications' to varying extents, but sometimes without the titular ascription to hospitals.

2. *Vat.* gr. 299 is an anthology of medical writings dating from the later fourteenth century. Within a long concluding medical compilation (of around 180,000 words) it contains five remedies ascribed to three named physicians of the Mangana hospital, founded in the mid-eleventh century,[14] and one other remedy ascribed to a named but otherwise unknown doctor, for whom no institutional affiliation is given. The three hospital physicians are: (a) Stephanos, *archiatros* (chief physician) and *aktouarios* (court physician);[15] (b) Abram 'the Saracen', *aktouarios* and *basilikos* (imperial) *archiatros*; and (c) Theodore, *iatros* (physician) at the Mangana. There are six other passages ascribed only to the Mangana hospital, with no physician named. These are dispersed over about a half of the compilation but form only a tiny proportion of the whole. A further six passages in the same remedy collection correspond to parts of the collection in *Vat.* gr. 292 (no. 1, above) in which they are said to be derived from 'the great hospitals'.

3. The fifteenth-century *Par.* gr. 2194 includes eight remedies ascribed to Michael, *aktouarios* of the otherwise undocumented Mauraganos (*recte* Maurianos?) hospital. These six remedies are found in a text headed, in a hand that differs from that of the copyist, *dynameron xenonikon dia peiras* ('On the potency of hospital prescriptions found by experience'). That text is succeeded by another similar brief collection entitled, even more simply, *xenonika* (from the main Greek term translatable as hospital, *xenon*). So far as is currently known, none of the hospital-related material found here survives in any other manuscript.

4. The *Vind. med.* gr. 48, from the late thirteenth century, has a text at-
    tributed in its title to Romanos, *kouboukleisios* (an imperial honorific)
    of the Great Church (Hagia Sophia) and *protomenutes* (chief physician)
    of the imperial Myrelaion Hospital in Constantinople.[16] Fragments of
    this text survive in only two other manuscripts. The title *kouboukleisios*
    disappeared after the tenth century, and the Myrelaion hospital was re-
    founded by the emperor Romanus Lecapenus in the mid-tenth century.[17]
    Romanos *kouboukleisios* cannot be dated any more precisely than that.
5. The text attributed to Romanos is actually only the first half of a much
    longer work. Its second half survives separately, in the *Laur.* plut. 75, 19,
    under a different author's name, as the *Apotherapeutike* of one Theophi-
    los, in which the material is said to be drawn from hospital books (*xe-
    nonikon biblon*). *Apotherapeutike* is an odd term, but its sense of 'remedy
    list' is clear enough.[18]

    Both these two parts – Romanos's and Theophilos's – contain pas-
    sages similar to parts of Vat. gr. 299 (no. 2 above) where the hospital
    treatments are attributed to the Mangana hospital.
6. Manuscript *Laur.* plut. 7, 19, of the thirteenth to fourteenth centuries, is
    a collection mainly of theological works. Like nine other manuscripts,
    it contains a text (mostly, but not always, the same text) with the title:
    'Therapeutic medical treatments by various doctors set in order accord-
    ing to the defined procedure of the *xenon*'. This is a short piece of some
    2,750 words. In none of its versions does it live up to the orderliness
    implied in its title. It includes abbreviated versions of remedies recorded
    in four other manuscripts under the name of John *archiatros*,[19] in one
    other manuscript under that of Galen, and in a sixth, under both names.
    More on the 'therapeutic medicines' below.

Overall, then, we have five or six texts, known to us from eighteen manuscripts, which have hospital connections made explicit in their titles or their
contents. To them can be added two manuscripts (*Par.* gr. 2315 and 2510) that
were copied for hospitals, one manuscript (*Scorialensis* Y.III.14) dedicated to
a hospital by its scribe George (all three of these from the fourteenth century),
and perhaps three or four others that may have been owned by a hospital in the
late Byzantine period, including such 'luxury products' as the 'Niketas codex'
and the re-bound 'Vienna Dioscorides'.[20] Some fifteenth-century humanist
feats of Galenic collecting and scholarship may have had a hospital setting in
the Kral Xenon in Constantinople, but they are as far removed from patients'
immediate clinical needs as they are from the style of the *iatrosophion*.[21]

III

As for the Islamic side: there was a genre of medical formularies (or pharmacopoeias, or dispensatories), written collections of compound remedies – the

aqrabadhin. Within that body of writings we find at least three works explicitly redacted for use in the *bimaristan* (hospital).

1. Sabur ibn Sahl (d. 869) was a Nestorian Christian physician from Gondeshapur in Iran, where he may have held a post in the city's famed local hospital.[22] He became a court physician to the Abbasid Caliph al-Mutawakkil and his successors. His formulary survives in three different versions of varying length, known to philologists appropriately as the short, middle, and long versions. It is noteworthy in passing that the unique surviving manuscript of the short one (*Berol. or. oct.* 1839, copied around 900) shows signs of extensive use: thumb imprints on the cover, reading marks of wax on several leaves, and numbering of quires and folios as 'finding aids' perhaps added early in the manuscript's life.[23] Overall these different versions survive in five manuscripts dating from the tenth to the seventeenth century or even later. It is not clear which version most faithfully reflects Sabur's original, perhaps written in Syriac. Nor can it even be known whether any of the surviving redactions were made during his lifetime. In the mid-eleventh century, someone produced a fourth version: a revised, rearranged, abridged text explicitly entitled: 'The formulary of Sabur according to the 'Adudi hospital, a synopsis of Sabur's formulary on the composition of drugs, [in] sixteen chapters' (one chapter fewer than the small version but drawing on both small and large redactions). The 'Adudi was the hospital founded in Baghdad on the west bank of the Tigris by the Buyid ruler 'Adud al-Daula. It opened in the year of his death, 982. The version made for it is represented in a unique manuscript, dated 1341, the work of a copyist not entirely at ease with what was presumably being dictated to him: *Munich Staatsbibliothek* arab. 808,2. I shall come back to Sabur and this hospital text below.

Some circumstantial evidence suggests that the hospital formulary under his name became, if not standard, then widespread in the major hospitals of Baghdad, perhaps of the caliphate. The court and hospital physician al-Kaskari who worked in tenth-century Baghdad wrote in the prefatory remarks to his medical compendium:

> In each chapter I have limited myself to a description of the pastes
> [. . .] pills, pastilles, liquids, collyria [. . .] dressings, and other things in
> Sabur's Dispensatory to which people resorted in the hospitals. I compared this with the manuscripts in the hospitals dealing with this.[24]

In his *Fihrist* the bio-bibliographer Ibn al-Nadim (d. 995–998) corroborates the information that Sabur's work was used in hospitals as well as apothecary shops.[25]

2. Ibn al-Tilmidh (b. *c.*1065 in Baghdad, d. 1154 or 1165) was another Christian doctor who worked in the 'Adudi hospital.[26] He rose to be chief physician

there as well as court doctor to the Caliph al-Muqtadiʿ. Written in the 1140s, his formulary became, according to the later biographical dictionaries, the default pharmacopoeia in the hospitals of Baghdad, replacing that of Sabur.[27] This formulary survives in two recensions, long (20 chapters) and short (13). A version of the short text seems also to have been adopted as a hospital formulary. The main, long version comes to us in at least five manuscripts ranging in date from *c.*1200 to *c.*1600. According to the subtitles of some of these it was 'compiled from a number of [other] formularies'.

3. Finally in this roster of authors of hospital *aqrabadhinat* comes the (Karaite) Jewish apothecary Ibn Abi al-Bayan (d. *c.*1236).[28] He too was a court physician, and treated Saladin's successor al-ʿAdil. He was director of the Nasiri hospital in Cairo and composed his *Dustur al-bimaristani* for use in it. It survives in some twelve manuscripts, which represent two different versions, dating from around 1200 to 1600, and was perhaps based on earlier compilations already maintained in the Cairo hospital.[29]

IV

With the 'cast' of texts assembled, we can turn to the business of comparison.

Even a brief review of the material in Arabic immediately suggests differences from the Byzantine corpus. First, at the simple level of the progress of scholarship, on the Islamic side there are editions and translations at our disposal, as well as a significant if small secondary literature (which is one reason why I have given less detail of Arabic than of Greek manuscripts). Even if some of the editions are very recent, this discursive literature has been building up over a number of years. That state of affairs contrasts with the virtually solitary work of David Bennett.[30] To some extent the contrast reflects the far greater degree of philological and historical attention given to Islamic medicine in general, by comparison with the neglect from which Byzantine medicine has quite generally suffered. Many of the major Greek texts languish unedited, not to mention the *iatrosophia*. There are some studies of individual authors and writings but no modern synthesis.[31]

The contrast owes far more, however, to the fact that the manuscript traditions of the Islamic works in question are *relatively* easy to establish, at least in broad outline. For all the individual variation of particular witnesses, they fall into distinct recensions each with its own stemma. We find named authors, with biographies known even if only in stark outline. The authors are often active at court. They also hold high rank in specific hospitals that have their own documented histories, two in Baghdad, one (in the case of Ibn Abi al-Bayan) in Cairo. Their writings are specifically redacted for use in these hospitals. They display a firm editorial hand. They cite their sources, but they also rework them. There are some vignettes in narrative evidence of the actual use of their work. Each author's text seems to achieve 'market dominance' in its region. That dominance lasts for centuries in the cases of Sabur ibn Sahl and Ibn al-Tilmidh. Ibn al-Bayan was surpassed in popularity rather more quickly, by the Jewish apothecary al-Kuhin al-'Attar. But then the latter's *Minhaj al-dukkan* (Management of the [Pharmacist's] Shop) of about 1260 continued in use for 400 years, until the 1660s.[32] The status of hospital medicine within the whole genre of the pharmacopoeia is attested by the way al-Kuhin al-'Attar explicitly removed hospital references when transplanting material from his principal sources, which included Sabur and Ibn al-Tilmidh.[33] He was trying, almost against the odds, to replace the perspective of a hospital doctor with that of an apothecary.

Nothing like this can be said of the Byzantine corpus. Its 'authors' or compilers are anonymous, pseudonymous, or at best obscure. Their careers, such as they may have been, are lost to us. Though some parts of the corpus purport to have a specific hospital association (e.g. with the Mangana), the actual hospitals in which the texts may have been used are unknowable. The textual history of the material is immensely complex. Writings combine and recombine, changing title and ascribed authorship. If the Islamic material presents a stiff but ultimately surmountable challenge, that from Byzantium is an editor's nightmare. Overall, little can be surmised about where or when the texts were deployed. There is certainly no clear succession of dominant writings.

The Islamic corpus is probably larger in its page extent than the Byzantine one. I estimate that, in his work, David Bennett is discussing something of the order of 200–230 pages of manuscript material, including some overlaps in content and the whole of the Romanos/Theophilos text, but not counting wholesale duplication. (Of course this takes no account of variation in script and folio size. My point is simply that the aggregate is nearer to 200 than to 10 or to 800 pages.) I also estimate very crudely that this is a slightly smaller aggregate than the three main authors writing in Arabic for hospitals combined. While there are occasional signs that other hospital formularies than the works of those three were created and preserved in Islamic hospitals, perhaps anonymously,[34] it seems likely nonetheless that those works surviving in Arabic are most of the iceberg, not just the tip.

That iceberg, to continue the metaphor, is quite substantial in relation to the ice shelf from which it has become 'calved'. Ullmann's survey of the medieval literature of pharmacy composed in Arabic[35] (that is, not counting translations of Galen or Dioscorides) allows us to situate the work of our three hospital writers within a larger corpus of only some twenty-three authors, who wrote either freestanding works or included major sections on complex remedies within larger treatises (as did Ibn Sina with the *Canon*). I do not know of a comparable survey of the Greek manuscript material, but I doubt that the 'Bennett corpus' would loom anything like as large within it.

To approach the question of relative proportion in a different way: the scale of the Byzantine material should be set against the estimated aggregate of 2,200 medical manuscripts surviving in European libraries (although that includes some post-Byzantine material).[36] The numbers of hospital manuscripts could of course be inflated a little. The Byzantine iceberg may well have been deeper than the Islamic one. Many manuscripts that once existed will have succumbed to ordinary wear and tear, let alone the Fourth Crusade or the Ottoman onslaught. Hospital material can survive without its title. And more hospital texts doubtless remain to be discovered, hiding behind misleading or inadequate catalogue entries. Yet there are limits to the number of hypothetical manuscripts that can plausibly be added. For material can gain as well as lose its xenon ascription in the unpredictable course of copying and recopying. However we exercise the imagination, the number of hospital manuscripts that were produced in Byzantium must remain a very small proportion – a fraction of one per cent – of the entirety of medical writing. We must envisage a tiny corpus as far as the Byzantine Middle Ages are concerned.[37]

On the Islamic front, again I do not know of any estimate of the total surviving bulk of the manuscripts to set alongside that for the medieval Greek corpus. Ullmann's second index to his survey of *Die Medizin in Islam* lists over 1,000 Arabic and Persian book titles, including translations. While some are no longer extant, it is a fair estimate that many of those that are, perhaps the majority, survive in more than one manuscript. Simply as a percentage of the total, then, the Arabic hospital texts are probably as insignificant in relative bulk as the Greek.

Any such statistic fails, however, to take account of the relative prestige of the two corpora. The Arabic texts may represent only a sub-genre of the type of writing called *aqrabadhin*, but that genre is more distinct than that of the *iatrosophion*. A few Greek hospital texts were given the sobriquet *xenonika*, but hardly to the extent that implied the recognition of a new kind of medical writing. The medical world of the great hospitals in Baghdad or Cairo is a world in which court and hospital practice seem perfectly compatible for elite physicians, whatever medicine they actually dispensed in the hospitals. We have no such evidence for regular links between Byzantine hospital doctors and the imperial court.[38]

On the other hand, the medical standing of Byzantine hospitals should not be underestimated. Consider the sheer longevity of the tradition of hospital writing. What survive for us are mostly later medieval copies of ninth- to eleventh-century texts. And some of the *xenonika*, like the Arabic hospital formularies, continued to be copied into the sixteenth century. Given the cost of the materials and the skills required for the making of the least pretentious codex, this longevity is some tribute to the perceived value of hospital remedies. Considerable stature must have attached to these remedies and treatments. This is a medical world in which texts mutate with each copying. A title, if there is one, becomes an assertion of value rather than a certificate of authenticity. Witness the remedies which are now attributed to a hospital, now to John *archiatros*, now to Galen. What matters in the present context is not which (if any) of those ascriptions is the right one. Nor is it whether a given remedy generally originated, or was used, in a hospital. What is significant, rather, is that, at some stage in the remedy's manuscript career, someone – sponsor or copyist – thought that the hospital ascription was an appropriate measure of value. A hospital remedy is as good (so the manuscripts imply) as one supplied by Galen. A hospital *archiatros* is as good an authority as any of the other possible names that might be attached to a treatment. And this is so even in the later medieval period, when there were fewer Byzantine hospitals and it is far from clear that even the 'great ones' continued to function on the same scale after the Latin conquest ended.[39] By the same token, hospital texts – when they are labelled as such – keep very good company in the medical anthologies that have preserved them. They can be found associated with all the 'big names' from Hippocrates to John *aktouarios*, one of the last of the stellar Byzantine physicians.

V

So far the texts have been viewed from the outside: their profiles within the total pool of manuscripts, within established genres, within their social setting in hospital and court. The inside, the contents, need scrutiny.

Some common features first. It should already be evident that there is nothing special about hospital medicine in either Byzantium or Islam. These texts can be redactions of medical writings for general use. That is precisely because the hospital, whether Byzantine xenon or Islamic *bimaristan*, is not a place for great medical innovation, even though, as Pormann has suggested for early Islam, it may be a place of experiment, of limited, un-'controlled' treatment trials. (On the Islamic side, at least, as noted earlier, a difference recognized at the time was not between hospital and non-hospital but between the approaches to dispensing medicine of a physician and an apothecary.)[40]

Not until the nineteenth century, after all, will hospitals anywhere begin to provide a type of medicine that could not be had outside 'the clinic'. Again, as a common feature it should be remarked that both bodies of information about drugs and remedies, the Greek and the Arabic, depend to a considerable extent upon a classical Greek past, in which the names of Galen and Dioscorides loom large. Finally, on neither side of the religious division do the texts, because of their practical emphasis, generally include background theory of humours or complexions, semiology, or reference to the condition of the patient. This is a relatively simple kind of medical writing.

Differences as well as commonalities must be registered, however. To bring them out I shall focus the comparison on just two texts. They are the short Greek piece (*c.*2,750 words) headed 'Therapeutic medical treatments by various doctors set in order according to the defined procedure of the *xenon*', **T** for brevity, and the hospital redaction of Sabur (**S**), which bears the title (following Kahl's translation), 'The formulary of Sabur according to the copy of the 'Adudi hospital, [being] a synopsis of Sabur's dispensatory on the composition of drugs, [in] sixteen chapters'. This recension (to recall) survives uniquely in a thirteenth-century manuscript but was dated by Degen and Ullmann to the mid-eleventh century (presumably before the flood that partially destroyed the hospital in 1045).[41] **T** survives in ten manuscripts dating from the thirteenth to the sixteenth centuries, but Bennett, following Litavrin, is inclined to date its compilation to around the mid-eleventh century also.[42] The two texts are thus more or less contemporary.

The most immediate difference between them lies in their organization, which is characteristic of their respective medical cultures and the hospital texts of each. **T** is arranged in the traditional head-to-foot order, at least for its first 46 remedies, after which a miscellaneous supplement seems to follow:[43]

Head

1 For a sharp pain in the head
2 For a pain on one side of the head or face
3 For a pain in the head and one side of the head
4 For a feverishly hot head
5 Decoction for use in cases of giddiness
6 Head lotion

Eyes

7 An eye remedy
8 For trachoma of an eye
9 For cases of itching affecting the eyes
10 For a discharge from the eyes

Nose

11 For a nosebleed
12 For dryness of the nose

Mouth

13 A mouthwash
14 For ulceration of the mouth
15 Toothpaste
16 For haemoptysis
17 For pain in the tongue

Intestines

18 A laxative epithem
19 Affections of the bowels
20 For induration of the intestines

21 Affections of the liver, and pleurisy
22 For the liver
23 Poultices for sufferers from pleurisy
24 For a liver affection
25 For stomach pain
26 A plaster [strictly an epithem] for stomach pain and every affection aris-
    ing from there
27 For affections of the spleen
28 An epithem for the spleen
29 About embrocations for the spleen
30 For all internal pain and poisoning
31 Kidney affections
32 A fomentation for kidney affections
33 Diuretics
34 An enema for sciatica

Skin lesions
35 For sores on the privy parts
36 For cases of an external sore on the private parts
37 For every kind of induration
38 Counter-irritant plasters
39 An ointment for injuries
40 A medicinal ointment
41 For an excrescence of the flesh
42 A method of fomentation of the flesh
43 For a haemorrhage

Feet
44 For swollen feet
45 For gout
46 For a callosity
    [end of head to foot organization]

Fever
47 For shivering fits

Emetics
48 Emetics

Inflammations
49 For external haemorrhoids
50 For buboes and the plague

Purges

51 Galen's purgative pills
52 Purgative for those suffering from the dropsy
53 Prescription for purging of phlegm

Ears

54 For the mucous discharge which some call *glyky*, whatever its origin (mastoiditis)
55 Ear remedies for blockage of the ears

Throat and lungs

56 Affections of the uvula; for cases of the enlargement of the uvula
57 Gargles
58 Cough remedies
59 The Linctus
60 Remedies for shortness of breath

Skin lesion

61 For a suppuration (spreading) from head to hands or feet or any other limb

Digestion

62 A dry powder for the stomach to be taken with wine
63 For those who do not keep down their food
64 A desiccative compound efficacious for a flux from the head

Miscellaneous lesions

65 For a scald from hot water
66 For pruritis

St Gregory's Salt

67 A salt prepared by Gregory the Theologian

Antidotes

68 On the great decoction of the *xenon*
69 The great decoction of Athanasios
70 Antidotal drugs

S by contrast, in common with most *aqrabadhinat*, is arranged predominantly by kind of drug:[44]

1	Pastilles	10	Stomachics
2	Lohochs	11	Hierata
3	Beverages and robs	12	Decoctions and pills
4	Oils	13	Preserves
5	Cataplasms	14	Preparing and testing theriac
6	Enemas	15	Treating teeth and gums
7	Powders	16	Uses and properties of animal parts
8	Collyria		
9	Liniments		Addenda: 49 compounds

Note that only chapter 15 on teeth and gums is 'topically' headed. Note also that madness is not represented, despite the emphasis on its treatment in many medieval Islamic hospitals.[45] We should also register the unsystematic addenda, comparable in that respect to **T**, but here (rather oddly for a hospital) mostly concerned with sexual hygiene or cosmetics.[46]

The structure of the remedies also differs between the two texts. Remedies in **T** have a short purposive title followed by a list of possible ingredients, mostly unquantified, and with few directions for administration. **T** is a piece of writing that, if really to be used clinically, allows for (indeed, depends upon) the experience of the doctor in deciding quantity and ingredients according to availability and need. In contrast, as Kahl summarizes, **S** proceeds fairly regularly by name and/or category of drug, range of application, ingredients with doses, instructions for combining ingredients, and directions for use. One could speculate that this would have worked better in a larger hospital with a staff of assistants, not necessarily medically trained, who might dispense remedies under a physician's supervision. When it opened, the 'Adudi hospital reportedly had 25 doctors, including oculists, surgeons, and bone-setters. The Byzantine texts, on the other hand, are more redolent of small hospitals that were each essentially one-person 'outfits'.[47]

The number of remedies marks a further difference between **T** and **S**: over 100 in **T** – where a single title may encompass a number of remedies – but 292 in **S**, albeit a text at least four times as long.[48] Gastrointestinal problems predominate in both, not surprisingly: 21 per cent, Kahl estimates, in **S**; 25 per cent in **T**, according to Bennett. Eye diseases rate surprisingly few mentions: 4.4 per cent (Kahl), 5.7 per cent (Bennett, using the fullest manuscript witness to **T**). Some ingredients are common to both: barley, celery, cinnamon, ginger, gum Arabic, honey, Indian spikenard, mastic, pepper, pomegranate, rose saffron, vinegar, water, and wine. But the wider range in **S** reflects the openness of the Islamic world to inter alia Indian and Chinese 'imports'.[49] **S** employs 411 simples while **T** uses 212 (including some ingredients in alternative guises, e.g. arsenic and orpiment). Most of **S**'s preparations are compounds. (Remedy 9 in chapter 1 of **S** invokes 17 ingredients for a pastille.) By contrast the majority (80) of the remedies in **T** contain between 1 and 4 ingredients; 23 recipes have between 5 and 8; and only the remaining 6 have more than 8 ingredients.

In **T**, according to Bennett, 74 per cent of the ingredients are vegetable, compared to 67.4 per cent in **S**, which as well as vegetable and mineral remedies has its special section (chapter 16) on medicine from animal parts. With that in mind, compare their respective remedies for buboes:

> Take fermented dough three parts; borax, salt, pigeon droppings, and cock droppings one part in each. [This is] ground, strained, kneaded with olive oil, and used [applied?].

> From the outset, take a drink of natural brine with warm (water); when it has begun to take effect, boil a measure of lentils with water until it has been well infused, put the juice of the lentils into a linen cloth, and strain it, squeezing it well. [Now] put [the decoction] in another vessel and add to it honey and Indian nard and boil again. Give it as a drink to the patient since it expels every unhealthy state of the humours. Another remedy: there is a large-leafed plant that grows by rivers; give its well-steeped root as a drink, and boil as well as its [edible residue to eat].

Prejudice might suggest that the (still palatable to modern tastes) herbal/vegetable remedy is Islamic, the (stereotypically medieval) animal-based one Byzantine; the longer text Arabic, the shorter Greek. As it happens, the converse is true.[50]

VI

Comparison of this sort could be extended indefinitely. The Greek text, for example, has no equivalent of the Arabic section (redacted for a supposedly secular hospital) of *hierata*, remedies manifesting divine power. Yet, in general, no one who wants to assert the medical superiority of early Islamic hospitals over early Byzantine ones – superiority defined in terms of access to the full range of Galenic medical learning – is going to be shaken by what the foregoing juxtaposition (not just the pair of bubo remedies but the whole exercise of comparison) has suggested. Still, the Greek material has much to be said in its favour, too: it is clinically practical. We omit a whole dimension of medieval hospital history, and a whole dimension of the history of *iatrosophia* too, if we do not attend to it, and seek to place it in the widest comparative context.[51]

Notes

1 For the definition and outline history of the hospitals in question, see P. Horden, 'The earliest hospitals in Byzantium, western Europe, and Islam', *Journal of Interdisciplinary History* 35 (2005): 361–389 [reprinted as Ch. 2 in the present volume]; Horden, 'How medicalised were Byzantine hospitals?', *Medicina e*

Storia 10 (2006): 45–74; P. E. Pormann, 'Islamic hospitals in the time of al-Muqta-dir', in John Nawas (ed.), *Abbasid Studies*, II (Leuven, 2010), 337–381. See also D. Stathakopoulos, 'Disease and where to treat it: a Byzantine vade mecum', in B. Zipser (ed.), *Medical Books in the Byzantine World* (*Eikasmós: Quaderni bolognesi di filologia classica*, Studi Online 2, Bologna 2013), 19–33. What follows could not have been written without the unstinting assistance and advice of the late David Bennett.

2 For the definition of *iatrosophia* see V. Nutton, 'Byzantine medicine, genres, and the ravages of time', in Zipser, *Medical Books in the Byzantine World*, 7–18.

3 G. C. Pournaropoulos, 'Hospital and social welfare institutions in the medie-val Greek Empire (Byzantium)', in *XVIIe Congrès international d'histoire de la médecine,* I (Athens, 1960), 378, quoted by D. Constantelos, *Byzantine Philan-thropy and Social Welfare*, 2nd edn (New Rochelle, NY, 1991), 118.

4 T. Miller, 'Charitable institutions', in Elizabeth Jeffreys et al. (eds), *The Ox-ford Handbook of Byzantine Studies* (Oxford, 2008), 627, reflecting the overall argument of Miller, *The Birth of the Hospital in the Byzantine Empire*, 2nd edn (Baltimore, MD, 1997).

5 A. Sayili, 'The emergence of the prototype of the modern hospital in Medieval Islam', *Türk Tarih Kurumu Basimevi Belleten* 44 (1980): 279–286, cited by Leigh Chipman, *The World of Pharmacy and Pharmacists in Mamluk Cairo* (Leiden, 2010), 135.

6 P. E. Pormann and E. Savage-Smith, *Medieval Islamic Medicine* (Edinburgh, 2007), 101, with italics added; echoing Pormann, 'Al-Muqtadir' and other pa-pers by him (which is why I attribute the view to Pormann solely rather than to both authors). For the comparison of proportional hospital provision in tenth-century Baghdad with that of the whole of Pakistan in 1998, see Pormann and Savage-Smith, *Medieval Islamic Medicine*, 110. According to the on-line World Health Statistics 2010 Pakistan did indeed average 6 hospital beds per 10,000 of population in 2000–2009, placing it at very near the bottom in terms of world rankings. This statistic seems to tell us more about Pakistan than about Baghdad. [See now also Ahmed Ragab, *The Medieval Islamic Hospital: Medi-cine, Religion, and Charity* (Cambridge, 2015), the arguments of which I cannot always agree with and which needs more discussion than I can give it here.]

7 On that last-mentioned front see e.g. Leigh Chipman, 'How effective were cough remedies known to medieval Egyptians?', *Korot* 16 (2002): 135–157.

8 P. E. Pormann, 'Medical methodology and hospital practice: the case of fourth-/ tenth-century Baghdad', in P. Adamson (ed.), *In the Age of al-Farabi: Arabic Philosophy in the Fourth/Tenth Century* (London, 2008), 95–118.

9 See the contributions of Emilie Savage-Smith and Cristina Álvarez-Millán to *Social History of Medicine* 13 (2000): 293–306, 307–321.

10 *Pace* Pormann, 'Al-Muqtadir', 364.

11 M. Ullmann, *Islamic Medicine* (Edinburgh, 1978), 106.

12 B. Lewin, *Akrabadhin,* or *karabadhin,* in *Encyclopaedia of Islam 2* (the term derives from the Greek *grapheidion,* short treatise or register, via the Syriac). [See also O. Kahl, 'Aqrabadhin', *Encyclopaedia of Islam THREE,* http://dx.doi.org/10.1163/1573-3912_ei3_COM_22684 (accessed 28 July 2018).]

13 D. C. Bennett, '*Xenonika:* Medical texts associated with *Xenones* in the late Byzantine period', University of London PhD thesis 2003 [partially published, posthumously, as *Medicine and Pharmacy in Byzantine Hospitals: A Study of the Extant Formularies* (Abingdon, 2017)]. See also Miller, *Birth of the Hospital*, ch. 9. The summary that follows revises and corrects that in my paper, 'How medi-calised?', 60–62.

14 Miller, *Birth of the Hospital*, 149f., with P. Lemerle, *Cinq études sur le XIe siècle byzantin* (Paris, 1977), 273–283.

15 On the changing meaning of *aktouarios*, see *Oxford Dictionary of Byzantium*, 3 vols (Oxford, 1991), s.v.

16 On the *protomenutes*, see U. Criscuolo, 'Pour le texte du médecin Romanos', in A. Garzya (ed.), *Storia e ecdoctica dei testi medici greci: histoire et ecdotique des textes médicaux grecs* (Actes du colloque international Paris 24–26 mai 1994, Naples 1996), 113–131, at 114.

17 Miller, *Birth of the Hospital*, 113f.

18 On the text see also A. P. Kousis, 'The Apotherapeutic [*sic*] of Theophilos according to the Laurentian codex, plut. 75, 19', *Praktika tēs Akadēmias Athēnōn* 19 (1944): 35–45; A. M. Ieraci Bio, 'Sur une *Apotherapeutikē* attribuée à Théophile', in A. Garzya (ed.), *Storia e ecdotica dei testi medici greci* (Naples, 1996), 191–205.

19 See further B. Zipser, *John the Physician's Therapeutics* (Leiden, 2009).

20 Bennett, '*Xenonika*', appendix V, 440f., listing also post-Byzantine manuscripts ascribed to *xenones*. [On Niketas see now M. Bernabò (ed.), *La collezione di testi chirurgici di Niceta: Firenze, Biblioteca medicea laurenziana, Plut. 74.7. Tradizione medica classica a Bisanzio* (Rome, 2010). The above list excludes such manuscripts as Mount Athos, Iviron monastery (Ibereticus) 151, which was in the monastery's infirmary (as attested by an annotation on f. 18v) but probably only in the post-Byzantine period. I owe my knowledge of this manuscript to Petros Bouras-Vallianatos.]

21 Bennett, '*Xenonika*', 37, 62f., 81f., 124; Brigitte Mondrain, 'Jean Argyropoulos professeur à Constantinople et ses auditeurs médecins, d'Andronic Éparque à Démétrios Angelos', in C. Scholz and G. Makris (eds), *POLYPLEUROS NOUS: Festschrift für Peter Schreiner* (Munich, 2000), 223–249.

22 For what follows see M. Ullmann, *Die Medizin in Islam* (Leiden, 1970), 300f.; *Sabur ibn Sahl. Dispensatorium parvum*, ed. O. Kahl (Leiden, 1994); *Sabur ibn Sahl: The Small Dispensatory*, trans. O. Kahl (Leiden, 2003); O. Kahl, *Sabur ibn Sahl's Dispensatory in the Recension of the 'Adudi Hospital* (Leiden, 2008). [See also O. Kahl, 'The Prologue to Sābūr ibn Sahl's *Small Dispensatory*', *Journal of Semitic Studies* 57 (2012): 145–163; Ragab, *The Medieval Islamic Hospital*, 214–218.]

23 Kahl, *Small Dispensatory*, xi. [See also Chapter 10, this volume.]

24 Pormann, 'Al-Muqtadir', 346; Ullmann, *Medizin*, 300.

25 *Khitab al-Fihrist*, ed. G. Flügel, 2 vols (Leipzig, 1871, 1872), II, 297.

26 *The Dispensatory of Ibn at-Tilmid*, ed. O. Kahl (Leiden, 2007); Ullmann, *Medizin*, 306; Chipman, *World of Pharmacy*, 31f.

27 Kahl, *Ibn at-Tilmid*, 5.

28 Chipman, *World of Pharmacy*, 38–41; Ullmann, *Medizin*, 309.

29 Chipman, *World of Pharmacy*, 39; Ullmann, *Medizin*, 309. [E. Lev, L. Chipman, and F. Niessen, 'A hospital handbook for the community: evidence for the extensive use of Ibn Abī 'l-Bayān's *al-Dustūr al-bīmāristānī* by the Jewish practitioners of medieval Cairo', *Journal of Semitic Studies* 53 (2008): 103–118.]

30 See Bennett, '*Xenonika*', 34f., for previous work; also his contribution to *Social History of Medicine* 13 (2000): 279–291. See also A. Touwaide, 'Byzantine hospital manuals (*iatrosophia*) as a source for the study of therapeutics', in B. S. Bowers (ed.), *The Medieval Hospital and Medical Practice* (Aldershot, 2007), 148–173.

31 A Byzantine monographic equivalent to Pormann and Savage-Smith, *Medieval Islamic Medicine* is almost inconceivable in the present state of our knowledge; see meanwhile *Dumbarton Oaks Papers* 38 (1984), 'Symposium on Byzantine medicine'. [For a short summary in English see now T. S. Miller, 'Medical thought and practice', in A. Kaldellis and N. Siniossoglou (eds), *The Cambridge Intellectual History of Byzantium* (Cambridge, 2017), 252–268. Bibliographically more comprehensive: F. Daim (ed.), *Byzanz: Historisch-Kulturwissenschaftliches Handbuch* (Stuttgart, 2016), cols 1017–1050.]

32 Chipman, *World of Pharmacy*, 1.
33 Ibid. 19, 32f.
34 Ibid. 39f.
35 Ullmann, *Medizin*, ch. 15.
36 A. Touwaide, 'The corpus of Greek medical manuscripts: a computerised inventory and catalogue', in W. M. Stevens (ed.), *Bibliographic Access to Medieval and Renaissance Manuscripts: A Survey of Computerised Data Bases and Information Services* (New York, 1992), 75–92. [See now A. Touwaide, *A Census of Greek Medical Manuscripts: From Byzantium to the Renaissance* (London, 2016).]
37 Bennett, '*Xenonika*', 441.
38 The closest parallel would be the doctors attached to the Pantokrator hospital according to its *typikon* or foundation charter, who were not supposed to abandon their hospital duties in order to treat provincial aristocrats, however close to the emperor they might be: P. Gautier (ed.), *Revue des études byzantines* 45 (1987): 107, ll. 1305–1308, with Horden, 'How medicalised?', 54.
39 Miller, *Birth of the Hospital*, xvi–xviii, produces evidence, some of it perplexing or oblique, of doctors active in late Byzantine hospitals in the capital. For a thorough review see D. Stathakopoulos, 'Stiftungen von Spitälern in spätbyzantinischer Zeit (1261–1453)', in M. Bogolte (ed.), *Stiftungen in Christentum, Judentum und Islam vor der Moderne* (Berlin, 2005), 147–157.
40 Chipman, *World of Pharmacy*, 18f.
41 R. Degen and M. Ullmann, 'Zum Dispensatorium des Sabur ibn Sahl', *Welt des Orients* 7 (1973/1974): 241–258; flood: Pormann and Savage-Smith, *Medieval Islamic Medicine*, 98; the hospital was not rebuilt for another 23 years.
42 Bennett, '*Xenonika*', ch. 6, with app. IV; for dating of the compilation as represented in the earliest manuscript, see G. Litavrin, 'Malade et médecin à Byzance, XIe–XIVe siècles: remarques sur le cod. plut. VII 19 de la Bibliothèque de Lorenzo de' Medici à Florence', in E. Patlagean (ed.), *Maladie et société à Byzance* (Paris, 1993), 97–101, at 98.
43 Adapted from Bennett, '*Xenonika*', table 6.3 (p. 249).
44 Adapted from Kahl, *Recension of the 'Adudi Hospital*, 9.
45 M. Dols, *Majnūn: The Madman in Medieval Islamic Society* (Oxford, 1992), 112–135.
46 Kahl's defence (*Recension of the 'Adudi Hospital*, 9, n. 35) of this supplement's basic integrity with the main compilation, *contra* Degen and Ullmann ('Zum Dispensatorium des Sabur ibn Sahl') takes no account of that oddity.
47 Pormann and Savage-Smith, *Medieval Islamic Medicine*, 98.
48 I am especially grateful to David Bennett here for his help in compiling the statistics of **T**.
49 Kahl, *Recension of the 'Adudi Hospital*, 10f.
50 Ibid. 63, 165; Bennett, '*Xenonika*', app. IV, 63f.
51 A final forward-looking comparison: differences of scale and sophistication between Greek and Arabic material pale when both are juxtaposed to the 1,035 detailed recipes in the vernacular *ricettario* of the great hospital of Santa Maria Nuova, Florence, compiled in 1515. See J. Henderson, *The Renaissance Hospital: Healing the Body and Healing the Soul* (New Haven, CT, 2006), 297–335.

12

A CONTEXT FOR SIMON OF GENOA'S MEDICAL DICTIONARY (*CLAVIS SANATIONIS*)

Medicine at the papal court in the later Middle Ages

I

Among the numerous works of the great thirteenth-century polymath Ramon Llull is the prose romance *Blanquerna*, which has some claim to be considered the first novel in European vernacular literature.[1] Recounting how his eponymous hero becomes pope, Llull refers to 'un escriva en Arabic' at the papal curia, one of the great Christians of his age, seemingly a man with an international reputation for learning. It is possible that Llull was referring to Simon of Genoa. If so, it is welcome testimony. We otherwise know very little about Simon beyond what he divulges in the preface to the *Clavis*. He held benefices in Padua and Rouen, and became sub-deacon, chaplain, and personal physician to Pope Nicholas IV. He tells us that he travelled for almost 30 years gathering materials for his vast and magisterial glossary. He was still active in the early pontificate of Boniface VIII, completing his work before the death in 1296 of Campano of Novara, whom he thanks in the preface. And that is virtually all we know of his biography.[2] The details of Simon's clerical career and intellectual development – including the real extent of his knowledge of Arabic – remain controversial.[3] So also do the circumstances in which the *Clavis* was commissioned and prepared. Was this work the fruit of Simon's own initiative or, as seems more likely, of papal patronage? What were his sources and where did he find them, and who helped him in the endeavour beyond the local informants to whom he occasionally refers? Although the Simon Online project to study the *Clavis* has identified 37 or more of those sources, it is still not clear which libraries Simon used. Only one extant codex, the Laurentian Celsus (plut. 73,1),[4] has been identified as a manuscript that he read – although it is also possible that one or other of two extant Spanish witnesses to an Arabic translation of Dioscorides was among his resources.[5]

Given the limited evidence available so far of Simon's career and his purposes, understanding of his work can advance on only two fronts. One is philological: close study of the *Clavis*, its analogues and possible sources. That is the approach of the other contributions in this collection. They focus on texts. The alternative, sketched here as a preliminary, is contextual and focuses on people: on the social history of medicine and doctors at the papal court, mainly but not exclusively in the long thirteenth century from the election of Innocent III to the death of Boniface VIII.[6]

II

The starting point must be this. The pope is a man – unless of course one credits the legend of Pope Joan, which became an ingredient in anti-papal polemic around the mid-thirteenth century, stressing, not coincidentally, the pontiff as physical, sexual, and of course gendered being, with a desire for self-perpetuation (Kelly 1988, appendix; Paravicini-Bagliani 2000, 133). The pope may be the 'vicar of Christ', 'lower than God but higher than man', as Innocent III put it. The 'apex of the human race', he exercises *plenitudo potestatis*. Through the merits of St Peter, of whom each pope is the direct heir, he is, in certain circumstances, *impeccabilis*, and thus well on the way to being infallible (Ullmann 1970; Tierney 1972; Paravicini-Bagliani 2000, 9–10).

Yet the pope is also a mere mortal, destined for a short reign.[7] 'Why does the head of the Apostolic See never live for very long but reaches his last day within a short space of time?' enquired Peter Damian in response to an enquiry from Alexander II (r. 1061–1073), perturbed that none of his predecessors had survived for more than four or five years in office. Damian found no pontificate to have exceeded that traditionally attributed to St Peter, that is, 25 years. Bernard of Clairvaux was well aware of this, just under a century later, when he wrote to Eugenius III (r. 1145–1153): 'How many popes have you seen die in a just a short time? [...] the end of your office is not just certain but near.' 'Behold then two salutary ideas,' Bernard further wrote, resuming the theme in his *De consideratione*: 'consider that you are the pope, and consider that you are – not that you were – a miserable speck of dust.' The return of dust to dust was likely to follow quite soon after consecration. There were twenty-seven or so popes (and one anti-pope) between Urban II and Boniface VIII whose year of birth is known or can be hazarded with some confidence.[8] Eleven were enthroned in their fifties, seven in their sixties, and eight in their seventies or eighties. The only outsider in this gerontocracy is Innocent III, a mere thirty-eight years old at his election. Even for him, St Peter's twenty-five years might have seemed a far distant goal rather than a limitation. It is hardly surprising that no 'legitimate' pope surpassed that twenty-five-year milestone until Pius IX in 1871 (Paravicini-Bagliani 2000, 53).

The tension between pope and speck of dust, between the exalted office and the frail mortal who held it, could be eased by separating the two out. The anonymous theorist of York, who c.1100 more or less invented the notion of the 'king's two bodies', went further with the pope and awarded him three: supreme pontiff, above all men; human person, their equal; and sinful person, inferior to others, on a par with murderers and adulterers (Paravicini-Bagliani 2000, 67).

III

What attitude to medicine should such a tripartite figure take? St Bernard would have known the answer. A pope, like a monk, he might have said, should not allow himself to be treated with anything more than common herbs, if that (Ziegler 1998, 219, 224). For Bernard, the opinions of Galen and Hippocrates were to be held in contempt. Yet the papacy generally took a different view. Not many other pontiffs would have merited the criticism that the great Catalan physician Arnald of Villanova levelled at Boniface VIII, his most eminent patient: 'not zeal for Christ or health of souls ruled in him but [health] of bodies' (Paravicini-Bagliani 2000, 227). Yet Boniface represents only one extreme of a spectrum – as Bernard represents the other. The pope, like any other mortal, was free to enjoy the benefit of secular medicine, provided – as enjoined by the Fourth Lateran Council (canon 22) – he confessed his sins first and put the medicine of the soul above that of the body. Hippocrates and Galen were portrayed in the cathedral crypt at Anagni, probably at the behest of the canons there. These men in turn were closely connected with Innocent III and still more Gregory IX, under whom the court often moved to Viterbo for the summer (Paravicini-Bagliani 2000, 178, 187). The Augustinian theologian James of Viterbo (c.1255–c.1308) even opined that medicine would have been useful in Paradise, before sin, and thus sickness, arose (Ziegler 2001, 201–202). After all, the doctor's skill and means of curing alike came from God (*Ecclesiasticus* 38.1–4). Canon law restricted the practice of medicine only by those in major orders and living under a rule, and was meant to deter them from doing it for profit (Amundsen 1996, 227–235). Hence, for example, over a third of the practitioners known from medieval France (between the twelfth and fifteenth centuries) were members of the clergy (Ziegler 1998, 3).

Broken down by century, that proportion was probably at its highest in the twelfth century, and started to decline in the thirteenth. In 1219 Honorius III extended the scope of the prohibition from those living under a rule to a wider array of archdeacons, deacons, rural deans, and others holding benefices, and also to priests. But the measure was intended to protect the study of theology and was directed at medical learning more than at medical practice (Amundsen 1996, 231–233). Even Celestine V, who tried to prevent all clerics from practising medicine, exempted those whose cures were administered to family and friends or to others free, out of charity. Dispensations from all these measures could in any case be secured, and the measures' scope was soon reduced, essentially so that parish clergy were untouched by the canon law on this matter; reduced by – predictably – Boniface VIII. Hence then – the very tip of the clerical-medical iceberg – those major figures such as Teodorico Borgognoni, the surgeon who became a bishop, and above all Peter of Spain. Unless two distinct figures are being conflated by historians, Peter began as dean of Lisbon, perhaps went on to serve as personal physician to Gregory X (clear evidence on that is lacking), became archbishop of Braga, and finally, having been made cardinal, was elected pope as John XXI in 1276 (Paravicini-Bagliani 1991, 28–29, 32).

With such a progression possible, it is hardly remarkable that leading abbots and bishops should retain doctors, or that the papal court should attract and welcome many of the most distinguished of them. The unsurpassed scholarship of Paravicini-Bagliani has given us a detailed prosopogaphy of over 70 medical men known or conjectured to have had some association with popes and cardinals during the long twelfth century.[9] The list is 'end-heavy': more than a third of them (25) were active under Boniface VIII, other pontificates variously attracting only up to six names. Those who may have been specifically papal physicians range in number between one and three per reign, but again the tally rises under Boniface, to five. As with papal chaplains, who are being studied by Matthew Ross of University College, London, some associations between medical men and popes or cardinals are transient and ad hoc, some are very lasting. According to the Renaissance chronicler Filippo Villani, Taddeo Alderotti cured Honorius IV of some ailment, but that was his only recorded connection with the curia and it may not even be historical. At the other end of the spectrum, Campano of Novarra was active for some 30 years at court under four popes, from Urban IV to Boniface VIII, and William of Brescia served Boniface VII, Clement V, and John XXII.

These examples immediately indicate that many of the names involved are major figures in the general history of learned medicine in the period. To the list we can probably add Philip of Tripoli, Richard of Fournival, Teodorico Borgognoni, William of Moerbeke, Arnald of Villanova (Arnald perhaps the most significant for European medicine as a whole in this roster of luminaries), and of course, not least, Simon of Genoa. The papal court was obviously an attractive source of patronage. We note the interplay of medical and clerical careers, medical success leading to clerical preferment, as with Teodorico Borgognoni who probably rose to be papal penitentiary and chaplain on the strength of having cured Innocent IV's nephew. Campano of Novara clearly became very rich during his long service as astronomer/astrologer as well as doctor at the curia. He had a palace in Viterbo and his landed wealth was appraised at more than 12,000 florins (Paravicini-Bagliani 2000, 189). Paravicini-Bagliani's study of cardinals' wills shows more generally that their bequests to personal physicians usually outstripped in generosity those to other *familiares* (2000, 191; 1980). The rewards of service could take a variety of forms. Richard of Fournival was dispensed from the restriction of canon law so that he could practise surgery, as presumably at some point was Teodorico. Richard of Wendover (who may or may not be the same as Richard the Englishman) received an ivory cross from Gregory IX on his deathbed. Arnald of Villanova was given a gold cross by Boniface VIII. John of Procida gained political intercession over some property in Naples that he had lost by backing the wrong horse in the imperial succession dispute. His patient, a cardinal and future pope, wrote to the current pope, Clement IV, asking him to intercede with Charles of Anjou (Paravicini-Bagliani 2000, 191).

In the first half of the thirteenth century a substantial number of papal medical men may have been educated at Salerno, for example the cardinal John of St Paul (Paravicini-Bagliani 2009, 97–112). This connection weakens in the second half, as doctors seem more likely to have come from cities in the papal states. By the end of the century, perhaps from the 1280s, there may have been some teaching of medicine in the *Studium curiae*, and this could have provided an alternative reservoir of skill and talent (but the evidence is controversial and the details obscure: Paravicini-Bagliani 1991, 393–408).

One sign of the growing general esteem for medicine on the part of the thirteenth-century papacy is that doctors seem to become indispensable presences at the pope's deathbed (Paravicini-Bagliani 1991, 7–8). Another is that the remedies that doctors were believed, rightly or not, to have created for popes were celebrated as such in the wider manuscript literature of medical recipes (21–22, 24, 27, 49). Albertus Magnus was never a curial physician so far as is known, but that did not hinder the transmission of the *pillule mirabilis operationis* that he is credited with having made for Gregory IX (21).

IV

Some caveats need mentioning, nonetheless. Paravicini-Bagliani's prosopography, though of impeccable scholarship and wholly indispensable, is full of conjectural identifications, not least that of Peter of Spain and Pope John XXI. This is inevitable given the state of the evidence, and the author never disguises the fact. But it is still worth occasionally questioning the criteria of inclusion. Romuald very probably did become archbishop of Salerno, for example, but should he be listed as a doctor at the papal court on the strength of a line of verse by Giles of Corbeil saying he was admired by the curia as a medical writer and a 'patron of life'? Or, again, was Innocent III's doctor, Romanus, the same as the cardinal bishop whose sole recorded claim to medical expertise is his awareness of the rather basic notion that medicine heals by contraries? Should Adam of Kircudbright, chaplain to Urban IV, be listed when his medical fame is reportedly that he served as Robert the Bruce's doctor? Peter of Abano dedicated a treatise on poisons to a pope but we cannot tell which one; and although he claimed to enjoy papal favour it is not clear that he practised at the curia either.

We can pick out individual pieces of the jigsaw and show that they do not quite fit together. But the overall picture is still robust enough to convey the substantial presence of authorities on medical practice in and near the papal court. And that provides some context for Simon. In his medical activity he was one of many. He blends into the crowd of doctors clustering round popes and cardinals hoping for medical patronage and ecclesiastical preferment. In the longevity of his association with the curia he was unusual but by no means unique.

For us, however, Simon is known as a text more than as a person; and on this front, too, it is possible to sketch a context within which his decades of work on the *Clavis* come to seem, not less remarkable, but at least a little more explicable. This is not the place for detail; but, again from the fundamental work of Paravicini-Bagliani, it is clear that during the thirteenth century the papal court was increasingly a focus for a number of scientific interests – scientific in both the medieval and the modern senses.[10] Astronomy and geometry (Campano of Novarra), geography (David of Dinant), and optics are only some of the subjects read or written about at court. The concentration of expertise could be unrivalled: 'in the decade 1267–1277, Viterbo was the European capital of optics' (Paravicini-Bagliani 2000, 196–197, 209). That is thanks to the intersection, in the papal ambit, of the careers of William of Moerbeke, Witelo, John Peckham, and Peter of Spain, at Viterbo in the papal states, where the curia resided almost without interruption from 1260 to 1280 (2000, 173).

Medical writings, too, belong under this heading of scientific patronage. To give only the main topics and some key names associated with each in the curial world:[11] surgery (Teodorico), anatomy (David of Dinant again), food (at Viterbo, William of Moerbeke translated Galen on this, as later, in Rome, did Accursino of Pistoia), and regimen (John of Toledo; John of Capua, Peter of Spain, and most notably Arnald, whom Boniface more or less immured in a papal castle in order to focus his mind on the task of writing for him a regimen). Surgery, anatomy, regimen – these are topics in standard Galenic medicine of the period. But the papal court became a centre for speculation and writing about less predictable, even occult, topics. One of them was the question of how to delay the ill effects of old age and to prolong life. Instead of being cut short like St Peter, might the pope instead outdo Peter and even rival Methuselah? Involved here were alchemical remedies. It is no coincidence that Philip of Tripoli translated at the curia the pseudo-Aristotelian *Secreta secretorum* (*Secret of Secrets*) (Williams 2003, 114–121). Besides devoting considerable space to prolongation of life, this text, the most widely read 'Aristotelian' title of the Middle Ages, was a source for much of the thinking about alchemy, physiognomy, magic, and astrology of the thirteenth to fourteenth centuries. Those who insinuated that Peter of Spain/John XXI died suddenly despite boasting that he could prolong his life, presumably with an elixir, or that several cardinals quaffed potable gold, may have known more than we do about the extent and the seriousness of curial interest in alchemy.[12]

Simon and his *Clavis* can to some extent be understood against this background. For example, it is clear that he consulted alchemical treatises.[13] Yet he also stands out because of the magnitude of the task he set himself and the time he took to complete it. Here the analogy with Witelo's work on optics and Campano's on Euclid or on the planets may be just as relevant. Both scholars were committed to major synoptic undertakings. Perhaps Simon was aiming for a similar comprehensiveness.[14]

V

Why such a comprehensive approach? Why all the scientific and medical activity that fed into it? Why was the papal court a centre of patronage on this scale? Paravicini-Bagliani's answer, given at several points in his more recent work (e.g. 2000, xiv, 185), is simple: the impact of the new learning becoming available as Arabic texts were translated. The translation activity and the reception of learning in Arabic, especially works of Aristotle and Avicenna, can be documented quite amply at the thirteenth-century curia.[15] That fact is not self-explanatory. Such texts do not arrive of their own accord. They have to be identified as desirable and sought out, and then laboriously translated. If we see the various forms of exoteric and esoteric learning in which popes and cardinals of our period took some interest as merely reflex responses to a new fashion in philosophical medicine, we miss the sense of excitement, the fervour of the hunt for new therapeutic possibilities, that news of such possibilities engendered. Aged and decrepit cardinals, and still more popes, living (some of the time, when to do so was unavoidable) in a notoriously insalubrious city, had many reasons to encourage novel ideas and techniques. Aspiring curialist doctors had many reasons to offer such novelties. In other words, the explanation of the texts is to be sought in the history of the patients involved; it is not that the arrival of the texts explains the attitudes and enthusiasms of the patients.

This is by no means to deny that wider contexts may also have had some bearing. Interaction with, and emulation of, the imperial court of Frederick II should not be discounted (Paravicini-Bagliani 1991, xiii, 55–84). Nor should we forget that this century of natural philosophy, of 'scientific' celebration and investigation of the material world, was also the century of Catharism, with its denigration of that world: a heresy as evident in the Papal States as it was in the Languedoc, and slow to succumb to the inquisition (French and Cunningham 1996). Yet such wider concerns will have seemed secondary to Gregory IX, with his gallstones, or to Honorius IV, so crippled by gout that he needed a crutch for support when celebrating Mass (Paravicini-Bagliani 2000, 183, 194).

There was nothing very new about this. Paravicini-Bagliani treats his long thirteenth century as a self-contained period. For him, it begins in clear-cut fashion with Innocent III, the first pope for whom we know of a *medicus pape* – and a papal apothecary; the first pope to have discussed his own maladies at some length; the first pope to have acquired a house for his doctor near the Vatican palace (2000, 186–187; see also Ait 2013). These claims for outright novelty on Innocent's behalf would have surprised many of his predecessors. Popes had been consulting the most learned doctors they could find since the time of Gregory the Great in the late sixth century if not earlier (Horden 2009, 265). Of course, there were changes of scale. Chris Wickham's personal database of charters and documentary evidence, compiled as part of his research for a monograph on Rome and its environs, 900–1200, the period before that of Paravicini-Bagliani, finds some 32 medical men for the whole three centuries (personal communication [Wickham 2014]). That seems a small number in comparison, even though the database excludes narratives, which would surely yield more names. Yet it is not clear that changes in quality as well as quantity were under way as we move into the thirteenth century. Is a *medicus pape* necessarily more than a doctor who attends the pope, even if he lives in a 'tied cottage', or has he moved into a new category of 'papal physician'? The Latin is ambiguous. Granted, in the thirteenth century the credentials that an aspiring doctor derived from acquaintance with the new Arabic-derived learning would have made some difference. But we need to ask what sort of medicine was regularly dispensed to ageing pontiffs and their courtiers? Was it elixirs of life or something more basic? For evidence we have to look forward a little into the Avignon period, where the comings and goings of doctors at the curia can be documented in a similar way (Pansier 1909; Guillemain 1962). And to get a little nearer to the papal sickbed in that period we can sometimes turn to catalogues of *experimenta* – tried and tested remedies, rather than experiments in the modern sense, but 'experimental' in that no one knew how or why they worked. Their claim to repeated use lay in their effectiveness.

Arnald of Villanova recorded 73 successful 'experimental' treatments that he conducted on named individuals at or around the papal court in Avignon between 1305 and 1311 (McVaugh 1971). Although the treatments include use of gems, gold, mercury, and alcohol, Arnald's remedies depend mostly on vegetable ingredients, and are simple – far more so than those he expounded (to impress colleagues or patrons?) in many of his theoretical works. And some of the ailments he addresses (in patients of both sexes) hardly seem worthy of the foremost 'consultant' of his time. They include haemorrhoids, wrinkles, hair loss, and fleas, as well as amnesia, chronic headache, indigestion, swellings – and toothache.

Another *experimentum* for toothache. Once the lord pope [Clement V, the collection's dedicatee] had a pain in his jaw [...] One of his teeth had a cavity and there a worm tossed to and fro. When the worm stirred within the tooth the aforementioned lord suffered greatly, so that he could neither drink nor sleep. After I had carefully inspected it, I easily administered a remedy [...] I caused to be gathered a certain herb called camomile in the vernacular. (McVaugh 1971, 113; trans. Wallis 2010, 402)

Arnald fumigated the pontiff's mouth with smoke from heated camomile seeds and the worm dropped out. If this is generally what we would have found at the pope's bedside, it may come as a surprise after all the arcane learning with which the court has been associated. But it would not have surprised twelfth-century physicians. There may be more continuity between twelfth and thirteenth centuries than Paravicini-Bagliani supposes; and that continuity too would be a further part of the explanation for the medical history of the curia during the period in which Simon was active. There was a more long-standing tradition of medical patronage behind it.

VI

'Try anything once' – or, indeed, repeatedly. That might have been the unofficial papal motto where health and illness were concerned. *Experimenta* and basic herbal remedies at one end of the spectrum, the most recherché alchemical techniques at the other. One clear example of this 'no holds barred' approach is the frequency with which popes of the later Avignon period, the Great Schism, and after happily resorted to Jewish doctors (as did archbishops, bishops, abbots, and priests below them).[16] Hebrew sources alone claim that Master Gaio (Isaac ben Mordecai) served as doctor to Nicholas IV, and that seems too early by comparison with the plentiful evidence from later on. But Boniface IX, for example, had two Jewish physicians in attendance. Such men were learned and skilful, and they were available in abundance. For this was the period when, following the various expulsions from northern kingdoms, the concentration of Jewish doctors in Provence and adjacent regions was at its greatest.

If all else fails, try magic. Papal magic seems to belong under the heading of the slanders and trumped-up charges made, at various points in the later Middle Ages and Renaissance, against popes and anti-popes alike. But there is more to the subject. Popes in an earlier period than ours here had worn apotropaic bells attached to the hem of their vestments (Maguire 1997, 1038–1039). At his posthumous trial Boniface VIII was alleged to have received an *idolum* containing a diabolical spirit from Taddeo Alderotti (Paravicini-Bagliani 1991, 36). Yet it is likely that Arnald of Villanova really did present the same pope with a talisman in the form of a gold seal for use against his kidney stones (McVaugh 1993, 162–163). Around 1315 the future pope Clement VI copied out an illicit form of divination by name (onomancy) (Boudet 2006, 43).[17] John XXII fulminated in a letter of 1318 against a network of spirit conjurors, but he was frank about the fact that they included several people residing at his own court (Maxwell-Stuart 2005, 84–86; for context Boureau 2006). And so on. Later, the genuine interest of Benedict XIII and his circle in alchemy, astrology, and Joachimite prophecy could have provided the kernel for the fantastic charges of witchcraft and necromancy brought against him at the Council of Pisa in 1409 (Harvey 1973).

The history of the connections between popes and medicine in the long thirteenth century, the century when papal monarchy was at its apogee, could be pursued further in many directions: for example, hospital foundation, the medicalizing of canonization procedures, concern with autopsy and dissection and with division of the corpse for burial.[18] None of these, though, would shed particular light on Simon of Genoa and his *Clavis*. We can try to set him in a wider curial context and a longer history of papal patronage of science and medicine. Yet he remains an elusive figure, whose work we are only just beginning to understand.

Notes

1 [For clarity I have inverted the title of this paper from the original 'Medicine at the Papal Court in the Later Middle Ages: A Context for Simon of Genoa'. It is a contribution to the larger project of 'Simon Online', simonofgenoa.org, directed by Barbara Zipser.] Paravicini-Bagliani (1991), 184–185. It will be clear that I am heavily indebted throughout to this author's fundamental works on the thirteenth-century popes and the papal court (1991; 2000; 2009), and differ from them only on minor points of emphasis and interpretation. I am also extremely grateful for advice and references to Charles Burnett, Jo Edge, Klaus-Dietrich Fischer, Monica Green, Vivian Nutton, Jennifer Rampling, Matthew Ross, Chris Wickham, and Barbara Zipser. In what follows I have kept annotation to a minimum, just citing works that give full details of the people, texts and editions referred to. Names of historical figures have generally been Anglicized unless the original form is well known.
2 Paravicini-Bagliani (1991), 191–197, 247–251; (2000), 190–191.
3 For Simon's contact with Arabic speakers, see Zipser (2013), 150. Bhayro (2013) takes a far dimmer view than did Llull of Simon's competence in the language. See also Cronier (2013), 91–94. For the limited knowledge of Arabic at the papal court in Simon's time, see Paravicini-Bagliani (1991), 180–181, 186–189.
4 Billanovich (1975), 328 n. 18, a reference I owe to Klaus-Dietrich Fischer.
5 Cronier (2013) for further detail.
6 For detailed and accurate brief entries on all popes of the period, see Kelly (1988).
7 For what follows see Paravicini-Bagliani (2000), 11–13.
8 The figures that follow are based on data in Kelly (1988).
9 Unless otherwise indicated, all details of papal doctors in the following paragraphs derive from Paravicini-Bagliani (1991), 3–51.

10 For what follows see Paravicini-Bagliani (1991), 14, 16, 23–24, 42, 48, 87–115, 119–124, 143–175, 161–165.
11 Paravicini-Bagliani (1991), 13, 16, 25, 32, 41–42.
12 Paravicini-Bagliani (2000), 210–211. For continuing curial interest in alchemy, see also 221, 249, 346n., with Crisciani (2002).
13 See *Clavis* entries for *Elcismatos, Muzadir,* and *Sponium*, to which Barbara Zipser kindly directed my attention.
14 I am indebted here to Charles Burnett.
15 For Simon's use of Arabic manuscripts see again Cronier (2013), 91–94; Paravicini-Bagliani (1991), 179–232.
16 For what follows see Shatzmiller (1994), 94–95, Siraisi (1990), 29, and now Esposito (2013).
17 A reference I owe to Jo Edge.
18 See e.g. Birch (1998), 141–143; [Keyvanian (2015), 80–85, 339–383;] Ziegler (1999); Park (2006), 47, 52.

Bibliography

Ait, I. (2013). Alla corte dei papi: gli speziali. In E. Andretta and M. Nicoud (eds), *Être médecin à la cour (Italie, France, Espagne, XIIIe–XVIIIe siècle)*, 35–48. Florence: Sismel/Galuzzo.

Amundsen, D. W. (1996). *Medicine, Society, and Faith in the Ancient and Medieval Worlds*. Baltimore, MD: Johns Hopkins University Press.

Bhayro, S. (2013). Simon of Genoa as an Arabist. In B. Zipser (ed.), *Simon of Genoa's Medical Lexicon*, 49–65. London: Versita.

Billanovich, G. (1975). Centri di trasmissione: Milano, Nonantola, Brescia. In *La cultura antica nell'Occidente latino dal VII all' XI secolo*, vol. I. Spoleto: Presso la Sede del Centro, 321–352.

Birch, D. (1998). *Pilgrimage to Rome in the Middle Ages*. Woodbridge: Boydell.

Boudet, J.-P. (2006). *Entre science et nigromancie: astrologie, divination et magie dans l'Occident médiéval*. Paris: Sorbonne.

Boureau, A. (2006). *Satan the Heretic: The Birth of Demonology in the Medieval West*, trans. T. Lavender. Chicago: University of Chicago Press.

Crisciani, C. (2002). *Il papa e l'alchemia: Felice V, Guglielmo Fabri e l'elixir*. Rome: Viella.

Cronier, M. (2013). Dioscorides excerpts in Simon of Genoa's *Clavis sanationis*. In B. Zipser (ed.), *Simon of Genoa's Medical Lexicon*, 79–97. London: Versita.

Esposito, A. (2013). Alla corte dei Papi: archiatri pontifici ebrei tra '400 e '500. In E. Andretta and M. Nicoud (eds), *Être médecin à la cour (Italie, France, Espagne, XIIIe–XVIIIe siècle)*, 17–33. Florence: Sismel/Galuzzo.

French, R. K., and Cunningham, A. (1996). *Before Science: The Invention of the Friars' Natural Philosophy*. Aldershot: Scolar.

Guillemain, B. (1962). *La cour pontificale d'Avignon (1309–1376): étude d'une société*. Paris: Boccard.

Harvey, M. (1973). Papal witchcraft: the charges against Benedict XIII. In D. Baker (ed.), *Sanctity and Secularity: The Church and the World*, 109–116. Oxford: Ecclesiastical History Society.

Horden, P. (2009). The late antique origins of the lunatic asylum? In P. Rousseau and M. Papoutsakis (eds), *Transformations of Late Antiquity: Essays for Peter Brown*, 259–278. Farnham: Ashgate [reprinted as Ch. 5 in the present volume].

Kelly, J. N. D. (1988). *The Oxford Dictionary of Popes*. Oxford: Oxford University Press.

Keyvanian, C. (2015). *Hospitals and Urbanism in Rome, 1200–1500*. Leiden: Brill.

Maguire, H. (1997). Magic and money in the early Middle Ages. *Speculum* 72(4): 1037–1054.

Maxwell-Stuart, P. G. (ed. and trans.) (2005). *The Occult in Medieval Europe, 500–1500*. Houndmills: Palgrave Macmillan.

McVaugh, M. (1971). The *experimenta* of Arnald of Villanova. *Journal of Medieval and Renaissance Studies* 1: 107–18.

McVaugh, M. R. (1993). *Medicine Before the Plague: Practitioners and Their Patients in the Crown of Aragon 1285–1345*. Cambridge: Cambridge University Press.

Pansier, P. (1909). Les médecins des papes d'Avignon (1308–1403). *Janus* 14: 405–434.

Paravicini-Bagliani, A. (1980). *I testamenti dei cardinali del Duecento*. Rome: Presso la Società.

Paravicini-Bagliani, A. (1991). *Medicina e scienze della natura alla corte dei papi nel Duecento*. Spoleto: Centro italiano di studi sull'Alto Medioevo.

Paravicini-Bagliani, A. (2000). *The Pope's Body*, trans. D. S. Peterson. Chicago: University of Chicago Press (first published 1994, *Il corpo del papa*, Turin: Einaudi).

Paravicini-Bagliani, A. (2009). *Il potere del papa: corporeità, autorappresentazione, simboli*. Florence: Sismel/Galluzzo.

Park, K. (2006). *Secrets of Women: Gender, Generation, and the Origins of Human Dissection*. New York: Zone.

Shatzmiller, J. (1994). *Jews, Medicine, and Medieval Society*. Berkeley: University of California Press.

Siraisi, N. G. 1990. *Medieval and Early Renaissance Medicine*. Chicago: University of Chicago Press.

Tierney, B. (1972). *Origins of Papal Infallibility, 1150–1350: A Study on the Concepts of Infallibility, Sovereignty and Tradition in the Middle Ages*. Leiden: Brill.

Ullmann, W. (1970). *The Growth of Papal Government in the Middle Ages: A Study in the Ideological Relation of Clerical to Lay Power*. London: Methuen.

Wallis, F. (ed.) (2010). *Medieval Medicine: A Reader*. Toronto: University of Toronto Press.

Wickham, C. (2014). *Medieval Rome: Stability and Crisis of a City, 900–1150*. Oxford: Oxford University Press.

Williams, S. J. (2003). *The 'Secret of Secrets': The Scholarly Career of a Pseudo-Aristotelian Text in the Later Middle Ages*. Ann Arbor: University of Michigan Press.

Ziegler, J. (1998). *Medicine and Religion c. 1300: The Case of Arnau de Vilanova*. Oxford: Clarendon Press.

Ziegler, J. (1999). Practitioners and saints: medical men and canonization procedures in the thirteenth to fifteenth centuries. *Social History of Medicine* 12(2): 191–225.

Ziegler, J. (2001). Medicine and immortality in terrestrial paradise. In P. Biller and J. Ziegler (eds), *Religion and Medicine in the Middle Ages*, 201–242. York: York Medieval Press.

Zipser, B. (2013). Simon Online, an alternative approach to research and publishing. In B. Zipser (ed.), *Simon of Genoa's Medical Lexicon*, 149–155. London: Versita.

13

SMALL BEER?

The parish and the poor and sick in later Medieval England

There were no rates for the poor even in my grandfather's days: but . . . the church ale at Whitsuntide did their business.

(John Aubrey)[1]

I

A story about Oscar Wilde at Oxford, told in variant versions all doubtless equally apocryphal, has him being orally examined in Divinity by the famous W. H. Spooner. Asked to construe from the Greek the passage in Matthew's gospel about Judas's betrayal of Christ for 30 pieces of silver, Wilde then ignored all requests to stop. 'Hush, hush,' he admonished Spooner, 'let us proceed and see what happened to the unfortunate man.'[2]

The first task of any study of parochial poor relief in the later Middle Ages is to recapture some of that ignorance of what happened next. We must try to forget that we know, or think we know, how the story will end – with the Old Poor Law of 1598 and 1601, the Law which was based on parish rates, and which broadly endured until 1834. That is, we have to avoid constructing a teleological narrative in which all roads lead to those Elizabethan statutes, and in which earlier forms of parish poor relief may be underestimated precisely because they were not statutory.

Doing that is hard. For medievalists, to look forward into the Tudor age is virtually inescapable. Despite the historical caesura of the Reformation, and the rarity with which scholars straddle a great historiographical divide,[3] the ecclesiastical histories of the fifteenth and sixteenth centuries cannot be discussed in isolation from one another – perhaps on any front, but least of all on that of poor relief. Whatever our rough starting date – 1200, 1300, or 1400 – our whole view of the topic is likely to be coloured by the fact that the parish emerges during the seventeenth century as the primary agent of poor relief.[4] We have to decide how far that emergence reflects a radical discontinuity with medieval poor relief or (as I shall argue here) more continuity than many historians have allowed. Moreover, both the nature of the evidence and the current state of scholarship enforce upon medievalists a degree of forward looking. Historians of the Tudor poor benefit from relatively detailed and voluminous evidence, a clear chronology, and reliable syntheses – from Miss Leonard's and the Webbs' to those of Paul Slack.[5] Medievalists interested specifically in the parish and the poor, by contrast, soon find that this is a subject visible, at best, fleetingly – always out of the corner of the eye.[6] We have only isolated pieces of evidence, from which we do not know how to extrapolate, and we have no agreed narrative of the relevant facets of parish history into which to insert them. We look with envy to the sharper and fuller picture yielded by the sixteenth century, and may be tempted into misreading it – for example, by assuming that things were changing in the early sixteenth century when they were, perhaps, simply becoming better documented. To raise that possibility is not to suggest that historians have exaggerated the enormity of economic and religious change in the sixteenth century, or the lasting impact of that change on the ways in which poverty was perceived and evaluated, and on the scale and overall 'depth' of poverty itself.[7] It is simply to propose that the Reformation, although decisive for the next three centuries of English poor relief, may, on this particular front, mask some degree of continuity with the later Middle Ages.

II

How to uncover and assess that continuity? And how to bring the study of the later Middle Ages and that of the early modern period into a more balanced relationship? The initial step is to break down the teleological narrative by which the Old Poor Law was the Tudor parish's sole destiny.

Of course, from the 1530s onwards the parish had figured largely in many of the various projects, experiments, and enactments of the royal Council, of Parliament, and of major civic authorities for the support of the deserving poor and the deterrence of able-bodied scroungers.[8] But we have rightly been warned, by Paul Slack, not to see these measures as a logical, cumulative progression towards compulsory parochial poor rates enforced by statute:

> A permanent welfare apparatus was being forged out of disparate local and legislative efforts . . . It must be admitted, however, that historians of the poor law . . . have sometimes been mesmerised by its local antecedents and its later development, and have been tempted to overstate both its insularity and the smooth inevitability of its legislative evolution.[9]

In 1598 the government was not responding to long-term trends in parish history or the economic conjoncture but to recent rebellions and impending famines and epidemics.[10] It was under pressure from traditionalists to hold back from a compulsory poor rate and from radicals to go beyond one. The novelty of the 1598 and 1601 statutes did not lie in their provisions, for the parish had been involved in poor relief since the 1530s and there had been compulsory levies since the 1540s. Rather, as Marjorie McIntosh has observed, it lay in the system's durability.[11] The age of experiment, in which the parish held a crucial but varying place, was formally over – but in the circumstances it might well have continued.

Even so, the parish's new statutory and (as it proved) permanent role was not actually achieved very quickly. Some parishes preserved traditional, voluntary almsgiving as their main support for the poor well into the seventeenth century. The geography of the Old Poor Law was extremely patchy. By the Restoration, it may have been *fully* effective in only a minority of English parishes and had made hardly any impact in Wales.[12] Moreover, nowhere did it render obsolete those long-established informal mechanisms of self-help and neighbourly charity that were crucial to the survival of the poor, especially those not 'on the parish'.[13] The Poor Law thus marked a less dramatic change in the overall character and relative importance of parochial relief than historians have often supposed.

Not only that: its uniqueness may also have been over-stressed. It blends to a considerable extent into the evolution of poor relief in early modern Europe. Granted, only England saw the (eventual) implementation of national compulsory poor rates. Yet similar schemes were attempted in Scotland and, obviously on a smaller scale, in some Danish, French, Swiss, and Italian cities, and were at least contemplated in Germany, Sweden, and the Spanish Netherlands.[14] The English statutes had been framed in an intellectual milieu much influenced by other European projects for the poor, and, in return, England had even managed one distinctive export to the continent – the workhouse.[15] We must abandon any notion that English parochial 'outdoor' relief can be sharply contrasted with the continental 'indoor' relief of large urban hospitals.[16] The differences between compulsory English rates and the published subscription lists of continental European parishes (or of immigrant communities in England) with their less formal pressures should also be blurred.[17] In the collection of revenue, statutory taxes are not everything. Customary mechanisms may be no easier to evade.

The early modern history of parochial poor relief thus needs modification in several ways that are significant for the medievalist. First, the implementation of the 1601 Poor Law was slow and, to begin with, geographically limited. Second, the Law was not, in practice, as distinctive within the wider European context as has conventionally been maintained. Finally, above all, the statutes fixing the parish as the unit of poor relief were a more contingent matter than narrative histories of poverty in the period often imply.

III

This is the background against which we must approach the big question of why Tudor (and later) poor relief was parochial at all. Was the parish its vehicle *faute de mieux*? Or did the parish have strengths that made it the obvious choice – strengths developed during the later Middle Ages?

On the negative side, it must be admitted at once that the Dissolutions of the 1530s and 1540s had left few alternative institutions of charity intact. The abolition of chantries and their associated 'stocks', of gilds and fraternities with their distributions to both members and non-members, of monasteries with their almonries, and of some half of the country's hospitals and almshouses was, in aggregate, a real loss to the poor. The whole framework of organized charity had to be rebuilt – and its only possible bases were private benefactions, craft associations, and the parish.[18]

The anthropologist C. R. Hallpike has claimed that, in social evolution, what survives is not the fittest but 'the mediocre'.[19] The parish has an aura of mediocrity about it. Not just the Church's main institutional survivor of the Dissolution, it was, perhaps, perceived as simply adequate to some of the tasks with which the worsening scale of Tudor poverty presented it. Only in London was a bigger and more sophisticated apparatus clearly needed.[20] The parish's statutory role in poor relief also owed something to its familiarity to those who framed the statutes. The Council and the municipal authorities did not automatically think in parochial terms, and were more worried about migrant sturdy beggars than the impotent poor. Members of parliament by contrast, suspicious of growing central interference, represented an in every sense more parochial world of small towns and villages, in which relief of the 'deserving' was an obviously pressing need.[21]

So much for the negatives. On a more positive note, it should be added that the parish had a long history that suited it for its role as the government's agent of poor relief. First, as is well known, by the close of the Middle Ages, parishes were already in many respects secular institutions. Although their secular role grew very significantly during the sixteenth century, that growth was from an already high base line. Parishes had been units of royal taxation since the twelfth century and, during the later Middle Ages, overtook hundreds and manors as organs of local government and administration.[22] Second, since at least the late thirteenth century, parishes had also known a long if intermittent history of self-imposed compulsory local rates, mainly but not exclusively for repairs to the fabric of the nave.[23] They were also familiar with quarterly rates to pay the wages of the parish clerk.[24] Parishioners were, therefore, used to schemes for apportioning among themselves shares of a financial burden and for raising payments that were virtually compulsory (since defaulters could be arraigned before an ecclesiastical court).

Most significantly for their long-term future, parishes had also, in the aftermath of the Black Death, been implicated in the government's concern to address the problem of the able-bodied poor, the future 'sturdy beggars', who were expected to be able to find work.[25] The Ordinance and Statute of Labourers of 1349/1351 forbade the giving of alms from any source to the able-bodied. The Act of 1388 ordered that beggars who were genuinely unable to work should be maintained by residents of the city or town in which they lived – or in which they had been born.[26] Even in 1388 the principle of local responsibility was not new, however, and its weight may already have fallen *de facto* on the parish – parish of current residence or, on some inchoate notion of 'settlement', parish of birth.[27]

Although the central government thus seems to have been leaning on the parish as one leading source of poor relief by the later fourteenth century, it remains extremely hard to establish quite how the parish responded. A comparison with parts of continental Europe is telling. For example, in the Low Countries and northern Italy especially, but also in Provence, there had since as early as 1200 been a vigorous tradition of 'poor tables': municipal schemes for the daily disbursement, through parishes, of food, money, and clothing to registered paupers.[28] In the 1280s and later, the 'father of the poor' in parishes in Valencia gave out small sums of money every week, and food and clothing on feast days.[29] In Florence *c.*1500 there may also have been *spedaluzzi*, mini-hospitals, offering a roof and bedding to local poor, financed by alms collected in church and served by parishioners.[30] All such examples are in apparent contrast to the less institutionalized, and far less clearly documented, activities of the English parish in the later Middle Ages. Not surprisingly, historians acknowledge its role briefly while moving hastily on to the archival *terra firma* of fraternities.[31]

IV

The first problem that historians face is lack of clear evidence. Bequests to the poor of the parish may be made in wills – our chief source for so much of later medieval social and religious life – but we shall often not know when that happens, because the paupers are simply named rather than identified by their penury.[32] Our second main source is churchwardens' accounts; and these seem to include very little about direct transfers to the poor until the early sixteenth century.[33] The appearance of such transfers at that time (for example in the London accounts of St Mary at Hill[34]) long precedes the Parliamentary statute of 1535–1536 by which churchwardens and two others were required to maintain a 'box' to receive parishioners' 'charitable and voluntarie almes' on Sundays and feast days. It is not to be explained in simple political terms as part of the government's campaign against sturdy vagabonds.[35] Before the early 1500s, churchwardens did not systematically account in this public way for disbursements to the needy, although, as we shall see, other fragmentary evidence suggests that some disbursements were indeed made.[36] Even when we move later into the sixteenth century, with all its attempted governmental regulation, huge lacunae still disfigure any overall picture we try to construct. For example, the Churchwardens' Accounts of St Mary's Lambeth reveal that the parish was running an almshouse in 1517–1518 (as it happens, the same year in which the alms box of St Mary at Hill makes its unheralded debut in its wardens' accounts).[37] We should obviously like to know much more about this parochial almshouse, but it is only mentioned in 1517–1518, and then it does not resurface in the accounts until well after the Reformation, in 1566–1567, when it needed repair.[38]

After wills and churchwardens' accounts, our third main point of entry into the religious and economic life of the late medieval parish is through episcopal or local visitation records. But here too, pending systematic scrutiny of a large number of unedited texts, historians find they are simply chewing over the same few morsels, uncertain what to make of them. For instance, an archidiaconal visitation of Oxfordshire in 1520 (or perhaps 1517) showed that 35 out of 193 parishes were reported as neglecting their poor. This has lent itself to an argument among historians, lasting for almost a century, about whether the glass is 82 per cent full (a large majority was doing a good job, and the rest were at least expected to do so) or 18 per cent empty (a significant minority was performing poorly).[39] What it has so far not led to is a search for comparable evidence from other areas even from within the same diocese.[40]

The difficulties of this subject of the parish and the poor are, however, not only those presented by the evidence. There remains a conceptual issue. What is the parish?[41] Or, perhaps, when is the parish? When is it more than a social framework or arena for action and a corporate agent in its own right?[42] What bodies or occasions are to count as manifestations of parochial charity? Consider some examples. Suppose the parish is successful in fostering or maintaining some degree of community (charity as it would have been called) in a village or town and the parishioner-members of that community engage in informal networks of mutual aid.[43] Is that parochial poor relief, or must institutions somehow be involved? Suppose local beggars beg their way through a parish doorstep by doorstep – that is, privately, in accordance with the 1388 statute – and parishioners respond out of a sense of collective obligation as well as individual philanthropy.[44] Is that parochial charity? Suppose churchwardens act as executors of parishioner's wills and thus distribute bequests to a few named poor within the parish or, because the will is explicit on the matter, to all the poor within the parish.[45] Is that parochial charity? Suppose the rector or vicar selects a few paupers to attend a funeral or chantry chapel and receive a dole,[46] or chooses recipients of the leftovers from bequests for the 'lights' that burned in front of altars and images.[47] Is that the parish in action? Suppose, as happened at Saffron Walden around 1400, a few local worthies establish almshouses 'with the unanimous consent and support' of the whole parish and vill; is that parochial charity or something narrower?[48] Finally, consider the impact on poorer parishioners of bequests for lights and stores by their wealthier fellows. The poorer were relieved of parochial obligations by the wealthier. Is that parish poor relief, albeit of an indirect kind?

The most formidable aspect of this problem of definition arises from the many ways in which 'the parish' overlapped with other institutions that can be seen as agencies of welfare provision. In the secular realm, the vill is one such. Some vills established their own funds from which local paupers were in effect relieved of all but a token tax obligation.[49] Inside the church, another overlapping institution is the chantry.[50] But the most obvious of these is the fraternity.[51] A third or so known fifteenth-century fraternities professed charitable purposes. Of these, in 1389, 10 per cent or more offered charity to non-members as well as their normal insurance to members, a proportion that would more than treble by the early sixteenth century.[52] Some fraternities maintained a common box.[53] The largest of the guilds of medieval Westminster ran an almshouse in which four places were reserved for the poor of the parish.[54] The question is: how did fraternity relate to parish? Did proliferation of fraternities undermine or enrich the parish as an institution and a collectivity?[55] Was it even fraternal rather than parochial welfare provision that prepared the way for Tudor arrangements?[56] In some cases membership of parish and fraternity almost exactly coincided; elsewhere the relationship was less straightforward.[57] But nowhere is it easy to say when the charity in question was *not* parochial, and should therefore be excluded from the present discussion. That is also true of the ways in which the personnel of the parish overlapped with those of fraternities and secular authorities.[58] The same person might be a church and a guild warden. Mayors and burgesses served as churchwardens, and their involvement in acts of charity might relate ambiguously to the offices they held.[59] Once again, we cannot easily say what is parochial and what is not. The ecclesiastical and the secular are inextricable.[60]

These are sticking points in the interpretation of contemporary evidence. We compound them, though, because of our imposition of our own categories. We want to distinguish the individual from the collective, the private from the public, the informal from the institutional. Later medieval parishioners did not think in this way – or, if they did use some equivalents of these categories, they defined them differently.[61] Parochial action focused on named individuals, well known to the 'actors'. The public institution of the almshouse was modelled on the home. Those in receipt of charity one year might be providers of it the next. None of this fluidity is readily accommodated by our seeking to tease out the parish *qua* parish as disburser of poor relief.

V

Given all these difficulties, evidential and conceptual, it is hard indeed to bring parish charity into focus. The material available permits no detailed local study. All that we can gain is some sense of the range of what parishes might do for their poor before the Reformation. That is, we can assemble individual instances without, in most cases, having any idea of how typical they were or how they might fit into a larger picture.

The oldest and perhaps most durable form of parochial charity was that of the priest. The quarter or third of tithes that the bishop should distribute to the poor was 'transferred' by the canonists to the parish priest by the eleventh century, when parishes were numerous enough to supplant the bishop's house as the pauper's likely first port of call.[62] The portion in question was, however, redefined by English synodal statutes. The council held at Lambeth in 1281, for instance, qualified the priest's obligation to provide hospitality, to needy travellers as well as the local poor: not a fixed proportion of tithe but 'as far as resources allow . . . so that at least extreme necessity among poor parishioners is relieved'.[63] The sums given were often small and many priests were, or professed to be, too poor to do very much.[64] (On the other hand, Chaucer's poor parson still managed donations to poor parishioners.)[65] Visitation records from the thirteenth and fourteenth centuries do not seem to register very widespread criticism of rectors for lack of charity.[66]

Later on the picture may have become more varied. In the rural deaneries of the diocese of Lincoln in 1517–1520, for example, including that for the Oxford archdeaconry referred to above, one finds 'omnia bene' recurring, which may reflect satisfaction with clerical charity – or may not, since we have no idea of respondents' expectations in individual cases. And there is even implicit praise of appropriators for maintaining poor relief: 'the parishioners [of West Wycombe] . . . say that all is well [omnia bene]. The prior and monastery of Bisseham annually distribute 6s. 8d. among poor parishioners.'[67] Yet, against a handful of such entries must be set over thirty in which rectors are accused of neglecting 'distribuciones' or the wider obligation of 'hospitalitas' – in one case for as long as sixteen years.[68] The fullness of the imaginary glass no longer seems so clear. On the other hand, when the Oxford area was revisited in 1530, no complaints about hospitality were recorded at all.[69] And the fact that such complaints could be made so vociferously, and that Parliament could act on the matter, as in 1391, discourages utter pessimism.[70] Lawsuits also show parishioners successfully asserting their claims to subvention at times when canonical obligations were being evaded. For example, in 1389 a Lincolnshire parish petitioned the church courts to compel its rector to restore an annual distribution of peas.[71] Complaints more generally show parishes (through their churchwardens) chasing absentee rectors, pluralists, and appropriators so as to recover charitable giving that had been neglected.[72] Such charity cannot have been an entirely empty excuse for legal action. If this kind of relief had dwindled to utter insignificance, its invocation in setting out the damage done by absenteeism and appropriation would have had little forensic force.[73] In 1330, the parishioners of the suitably named Seething in Norfolk took matters into their own hands and deflected tithes that should have gone to an appropriating hospital. They thus attacked one charity for damaging another, clearly not minded to accept the welfare promoted by a distant institution as a substitute for local action.[74]

It is not clear, then, that priestly charity had entered a terminal decline by the later Middle Ages. Brian Tierney concludes: 'In spite of its growing imperfections, it [sc. the canonical system of poor relief] survived into the sixteenth century to provide a foundation for the secular poor law of the Tudors.'[75] Indeed, to some extent Tierney's growing imperfections may be an 'optical illusion' created by the changing nature of the evidence. What survive from the earlier Middle Ages are *for the most part* canonical *prescriptions*. Only from later on can we read plentiful *descriptions* – descriptions of actual payments made and complaints about payments withheld or diverted. The gap between canonists' 'logic' (to echo Maitland's celebrated definition of law) and the 'life' of economic reality may always have been considerable, throughout the Middle Ages. Nor is it clear that, when we enter the period from which complaints survive, they were so numerous, or so widespread, as to imply the general dwindling of poor relief even in appropriated parishes. In the late fifteenth century, for instance, Salisbury Cathedral gave 5 per cent of its tithes and oblations from an appropriated parish back to that parish's poor.[76]

That could of course have been a local peculiarity. It is of some contextual significance that the clergy of Salisbury were rather conscientious about remembering the poor in their wills – more so, indeed, than were the local laity.[77] But elsewhere, even though the sums distributed by parish clergy were small, they could be supplemented by welfare provision from other parochial sources.

The most important of these may have been the parish collecting box. Canon law obliged parishioners to give alms to the poor above their tithes. Some parish box or 'charity pot' was one obvious way of discharging canonical obligation while leaving the task of distribution to others – most likely the churchwardens, although as we saw earlier, their accounts are largely silent on the matter before the early 1500s. Earlier evidence of such practice survives in diocesan legislation of John Carpenter, bishop of Worcester, issued in 1451. The churchwardens were to collect for the poor three times a year, on All Saints, Palm Sunday, and Pentecost, and they should either distribute the proceeds at once or hold them 'in commune pixide'.[78] This was presumably akin to the charitable 'stocks' or 'stores' also occasionally attested, funds from which the parish might lend or transfer cash, livestock, or land to the needy.[79] In All Hallows, London Wall, in 1459–1460, 2s. 6d. was received 'of men and wemen of the parysche for the charyte potte'.[80] Yet in 1469 the rector of St John Walbrook, London, had to bequeath £40 to establish a loan fund for his parishioners, which might not suggest that such reserves were commonplace.[81] In another London parish, St Dunstan in the East, however, testators were establishing money boxes of their own in the

253

1470s and again the early 1500s, for loans or gifts to the poor.[82] And they were doing so even though there was a 'church box' in 1506 if not earlier, and an unambiguously designated 'alms box' from at least the mid-1530s.[83]

After organized collections, which ought to have been central to parochial poor relief yet are surprisingly hard to document, come a variety of more sporadic measures. Chief among these may have been the administration of bequests, the portion of an estate that had to be left for charitable purposes. A Cambridge testator bequeathed 4d. to every household in his parish, presumably to be distributed by parish officials.[84] In 1473 a Bristol merchant, John Shipward, expected his rector to advise on the allocation of £10 that he left to supply bedding for the poor.[85] Examples such as these can readily be multiplied. But they tend to come more frequently from the end of the Middle Ages, and it is tempting to interpret that as a sign of real growth in the number or scale of benefactions.[86] Yet, just as wills can mislead the historian who relies too literally on their preambles or the nature of their bequests as an index of changing piety, so too can their changing availability distort our interpretation. Consider another example of a charitable bequest that required parochial distribution. A man and his wife leave the residue of their estate to provide dowries for poor girls. The girls are to be selected by the provost and three 'wise men' of the parish. The will comes from 1227, and it is Parisian (the first to survive from that city).[87] If we had English wills of a comparably early date, our view of medieval English lay charity might be very different in its emphases.

Under the same heading of bequests we must add the small sums distributed among the paupers in attendance at chantries or, sometimes in very great numbers, swelling the crowd and offering intercession at funerals, month's minds, and anniversaries.[88] Especially by the mid-fifteenth century, there could be frequent occasions on which the parish called on the impoverished 'rent-a-mourner'. In larger cities, many of the poor could scrape a living that way.[89]

A sixteenth-century parish almshouse was mentioned earlier.[90] It remains, however, an open question how often medieval parishes included an almshouse or hospital among their facilities for poor relief.[91] No documented English hospital is known to have been dependent on a parish before around 1300.[92] For the later Middle Ages Marjorie McIntosh has calculated that, between 1380 and 1469, parishes were involved with only 6 per cent of all hospitals or almshouses of which the 'governing body' is known. That figure rises to 13 per cent for the period 1470–1529, and reaches almost 15 per cent in the later sixteenth century.[93] The latter is not a statistically significant increase after the doubling of the second half of the fifteenth century, even though we must, of course, factor into the picture the loss of so many hospitals in the Dissolution.

The typology of parochial welfare must be rounded off with a miscellany. For instance, we occasionally hear of tenements on the perimeter of the parish churchyard that were let out or given to local paupers.[94] These could then sustain themselves, at least in part, through begging in the safety of the churchyard itself. Indeed the whole churchyard, not just the church door, was perhaps a more regularly significant area of customary parochial poor relief then we shall ever know.[95] The poor were sometimes buried there at parish expense, even though such a form of charity is seldom mentioned in wills or churchwardens' accounts. Here again the records of St Mary at Hill offer a tantalizing glimpse of what may have been commonplace: alms 'reserved toward beryalles of pure pepull'.[96]

Finally, ales. In the late seventeenth century, John Aubrey (as in our epigraph) looked back to his grandfather's day, before the introduction of the poor rate, when church ales did the job of supporting local indigents. The 'memory' may not have been entirely rose-tinted. The church ale, as a benefit 'booze-up', was usually directed at church fabric or even the middling sort of parishioner, and was restricted to times of good harvest (barley surpluses). But it might also yield profits that could be distributed to the needy at the end of the day or added to a parish 'store'.[97]

VI

Small beer? All these institutions, measures, or customs might even in aggregate not yield enough for the survival of an indigent parishioner, and the few historians who have worked at the topic have thus tended to deny anything more than symbolic significance to parochial poor relief. The crucial point is that, for the poor, parish subventions were only one element in the 'portfolio' that they had to build up. Not even in the seventeenth and eighteenth centuries did the poor rate engender a welfare 'monoculture'.[98] In the later Middle Ages, all the more, the parish was one actor among several in what has been called 'the mixed economy of care'. This 'economy' was by no means necessarily integrated. Nor was it always successful in keeping the poor from utter penury and a miserable death.[99] Witness the coroners' accounts of people found dead from starvation by the roadside. But 'mixed' it most certainly was; and this means that parochial charity must always be envisaged as part of a spectrum of overlapping agencies of relief. They overlapped, as we have seen, in their personnel; they overlapped also in their target beneficiaries, the deserving, impotent poor.[100] There was, in the post-Black Death later Middle Ages, little of the perceived need to find work for the apparently idle that would weigh so heavily on Tudor governments.[101]

For the sixteenth century, calculation of the relative proportions of the different 'sectors' is hard enough, even though at a certain point Slack can see the poor rate surpassing testamentary benefactions in volume.[102] For the later Middle Ages, overall estimates are generally impossible. It is true that Neil Rushton has recalculated the distributions to the poor attributed to monasteries, cathedrals, and colleges in the *Valor Ecclesiasticus*. At the

Dissolution, they are now thought to have been disbursing 7–9 per cent of their revenues: that is, three times more than previous estimates.[103] But that revelation is an isolated achievement wholly dependent on the Henrician survey. It gives us some idea of the relative monastic contribution to the mixed economy. The aggregate provision before the Reformation may have been as high as £13,000 – a figure that no other institutional sector is likely to have matched. Yet that is as far as we can go.

Contrast the far more difficult case of hospitals. Counting medieval hospitals, almshouses and the like is fraught with difficulty and is perhaps never tolerably accurate. On one hand, there may always have been more of them than we have so far discovered. For example, a recent survey of late medieval Norfolk and Suffolk increased the number of identifiable institutions by over 60 per cent.[104] Perhaps, further, there will always have been more than we can ever know about because the evidence simply does not survive. This may in turn, however, have been because they were fragile, ephemeral foundations. Thus, on the other hand, because hospitals could so quickly go out of business, there is always the danger that we shall overestimate how many functioned at any given time.[105] Still, McIntosh's calculation that 495 hospitals were functioning in the early 1400s and 584 in the early 1500s is likely to give the right order of magnitude. And on a reasonable assumption of the average number of inmates, and the total number of parishes in England (9,000), that would mean one person from every two parishes – at the most. For even as hospitals were increasing in total number, individual establishments were retrenching on poor relief and avoiding financial collapse by turning themselves into chantries.[106]

Guilds and fraternities may be a better bet for the statistically minded. Some statistics appeared above. By the early 1500s (to recall), around one third of confraternities and guilds offered charity to non-members. The problem is that we do not know how many fraternities there were nationally. We cannot determine how much of their charity was informal and thus circumvented their accounts. Nor do we know their total membership – which is important, because we can hardly discount their collective significance as a form of social insurance for poorer members.

Other sectors are not, however, amenable even to this minimal and tentative quantification. The arrangements made by manorial courts for orphans and elderly tenants or those unable to pay fines show that here was a source of support still lively towards the close of the Middle Ages; but little more can be said.[107] As for doorstep hospitality and charity, historians of the Tudors have sometimes posited a decline in that 'sector' as a part of the context for the growth of witchcraft accusations. (The elderly female beggar is refused help at the doorstep and goes away muttering; some later mishap in the family that she has called upon fuels suspicion that she is a witch.) The scenario seems, however, to have lost its appeal to historians of witchcraft, and has seldom been recognized by historians of charity. And if there was such a decline in charity, it did not necessarily start from a very high point in the late Middle Ages. We should be unwise to read back from the Tudor to (say) the Lancastrian age.[108]

Finally, we must register the 'informal sector' as it operated among more or less social equals: private ad hoc relief from family, neighbours, friends, non-resident kin, masters, landladies, better-off taxpayers. This, the largest sector (or so one guesses from comparative evidence), is the one about which least can be said by the medievalist, whose evidence is nearly all prescriptive and thus unreliable. Poor households were small and vulnerable to what has been called 'nuclear hardship'. Extra-domestic networks of credit and exchange were almost certainly widespread, but were not necessarily as large or as reliable as has often been supposed.[109]

Of course all these hypotheses about the various sectors of the mixed economy must be weighed against a socio-economic context of rising levels of general prosperity in the century and a half following the Black Death. There was probably much less demand for charity in the period $c.1350–1450$ than there had been in 1200 or 1300.[110] Many smaller parishes must have had only a few aged or impotent to watch out for – which makes the small disbursements of the parish if anything relatively more significant. Its role was indeed 'limited, but important' – rather than the other way round.[111]

VII

So far the poor have been taken to include the other category in my title, the sick. It is, however, worth allowing them to emerge from the shadows and to stand, or perhaps better to lie, on their own as a group of people whom the parish might help. Historians of the early modern period have come to realize that 'medical treatment and care formed an important part of poor relief and charity well before the so-called medicalisation of the eighteenth century'.[112] Such care was not restricted to poorhouses and hospitals but was available to those supported at home. In early modern rural parishes, as in municipalities, poor relief schemes could include payments to physicians, surgeons, or apothecaries. It could also take the form of employing one healthy recipient of relief to lodge and nurse another recipient who was ill.[113]

We shall not find any of this before the Poor Law or indeed before the Reformation. Just as there were, in medieval England, no equivalents of continental civic physicians retained to treat the poor, so the medieval parish employed no doctors.[114] Nor were English hospitals medicalized even to the limited extent that would be achieved in the sixteenth century. Indeed, no doctor is known to have been attached to an English hospital before the very end of the Middle Ages (in contrast, for example, to the major hospitals of north Italian cities).[115] A fortiori, none of the few hospitals run by parishes offered medical care. If such care was ever available to the poor it came through individual bequests, not corporate action. In 1480, for instance, a

London mercer left £5 a year for five years for a surgeon to treat the poor who could not afford 'lechcrafte'.[116]

The normal fees of educated physicians were indeed well beyond the means of the sick poor, and such physicians were in any case too few for any free treatment that they offered out of charity to have much impact.[117] Pilgrimage to a shrine even a modest distance away required major physical and financial effort and, in cases of serious illness, the support of friends.[118] Local 'empirics', wise women and cunning men, were more accessible than physicians, but still required some payment for their services.[119] Or so we may reasonably infer from the better-documented sixteenth century; relatively little can be known of their activities or clientele in later medieval times.[120]

What could the local church offer? The answer falls into three parts, of which the first and third may be surprising. The first part is the environment of the parish church: its healing relics if it had them, its devotional imagery, and its choral music (a much-neglected aspect of parochial life). All these in their differing ways might provide the spiritual uplift that, in both contemporary theology and medical theory, were held to be conducive to somatic health.[121]

The second part of the answer is the priest – not that we should imagine every parish priest to have had some basic medical knowledge. Priests were to visit the sick and bring them the sacraments whenever needed (by night or day), and they might occasionally take the incapacitated or paralysed into their own homes.[122] They were to instruct midwives in the techniques of emergency baptism of babies on the point of death, if necessary following Caesarian section. They might thus have acquired some rudimentary gynaecological knowledge.[123] And medieval midwives (of whom historians remain strikingly ignorant) might have offered advice on a wider range of problems than their usual designation suggests.[124] Yet, in England, we find nothing like the official parish midwives sometimes elected by the wives and widows of the parish in the diocese of Amiens in the mid-fifteenth century.[125] 'The parish priest, with his contacts outside the village, was expected to be knowledgeable in matters of health.'[126] So it was in Enlightenment France. In medieval England a few priests, of course, are known to have had some access to medical learning, and there may well have been many like them whose proficiency leaves scant trace. Some felt competent to diagnose cases of leprosy.[127] The Cambridge-educated rector of Dry Drayton in the early fourteenth century inherited a medical book.[128] In 1400, the rector of St Alphage's, Cripplegate, London, bequeathed 'all [his] medical books, *tam de phisica quam de cirurgia*'.[129] John Mirfield, a secular priest residing near St Bartholomew's Hospital in Smithfield in the fifteenth century wrote the *Breviarium Bartholomei*, a manual for medical self-help.[130] In 1424 John Ottryngton, 'alias Porter', chaplain of St John the Evangelist, Ouse Bridge, York, was even accused before the court of the dean and chapter of performing operations for breast cancer on women.[131] In such cases, even those of malpractice, the parishioners may have felt the benefit – although the London parson of St Leonard, Foster Lane, was arraigned by his own parishioners for 'killing many a man' with his pretended medical and surgical 'skills'.[132] Elsewhere, the rectorships, prebendaries, and the like held by identifiable medical practitioners were for the most part clearly just sources of income enhancement, rungs on the ladder to a lucrative practice at court or in a great household – and the parishioners were none the healthier.[133]

Like Christ whom he represented, however, the priest was, or was meant to be, a physician of souls. And this soul medicine, the third part of the answer to our question, is not to be dismissed as mere metaphor, as having nothing to do with the health of the (pauper) body.[134] The fathers of the Fourth Lateran Council had reminded the western Church that healing of the body could come only through prior healing of the soul.[135] The principal vehicle of this soul medicine was the sacraments, and especially the elevated host. As John Myrc wrote c.1400:

> For glad may that man be/That once in the day may him see; /For so much good doth the sight,/As Saint Au[gu]stine teacheth aright,/ That day that thou seeest God's body,/These benefices shallt thou have certainly;/Meat and drink at thy need,/None shall thee that day be greed;/. . . Sudden death that same day, /Thee dare not dread without nay;/ Also that day I thee plight/Thou shallt not lose thy sight.[136]

The later medieval doctrine of the *fructus, virtutes, utilitates,* 'medes', or 'merits' of the Mass is not to be marginalized from lay devotion as part of the 'the magic of the medieval Church'.[137]

The developments in doctrine and practice that were its essential context came in the twelfth and thirteenth centuries, and especially in the wake of Lateran IV.[138] They can be simply listed: transubstantiation; sacerdotal mediation; the reception of the Aristotelian idea of concomitance, whereby (in this case) Christ's flesh and blood were alike 'really present' in every bit of sacramental matter, and hence in the host alone; the withdrawal of the consecrated chalice from the laity (the chalice being even more accident-prone than the fragile host); elevation of the host after sacring, preceded by the attention-grabbing ringing of bells; the reduction of *reception* of the host to once a year, usually at Easter, for all but the Margery Kempes of this world; the widespread aspiration to *see* the elevated host at least daily. As Augustine had preached, Christ's body and blood bring 'health-bringing refreshment', *salubrem refectionem.*[139] That applied to the whole Mass. But thanks to the doctrinal developments just listed, the host, as Lydgate later phrased it, could be 'our chief preservative'.[140]

What specific physical benefits might the parishioner expect from beholding the elevated host? Myrc gives only one selection of possible answers.[141] To leave aside the obvious spiritual aids: on the day that you saw the host, some of the following might happen. You might feel enhanced hopefulness or diminished sorrow, an 'accident of the soul' held to be entirely therapeutic in medieval medical theory. You might experience a general restoration of health. You would have sufficient food or better digestion. You would be protected against misfortune. Your feet would be strengthened, as would your eyesight. While you were hearing Mass, the process of ageing would be halted – you would not become any more infirm. You would not have to fear sudden death – but, if somehow you did die, you would be in a state of grace. All this was rather more valuable than a Poor Law pension. And it came free.

The list of benefits varies, as do the patristic authorities to which they were bogusly attributed. But the material is all mainstream and widely diffused: sermons; poetry and songs, both Latin and vernacular; well-known instructional writing – besides Myrc, *The Lay-Folks' Mass Book* for example.[142] This is just one case of the, to us, unusual and often obscure ways in which the later medieval English parish might alleviate the condition of the needy. Its role was variegated and significant, even though, by itself, it often could not fully support its poor. They had to supplement any support they gained from the parish by drawing on other institutions and on their own 'social capital' – and that is broadly as true of the parish in 1550 or 1750 as it is of the parish in 1250 or 1450.[143]

Notes

1 John Aubrey, *The Topographical Collections*, ed. J. E. Jackson (Devizes, 1862), p. 10.

2 Matthew 26:14 or 27:36; R. Ellmann, *Oscar Wilde* (London, 1987), pp. 61–62.

3 E. Duffy, *The Stripping of the Altars: Traditional Religion in England 1400–1580* (New Haven, CT, 1992), is of course the great counter-example in religious history. For the parish see B. A. Kümin, *The Shaping of a Community: The Rise and Reformation of the English Parish c. 1400–1560* (Aldershot, 1996). On poor relief, there are few guides that comparably take the long view. M. McIntosh, 'Local Responses to the Poor in Late Medieval and Tudor England', *Continuity and Change* 3 (1988), 209–245, remains unique in detailed modern scholarship on its subject in print, and I am heavily in its debt. For context see P. A. Fideler, 'Introduction: Impressions of a Century of Historiography', *Albion* 32.3 [Symposium: The Study of Early Modern Poverty and Poor Relief] (Fall 2000), 381–407, and, now, his wide-ranging synthesis, especially helpful on the changing ideologies of poor relief, *Social Welfare in Pre-Industrial England: The Old Poor Law Tradition* (Basingstoke, 2006). See too M. McIntosh, *Controlling Misbehavior in England, 1370–1600* (Cambridge, 1998), and the debate on it in *Journal of British Studies* 37.3 (1998). N. J. G. Pounds, *A History of the English Parish: The Culture of Religion from Augustine to Victoria* (Cambridge, 2000), is helpful at a number of points. I am also much indebted to the regional study of M. Groom, 'Piety and Locality: Studies in Urban and Rural Religion in Surrey c.1450–c.1550', unpublished PhD diss. (University of London, 2001), ch. 3, on charity.

4 P. Slack, *Poverty and Policy in Tudor and Stuart England* (London, 1988), pp. 170–172; S. Hindle, *On the Parish? The Micro-Politics of Poor Relief in Rural England c. 1550–1750* (Oxford, 2004), p. 296. For an appreciation of Slack's book, to which I am greatly indebted in what follows, see Hindle, pp. 1–4; also Fideler, 'Introduction'.

5 E. M. Leonard, *The Early History of English Poor Relief* (Cambridge, 1900); S. and B. Webb, *English Local Government*, vol. VII: *English Poor Law History*, pt I: *The Old Poor Law* (London, 1927); Slack, *Poverty*; P. Slack, *From Reformation to Improvement: Public Welfare in Early Modern England* (Oxford, 1999). For other bibliography see Hindle, *On the Parish?*, pp. 1–2.

6 McIntosh, 'Local Responses'; the only other really comprehensive and thoughtful treatment of the spectrum of poor relief agencies in later medieval England known to me is C. Dyer, *Standards of Living in the Later Middle Ages: Social Change in England c. 1200–1520* (Cambridge, 1989, revised edn 1998), 234–257, 311–314. M. Rubin, *Charity and Community in Medieval Cambridge* (Cambridge, 1987), to which I am also indebted, deals mainly with ecclesiastical poor relief.

7 Keith Wrightson, *English Society 1580–1680* (London, 1982), pp. 121–148, and Slack, *Poverty*, pp. 22–32, 39, 42–55, remain fundamental. More recent literature is condensed in Fideler, *Social Welfare*, chs 1–3. Fideler nonetheless sees (p. 13) broad continuity in the 'system' of social welfare from fourteenth to eighteenth centuries.

8 Slack, *Poverty*, pp. 115–131; McIntosh, 'Local Responses', pp. 228–234; McIntosh, *Controlling Misbehavior*, pp. 88–96.

9 Slack, *Reformation*, p. 17. See also McIntosh, 'Local Responses', p. 209. Compare Kümin, *Shaping of a Community*, p. 248.

10 Slack, *Poverty*, p. 129.

11 McIntosh, 'Local Responses', p. 234.

12 Slack, *Poverty*, pp. 127–128, 170, 184 n. 38. Hindle, *On the Parish?* is more optimistic (pp. 234–235, 256), as is Fideler, *Social Welfare* (p. 140).

13 Hindle, *On the Parish?*, p. 92; Fideler, *Social Welfare*, pp. 134, 146, 193; I. W. Archer, *The Pursuit of Stability: Social Relations in Elizabethan London* (Cambridge, 1991), pp. 96–99, 178–182.

14 O. P. Grell and A. Cunningham, 'The Reformation and Changes in Welfare Provision in Early Modern Northern Europe', in *Health Care and Poor Relief in Protestant Europe 1500–1700*, ed. Grell and Cunningham (London, 1997), pp. 32–33. For France see e.g. P. Deyon, *Amiens, capitale provinciale* (Paris, 1967), p. 238 (annual tax for the poor from 1564). For an Italian example, see S. Cavallo, *Charity and Power in Early Modern Italy: Benefactors and their Motives in Turin, 1541–1789* (Cambridge, 1995), pp. 18–19. For other civic instances, see K. A. Lynch, *Individuals, Families, and Communities in Europe, 1200–1800: The Urban Foundations of Western Society* (Cambridge, 2003), pp. 132–134. For Scotland, see R. Mitchison, 'Poor Relief and Health Care in Scotland, 1575–1710', in *Health Care and Poor Relief*, ed. Grell and Cunningham, 220–233, and eadem, *The Old Poor Law in Scotland: The Experience of Poverty, 1574–1845* (Edinburgh, 2000), ch. 1.

15 Slack, *Reformation*, pp. 20–21; Grell and Cunningham, 'Reformation and Changes', p. 28.

16 *The Locus of Care: Families, Communities, Institutions and the Provision of Welfare since Antiquity*, ed. P. Horden and R. Smith (London, 1998), esp. pp. 11–12 and the contributions of S. Cavallo and M. Dinges. See also Cavallo, *Charity and Power*, pp. 22, 40–41, 98.

17 Grell and Cunningham, 'Reformation and Changes', p. 32.

18 J. J. Scarisbrick, *The Reformation and the English People* (Oxford, 1984), ch. 2; Slack, *Poverty*, p. 172, qualified by a superb local study, Carole Rawcliffe, *Medicine for the Soul: The Life, Death and Resurrection of an English Medieval Hospital* (Thrupp, 1999), pp. 190–198; McIntosh, 'Local Responses', pp. 225–228.

19 C. R. Hallpike, *The Principles of Social Evolution* (Oxford, 1986), p. 113.

20 Slack, *Poverty*, pp. 12–13.

21 Ibid. p. 131.

22 For what follows see Kümin, *Shaping of a Community*, pp. 48–50, 55–56, 247–248.

23 F. Pollock and F. W. Maitland, *The History of English Law Before the Time of Edward I*, second ed., vol. I (Cambridge, 1968), pp. 612–613; R. H. Helmholz, *The Oxford History of the Laws of England*, vol. I: *The Canon Law and Ecclesiastical Jurisdiction from 597 to the 1640s* (Oxford, 2004), pp. 470–473; Kümin, *Shaping of a Community*, pp. 48–50; Pounds, *English Parish*, p. 237. On the financial obligations of the lay parishioner more generally, see E. Mason, 'The Role of the English Parishioner 1100–1500', *Journal of Ecclesiastical History* 27 (1976), 17–29; R. C. Palmer, *Selling the Church: The English Parish in Law, Commerce, and Religion, 1350–1550* (Chapel Hill, NC, 2002).

24 McIntosh, 'Local Responses', p. 228; Kümin, *Shaping of a Community*, p. 49.

25 McIntosh, 'Local Responses', pp. 211–212, 214, 217. On the Tudor 'discovery' of the 'labouring poor', whose plight had been recognized only very occasionally during the Middle Ages, see Slack, *Poverty*, pp. 7–30, 65–66.

26 12 Richard II, c. 7.

27 By analogy, the labour legislation of 1349 had been anticipated in village by-laws for some time – since well before the Black Death. See C. Dyer, 'Work Ethics in the Fourteenth Century', in *The Problem of Labour in Fourteenth-Century England*, ed. J. Bothwell et al. (Woodbridge, 2000), pp. 32–33. See also McIntosh, *Controlling Misbehavior*, pp. 88–91.

28 Rubin, *Cambridge*, p. 244; Cavallo, *Charity and Power*, p. 25; M. Mollat, *The Poor in the Middle Ages: An Essay in Social History* (New Haven, CT, 1986), pp. 139–141, 154–155, 275–278.

29 J. Brodman, *Charity and Welfare: Hospitals and the Poor in Medieval Catalonia* (Philadelphia, 1998), p. 19.

30 A. D'Addario, *Aspetti della contrariforma a Firenze* (Rome, 1972), pp. 63–64, who, however, gives no archival references.

31 E. g. M. Rubin, 'The Poor', in *Fifteenth-Century Attitudes: Perceptions of Society in Late Medieval England*, ed. R. Horrox (Cambridge, 1994), pp. 169–170, 178.

32 Groom, 'Piety and Locality', p. 112. On the larger dangers of reading too much from, or into, wills, see C. Burgess, 'Late Medieval Wills and Pious Convention: Testamentary Evidence Reconsidered', in *Profit, Piety and the Professions in Late Medieval England*, ed. M. A. Hicks (Gloucester, 1990), pp. 14–33.

33 Groom, 'Piety and Locality', pp. 114, 116. For a summary list of surviving accounts, see Kümin, *Shaping of a Community*, appendix 1. On their limitations as evidence of the full range of parish activities, see C. Burgess, 'Pre-Reformation Churchwardens' Accounts and Parish Government: Lessons from London and Bristol', *English Historical Review* 117 (2002), 306–332, and ensuing debate with B. Kümin, vol. 119 (2004), 87–116.

34 *The Medieval Records of a London City Church (St Mary at Hill), AD 1420–1559*, ed. H. Littlehales, EETS 125 (London, 1905), p. 299, where it appears only because it is being 'raided'. On this parish see C. Burgess, 'Shaping the Parish: St Mary at Hill, London, in the Fifteenth Century', in *The Cloister and the*

World: Essays in Medieval History in Honour of Barbara Harvey, ed. J. Blair and B. Golding (Oxford, 1996), pp. 246–286.

35   27 Henry VIII, c. 25, item iv; for signs of its impact see McIntosh, 'Local Responses', n. 75. *Medieval Records of (St Mary at Hill)*, ed. Littlehales, p. 299: alms box for poor 1517–1518 (and p. 304: 1519–1520).

36   Note the growing role attributed to churchwardens by P. R. Schofield, *Peasant and Community in Medieval England 1200–1500* (Houndmills, 2003), p. 200.

37   *Lambeth Churchwardens' Accounts, 1504–1645, and Vestry Book 1610*, ed. C. Drew, Surrey Record Society 40, vol. I (Frome, 1940), pp. 24–25.

38   Ibid. p. 91.

39   G. G. Coulton, *Five Centuries of Religion*, 4 vols. (Cambridge, 1923–1950), III, pp. 210, 659–660; B. Tierney, *Medieval Poor Law: A Sketch of Canonical Theory and its Application in England* (Berkeley, CA, 1959), p. 128; cf. pp. 89–92; McIntosh, 'Local Responses', p. 220.

40   On visitation records, see *The Records of the Medieval Ecclesiastical Courts*, part II: *England*, ed. C. Donohue (Berlin, 1994). Such material can be sampled in translation in *Pastors and the Care of Souls in Medieval England*, ed. J. Shinners and W. J. Dohar (Notre Dame, 1998), esp. ch. 7 C.

41   Compare K. French, *The People of the Parish: Community Life in a Late Medieval Diocese* (Philadelphia, 2000), ch. 1.

42   Kümin, *Shaping of a Community*, p. 61; McIntosh, 'Local Responses', p. 220; Rubin, *Cambridge*, pp. 237–238.

43   For hints of a female parochial network, see P. J. P. Goldberg, 'Women in Fifteenth-Century Town Life', in *Towns and Townspeople in the Fifteenth Century*, ed. J. A. F. Thompson (London, 1988), p. 113.

44   For a possible example see P. H. Cullum, '"For Pore People Harberles": What Was the Function of the Maisonsdieu?', in *Trade, Devotion and Governance: Papers in Later Medieval History*, ed. D. J. Clayton et al. (Stroud, 1994), p. 47.

45   Kümin, *Shaping of a Community*, p. 61; McIntosh, 'Local Responses', n. 51.

46   For a bequest of property to maintain a chantry and weekly payments to three poor parishioners, see e.g. *Calendar of Wills Proved and Enrolled in the Court of Hustings, London 1258–1688*, ed. R. R. Sharpe, vol. II (London, 1890), p. 570.

47   J. Oxley, *The Reformation in Essex to the Death of Mary* (Manchester, 1965), p. 59, cited by Kümin, *Shaping of a Community*, p. 148.

48   F. W. Steer, 'The Statutes of Saffron Walden Almshouses', *Transactions of the Essex Archaeological Society*, n.s. 25 (1955–1960), pp. 161, 167.

49   C. Dyer, 'The Medieval English Community and its Decline', *Journal of British Studies* 33 (1994), p. 416; idem, *Standards of Living*, pp. 256, 314; idem, *An Age of Transition? Economy and Society in England in the Later Middle Ages* (Oxford, 2005), p. 240.

50   Burgess, '"A Fond Thing Vainly Invented": An Essay on Purgatory and Pious Motive in Later Medieval England', in *Parish, Church and People: Local Studies in Lay Religion, 1350–1750*, ed. S. J. Wright (London, 1988), p. 73; Kümin, *Shaping of a Community*, 160–161; Dyer, *Standards of Living*, pp. 246–247, 312.

51   P. J. P. Goldberg, *Medieval England: A Social History 1250–1550* (London, 2004), ch. 5.

52   McIntosh, 'Local Responses', pp. 214–215, 220. K. Farnhill, *Guilds and the Parish Community in Late Medieval East Anglia, c. 1470–1550* (Woodbridge, 2001), p. 75, argues that McIntosh's figures for charity to non-members quoted above are too low. See also Kümin, *Shaping of a Community*, p. 151. Forms of fraternal charity are illustrated in G. Rosser, 'Going to the Fraternity Feast: Commensality and Social Relations in Late Medieval England', *Journal of*

British Studies 33 (1994), pp. 436–437. C. Barron, 'The Parish Fraternities of Medieval London', in *The Church in Pre-Reformation Society: Essays in Honour of F. R. H. Du Boulay*, ed. C. Barron and C. Harper-Bill (Woodbridge, 1985), pp. 13–37, suggests at p. 27 that much charity bypassed the fraternity accounts.

53 Ibid. p. 15 n. 9 (London example of 1388).

54 G. Rosser, *Medieval Westminster 1200–1540* (Oxford, 1989), p. 320.

55 French, *People of the Parish*, pp. 12, 127; Groom, 'Piety and Locality', pp. 158–159; Farnhill, *Guilds*, p. 168; S. Brigden, 'Religion and Social Obligation in Early Modern London', *Past and Present* 103 (1984), p. 106. See esp. Rosser, 'Communities of Parish and Guild in the Late Middle Ages', in *Parish, Church and People*, ed. Wright, p. 29, for a vivid example of a fraternity that saved a parish from extinction; also pp. 33–34, and the same author's 'Parochial Conformity and Voluntary Religion in Late-Medieval England', *Transactions of the Royal Historical Society*, 6th ser., 1 (1991), 173–189.

56 Barron, 'Parish Fraternities', pp. 34, 36–37.

57 Compare the charitable parish fraternity described by J. Henderson, 'The Parish and the Poor in Florence at the Time of the Black Death: The Case of S. Frediano', *Continuity and Change* 3 (1988), 247–272. Rosser, 'Communities of Parish and Guild', pp. 39–40.

58 Rosser, 'Crafts, Guilds and the Negotiation of Work in the Medieval Town', *Past and Present* 154 (1997), 141–163.

59 A. D. Brown, *Popular Piety in Late Medieval England: The Diocese of Salisbury 1250–1550* (Oxford, 1995), p. 189.

60 Kümin, *Shaping of a Community*, p. 53.

61 McIntosh, 'Local Responses', p. 212.

62 Tierney, *Medieval Poor Law*, pp. 70, 76; F. Heal, *Hospitality in Early Modern England* (Oxford, 1990), pp. 224, 227–228.

63 *Councils and Synods . . . (1205–1313)*, ed. F. M. Powicke and C. R. Cheney (Oxford, 1964), pp. 907–908 (c. 11), with Tierney, *Poor Law*, p. 78; Rubin, *Cambridge*, pp. 239–241.

64 Dyer, *Standards of Living*, pp. 247–248. See also R. N. Swanson, 'Standards of Livings: Parochial Revenues in Pre-Reformation England', in *Religious Belief and Ecclesiastical Careers in Late Medieval England*, ed. C. Harper-Bill (Woodbridge, 1991), pp. 151–196, esp. 179–183.

65 *Canterbury Tales*, General Prologue, 488–9. Tierney, *Medieval Poor Law*, pp. 92–97, on the incomes of vicars and the average amounts left for hospitality; pp. 98–104, on synodal and episcopal enforcement of charitable obligations of appropriators or absentees.

66 Tierney, *Medieval Poor Law*, pp. 104–106.

67 *Visitations of the Diocese of Lincoln 1517–1531*, ed. A. Hamilton Thompson, 3 vols (Hereford, 1940–1947), I, p. 35. The Oxford archdeaconry material is on pp. 119–140.

68 Ibid. I, p. 41; cf. pp. 16, 25, 37, 42–53, etc.

69 Ibid. II, pp. 32–69.

70 15 Richard II, c. 6. Compare P. Marshall, *The Catholic Priesthood and the English Reformation* (Oxford, 1994), pp. 188–190; Heal, *Hospitality*, pp. 242–245.

71 Visitation of 1389 cited by W. O. Ault, 'Manor Court and Parish Church in Fifteenth-Century England: A Study of Village By-Laws', *Speculum* 42 (1967), p. 65. Helmholz, *Oxford History*, 409, is less optimistic overall.

72 Tierney, *Medieval Poor Law*, pp. 71–72, 121, 129. For context see Marshall, *Catholic Priesthood*, pp. 177–185.

73 Dyer, *Standards of Living*, p. 247; Tierney, *Medieval Poor Law*, pp. 107–108, 128, arguing against any overall diminution towards the close of the Middle Ages.

Note also P. Heath, *The English Parish Clergy on the Eve of the Reformation* (London, 1969), p. 141, for an instance in which the burden of hospitality supposedly compelled a priest's non-residence.

74 Rubin, *Cambridge*, p. 243. Compare Ault, 'Manor Court', pp. 65–66.

75 Tierney, *Medieval Poor Law*, p. 128. Contrast Schofield, *Peasant and Community in Medieval England*, pp. 194, 200.

76 Brown, *Popular Piety*, p. 196.

77 Ibid.

78 R. M. Haines, 'Bishop Carpenter's Injunctions to the Diocese of Worcester in 1451', *Bulletin of the Institute of Historical Research* 40 (1967), p. 206. For bequests to the poor man's box in Consistory Court wills of the same diocese 1509–1547 (a rarity), see C. Peters, *Patterns of Piety: Women, Gender, and Religion in Later Medieval and Reformation England* (Cambridge, 2003), p. 55.

79 McIntosh, 'Local Responses', p. 220; Slack, *Poverty*, p. 114.

80 *The Churchwardens' Accounts of the Parish of AllHallows, London Wall . . . (AD 1455–1536)*, ed. C. Welch (London, 1912), p. 7.

81 BL, Add. MS 73945. For this and other examples, see C. M. Barron, *London in the Later Middle Ages: Government and People 1200–1500* (Oxford, 2004), p. 278, n. 65.

82 TNA, PCC, Prob. 11/6, ff. 216v–218v (John Garstang, 22 April 1477); 11/14, f. 250v (Mathew Ernest, alias Metyngham, 27 March 1505). I owe my knowledge of the St Dunstan material cited in this and the next note to the kindness of Jennifer Ledfors.

83 Ibid., 11/15, f. 93 (Thomas Warley, 26 October 1506); 11/25, f. 40v (John Thretforde, 20 November 1536); Guildhall MS 4887, f. 72 (Churchwardens' Accounts, 4 November 1537). For poor boxes in London parishes after the Dissolution, see also *London and Middlesex Chantry Certificate 1548*, ed. C. J. Kitching, London Record Society 16 (London, 1980), nos. 17, 21.

84 Rubin, *Cambridge*, p. 245, n. 48.

85 *Notes or Abstracts of the Wills contained in . . . the Great Orphan Book . . . at Bristol*, ed. T. P. Wadley (Bristol, 1886), p. 158 (no. 264).

86 As by W. K. Jordan in numerous works. See Hindle, *On the Parish?*, pp. 98–99, and Archer, *Pursuit of Stability*, pp. 163–182, for bibliography and critique.

87 S. Farmer, *Surviving Poverty in Medieval Paris: Gender, Ideology and the Daily Lives of the Poor* (Ithaca, NY, 2002), pp. 34–35, with 171–172.

88 McIntosh, 'Local Responses', p. 220; Burgess, '"Fond Thing"', p. 77; Brown, *Popular Piety*, p. 197. Note e.g. the distribution of bread, ale, and cheese to the parish poor in the context of an obit at St Mary at Hill in 1492: *Medieval Records of . . . (St Mary at Hill)*, ed. Littlehales, p. 192. For later London examples see C. S. Schen, *Charity and Lay Piety in Reformation London 1500–1620* (Aldershot, 2002), pp. 54–57; also Duffy, *Stripping*, pp. 360–364.

89 R. N. Swanson, *Church and Society in Late Medieval England* (Oxford, 1989), p. 303; Fideler, *Social Welfare*, pp. 44–46. Compare B. Geremek, *The Margins of Society in Late Medieval Paris* (Cambridge, 1987), pp. 186–189.

90 At n. 37. For the 1540s see *London . . . Chantry Certificate*, ed. Kitching, no. 152, for rooms underneath the church hall of St Clement Danes used rent-free by the poor.

91 See e.g. *The Pre-Reformation Records of All Saints', Bristol*, ed. C. Burgess, vol. III, Bristol Record Society 56 (Bristol, 2004), p. 52, no. 29 (Joan Pernaunt), c. 10. Kümin, *Shaping of a Community*, p. 61, gives just two examples. See also Brown, *Popular Piety*, pp. 189, 197; Dyer, 'English Medieval Village Community', p. 416.

92 S. C. Watson, *'Fundatio, ordinatio* and *statuta*: The Statutes and Constitutional Documents of English Hospitals to 1300', unpublished DPhil dissertation

(University of Oxford, 2003). I am also grateful to Max Satchell for confirmation from his work in progress mapping medieval English hospitals.

93 M. McIntosh, 'Poverty, Hospitals, and Almshouses in England, 1350–1598', unpublished paper read at York University, 30 May 1991, table 4C. I am most grateful to the author for giving me a copy of the paper and for allowing me to cite it here.

94 Two examples: Cullum, '"And Hir Name was Charite": Charitable Giving by and for Women in Late Medieval Yorkshire', in *Woman Is a Worthy Wight: Women in English Medieval Society c. 1200–1500*, ed. P. J. P. Goldberg (Stroud, 1992), p. 199; Dyer, 'English Medieval Village Community', p. 416.

95 Just as, if parishioners were not restrained, it could be an arena for markets, court cases, and entertainments: *Pastors and the Care of Souls*, ed. Shinners and Dohar, p. 150, translating William of Pagula's *Oculus sacerdotis*.

96 *Medieval Records of (St Mary at Hill)*, ed. Littlehales, p. 284; Cullum, '"And Hir Name"', p. 196.

97 J. M. Bennett, 'Conviviality and Charity in Medieval and Early Modern England', *Past and Present* 134 (1992), pp. 28–30, with critique by M. Moisà, 'Debate ...', *Past and Present* 154 (1997), 223–234, and Bennett's telling 'Reply', 235–242.

98 See e.g. J. Broad, 'Parish Economies of Welfare, 1650–1834', *Historical Journal* 42 (1999), 985–1006; L. Botelho, *Old Age and the English Poor Law, 1500–1700* (Stroud, 2004); Hindle, *On the Parish?*, p. 454.

99 Horden, 'A Discipline of Relevance: The Historiography of the Later Medieval Hospital', *Social History of Medicine* 1 (1988), 359–374; J. Lewis, 'Family Provision of Health and Welfare in the Mixed Economy of Care in the Late Nineteenth and Twentieth Centuries', *Social History of Medicine* 8 (1995), 1–16.

100 On the medieval elaboration of the distinction between deserving (impotent) and undeserving (able-bodied) recipients of relief, see B. Harvey, *Living and Dying in England 1100–1540: The Monastic Experience* (Oxford, 1993), pp. 8–9, with helpful references. Also Dyer, *Standards of Living*, p. 237, rightly warning against placing the beginnings of discrimination in almsgiving too late in the Middle Ages. See also, in that vein, Duffy, *Stripping*, p. 363.

101 Slack, *Poverty and Policy*, pp. 29–30.

102 Ibid. p. 172.

103 N. S. Rushton, 'Monastic Charitable Provision in Tudor England: Quantifying and Qualifying Poor Relief in the Sixteenth Century', *Continuity and Change* 16 (2001), 9–44; Rushton and W. Sigle-Rushton, 'Monastic Poor Relief in the Sixteenth Century', *Journal of Interdisciplinary History* 16 (2001), 193–216. See also Harvey, *Living and Dying*, ch. 1; Dyer, *Standards of Living*, pp. 311–312.

104 E. Phillips, 'Charitable Institutions in Norfolk and Suffolk c.1350–1600', unpublished PhD diss. (University of East Anglia, 2001), p. iv.

105 C. Rawcliffe, *The Hospitals of Medieval Norwich* (Norwich, 1995), p. 149; Cullum, '"For Pore People Harberles"'; Dyer, *Standards of Living*, p. 244.

106 McIntosh, 'Local Responses', pp. 216, 222–223; McIntosh, 'Poverty, Hospitals, and Almshouses', typescript p. 25.

107 For remission of manorial court fines *quia pauper*, see e.g. E. Wedemeyer Moor, 'Aspects of Poverty in a Small Medieval Town', in *The Salt of Common Life: Individuality and Choice in the Medieval Town, Countryside, and Church*, ed. E. B. DeWindt (Kalamazoo, MI, 1995), pp. 117–156. The manor and the poor is touched on by Z. Razi, 'The Myth of the Immutable English Family', *Past and Present* 140 (1993), pp. 12–14. For retirement contracts, see R. M. Smith, 'The Manorial Court and the Elderly Tenant in Late Medieval England', in *Life, Death, and the Elderly: Historical Perspectives*, ed. M. Pelling and R. M. Smith

(London, 1991), pp. 39–61. For the physically and mentally incapacitated, E. Clark, 'Social Welfare and Mutual Aid in the Medieval Countryside', *Journal of British Studies* 33 (1994), 381–406, at pp. 388–390. For wider context, see *Medieval Society and the Manor Court*, ed. Z. Razi and R. M. Smith (Oxford, 1996), p. 31, for a bibliography of highly pertinent articles by E. Clark.

108 A. Macfarlane, *Witchcraft in Tudor and Stuart England* (London, 1970), ch. 12; K. Thomas, *Religion and the Decline of Magic* (Harmondsworth, 1973), chs 16 and 17. See now J. Sharpe, *Instruments of Darkness: Witchcraft in Early Modern England* (London, 2001). On the supposed decline of face-to-face charity, see I. W. Archer, 'The Charity of Early Modern Londoners', *Transactions of the Royal Historical Society* 12 (2002), pp. 242–243; Hindle, *On the Parish?*, pp. 20, 104–120 – neither mentioning witchcraft. Also Dyer, *Standards of Living*, pp. 248–249, 256–257.

109 Clark, 'Social Welfare and Mutual Aid'; Razi, 'Myth', p. 14; Moisà, 'Debate', pp. 229–232; Horden, 'Household Care and Informal Networks: Comparisons and Continuities from Antiquity to the Present', in *Locus of Care*, ed. Horden and Smith, pp. 42–43; Farmer, *Surviving Poverty in Medieval Paris*. Note also (too little known in this context) W. C. Jordan, *Women and Credit in Pre-Industrial and Developing Societies* (Philadelphia, 1993), esp. pp. 27–42. More can be done with early modern evidence. See I. Krausman Ben-Amos, 'Gifts and Favors: Informal Support in Early Modern England', *Journal of Modern History* 27 (2000), 295–338; Hindle, *On the Parish?*, p. 20, ch. 1.

110 McIntosh, 'Local Responses', p. 213; McIntosh, *Controlling Misbehavior*, pp. 81–83, 192; Barron, *London in the Later Middle Ages*, p. 301.

111 Kümin, *Shaping of a Community*, p. 61.

112 Grell and Cunningham, 'Reformation and Changes', p. 2.

113 For a rural Tudor example, see E. Duffy, *The Voices of Morebath: Reformation and Rebellion in an English Village* (New Haven, CT, 2001), pp. 12, 185. Major urban studies: M. Pelling, 'Healing the Sick Poor: Social Policy and Disability in Norwich, 1550–1640', in Pelling, *The Common Lot: Sickness, Medical Occupations and the Urban Poor in Early Modern England* (London, 1988), pp. 79–102; M. K. McIntosh, 'Networks of Care in Elizabethan English Towns: The Example of Hadleigh, Suffolk', in *The Locus of Care*, ed. Horden and Smith, p. 78; A. Wear, 'Caring for the Sick Poor in St. Bartholomew's Exchange, 1580–1679', in *Living and Dying in London* (*Medical History*, supplement no. 11), ed. W. F. Bynum and R. Porter (London, 1991), pp. 41–60. For a later period, see S. Williams, 'Practitioners' Income and Provision for the Poor: Parish Doctors in the Later Eighteenth and Early Nineteenth Centuries', *Social History of Medicine* 18 (2005), 159–186.

114 See e.g. D. Jacquart, *Le milieu médical en France du XIIe au XVe siècle* (Paris, 1981), pp. 131–137; V. Nutton, 'Continuity or Rediscovery? The City Physician in Classical Antiquity and Mediaeval Italy', in *The Town and State Physician in Europe from the Middle Ages to the Enlightenment*, ed. A. W. Russell (Wolfenbüttel, 1981), pp. 24–34.

115 M. Carlin, 'Medieval English Hospitals', in *The Hospital in History*, ed. L. Granshaw and R. Porter (London, 1989), pp. 29–31.

116 J. A. F. Thompson, 'Piety and Charity in Late Medieval London', *Journal of Ecclesiastical History* 16 (1965), p. 187.

117 C. Rawcliffe, 'The Profits of Practice: The Wealth and Status of Medical Men in Later Medieval England', *Social History of Medicine* 1 (1988), p. 66.

118 R. C. Finucane, 'Pilgrimage in Daily Life: Aspects of Medieval Communication Reflected in the Newly-Established Cult of Thomas Cantilupe (d. 1282) . . . ,' in *Wallfahrt und Alltag in Mittelalter und früher Neuzeit* (Vienna, 1992), p. 175.

119 C. Rawcliffe, 'Curing Bodies and Healing Souls: Pilgrimage and the Sick in Medieval East Anglia', in *Pilgrimage: The English Experience from Becket to Bunyan*, ed. C. Morris and P. Roberts (Cambridge, 2002), p. 113.

120 Thomas, *Religion and the Decline of Magic*, ch. 7; see also O. Davies, *Cunning-Folk: Popular Magic in English History* (London, 2003), pp. 86–89.

121 C. Rawcliffe, 'Medicine for the Soul: The Medieval English Hospital and the Quest for Spiritual Health', in *Religion, Health and Suffering*, ed. J. R. Hinnells and R. Porter (London, 1999), pp. 316–338, much of which could apply to parish churches. For liturgical 'music therapy', see Horden, 'Religion as Medicine: Music in Medieval Hospitals', in *Religion and Medicine in the Middle Ages*, ed. P. Biller and J. Ziegler (Woodbridge, 2001), pp. 135–153. For parish church music, see C. M. Barron, 'Church Music in English Towns 1450–1550: An Interim Report', *Urban History* 29 (2002), 83–91; B. Kümin, 'Masses, Morris and Metrical Psalms: Music in the English Parish, c. 1400–1600', in *Music and Musicians in Renaissance Cities and Towns*, ed. F. Kisby (Cambridge, 2001), pp. 70–81; and M. Williamson, 'Liturgical Music in the Late Medieval English Parish: Organs and Voices, Ways and Means', in C. Burgess and E. Duffy (eds), *The Parish in Late Medieval England* (Donington, 2006), pp. 177–242. For a sophisticated analysis of 'healing art' (murals) in a French (Saint-Aignan-sur-Cher) parish church *c*.1200, see M. Kupfer, *The Art of Healing: Painting for the Sick and the Sinner in a Medieval Town* (University Park, PA, 2003). Note also R. Marks, *Image and Devotion in Late Medieval England* (Stroud, 2004), pp. 100–102.

122 E.g. *Councils and Synods*, ed. Powicke and Cheney, p. 268, no. 3 (Statutes of Robert Grosseteste); Marshall, *Catholic Priesthood*, pp. 191–193; Thomas of Monmouth, *The Life and Miracles of St William of Norwich*, ed. A. Jessopp and M. R. James (Cambridge, 1896), p. 242: priest houses and feeds woman doubled up with curvature of spine.

123 John Myrc, *Instructions for Parish Priests*, ed. E. Peacock, EETS 31 (London, 1868), pp. 3–4; M. Green, 'Obstetrical and Gynaecological Texts in Middle English', *Studies in the Age of Chaucer* 14 (1992), p. 57.

124 Green, 'Documenting Medieval Women's Medical Practice', in *Practical Medicine from Salerno to the Black Death*, ed. L. García-Ballester et al. (Cambridge, 1994), pp. 338–341.

125 A. Saunier, 'Le visiteur, les femmes et les "obstetrices" des paroisses de l'archidiaconé de Josas de 1458 à 1470', in *Santé, médecine et assistance au Moyen Âge. Actes du 110e Congrès national des sociétés savantes, section d'histoire médiévale et de philologie*, vol. I (Paris, 1987), pp. 43–62.

126 J. McManners, *Death and the Enlightenment* (Oxford, 1981), p. 27. See also R. Heller, '"Priest-Doctors" as a Rural Health Service in the Age of Enlightenment', *Medical History* 20 (1976), 361–383.

127 C. Rawcliffe, 'A Case of Imputed Leprosy at Sparham, Norfolk', in *Much Heaving and Shoving: Late-Medieval Gentry and their Concerns, Essays for Colin Richmond*, ed. R. Horrox and M. Aston (Lavenham, 2005), pp. 145–157; eadem, *Leprosy in Medieval England* (Woodbridge, 2006), ch. 4, generously shown to me in advance of publication.

128 F. Getz, *Medicine in the English Middle Ages* (Princeton, NJ, 1998), p. 18 (Walter de Barton).

129 R. A. Wood, 'A Fourteenth-Century London Owner of *Piers Plowman*', *Medium Aevum* 53 (1984), 83–90, at p. 89 (William Palmere). See further Barron, *London in the Later Middle Ages*, p. 288.

130 Getz, *Medicine in the English Middle Ages* (Princeton, NJ, 1998), pp. 49–53.

131 P. Stell, *Medical Practice in Medieval York*, Borthwick Papers 90 (York, 1996), pp. 9, 28–29 (transcription).

132 Barron, *London in the Later Middle Ages*, p. 288; see also p. 280.

133 Rawcliffe, 'Profits of Practice', p. 70. I have not yet found any 'non-careerist' parish-priest physicians in C. H. Talbot and E. A. Hammond, *The Medical Practitioners in Medieval England* (London, 1965), or its supplement by F. Getz in *Social History of Medicine* 3 (1990), 245–283. This is hardly surprising since, like female healers, such men would generally fall beneath the notice of much surviving documentation.

134 Horden, 'Religion as Medicine'; idem, 'A Non-Natural Environment: Medicine Without Doctors and the Medieval European Hospital', in *The Medieval Hospital and Medical Practice*, ed. B. Bowers (Aldershot, 2007), pp. 133–145.

135 Canon 22, in *Decrees of the Ecumenical Councils*, ed. N. P. Tanner, 2 vols (Washington, DC, 1990), I, pp. 245–246.

136 Myrc, *Instructions*, p. 10, ll. 312–325 modernized.

137 Thomas, *Religion and the Decline of Magic*, p. 39.

138 For what follows see M. Rubin, *Corpus Christi: The Eucharist in Late Medieval Culture* (Cambridge, 1991), esp. pp. 62–63, 108, 229, 231; Duffy, *Stripping*, pp. 95–100; Marshall, *Catholic Priesthood*, pp. 41–43.

139 *Sermon* 131.1, in *Patrologia Latina*, vol. 38, cols 729–730.

140 'The Virtues of the Mass', in *The Minor Poems of John Lydgate*, ed. H. Noble MacCracken, EETS extra series 107 (London, 1911), pt 1, p. 88, l. 24.

141 For what follows see A. Franz, *Die Messe im deutschen Mittelalter: Beiträge zur Geschichte der Liturgie und des religiösen Volkslebens* (Freiburg im Breisgau, 1902, repr. Darmstadt 1963), pp. 36–72. Such material also appears in amulets based on the length of Christ's body, looking at or wearing which brings spiritual and material benefits. See C. F. Bühler, 'Prayers and Charms in Certain Middle English Scrolls', *Speculum* 39 (1964), pp. 274–275.

142 *The Lay Folks Mass Book or the Manner of Hearing Mass*, ed. T. F. Simmons, EETS 71 (London, 1879), p. 131, and commentary pp. 366–371.

143 M. McIntosh, 'The Diversity of Social Capital in English Communities, 1300–1640 (with a Glance at Modern Nigeria)', in *Patterns of Social Capital: Stability and Change in Historical perspective*, ed. R. I. Rotberg (Cambridge, 2001), pp. 138–140. I am enormously indebted to Marjorie McIntosh and George Bernard for commenting on this essay in draft, and especially to Caroline Barron and Clive Burgess, both of whom not only read the draft but supplied references too numerous to acknowledge individually. I am also greatly obliged to John Henderson for advice on matters Italian.

POSTSCRIPT

This paper dates from the early years of the millennium. It was written for a collection of studies on 'The Parish in Late Medieval England'. The collection included discussions of parish clergy, their learning, their patrons, parishioners in general terms, choirs and liturgy, drama, material culture, and so forth. I thought – as, happily, did the editors – that it would be helpful if the parish were also represented as a potential source, or at least venue, for poor relief (a subset of the far larger medieval category of 'charity' or 'alms') and for healing (wider than, perhaps different from, 'medicine'). I started by suggesting that we should pretend we did not know what was to happen under Tudor legislation and the Old Poor Law. We should look, without Whiggery or teleology, at the later medieval parish in its own terms. We should see what could be said in its favour as a place of material support and healing for the needy. The required context was not so much what would happen next but *medieval* comparisons from continental Europe, where available, and the wider background of the 'mixed economy' of care. All the same, some discussion of the question of continuity across the Reformation period was inevitable: did the parish become the vehicle for Tudor poor relief *faute de mieux*, as the 'last institution standing' after the various Dissolutions, or did it have something positive to be said in its favour in virtue of its long history of irregular but not negligible support in a variety of ways not derived from taxation?

I had no intention to offer up the pre-Reformation parish as a welfare paradise, an unsung corner of merry England. Yet perhaps the picture is too rosy. I stressed the glass a quarter full rather than three-quarters empty. The surviving evidence will not allow us to settle the matter, especially since we do not know what relevant transfers passed unrecorded in churchwardens' accounts. And at the time of writing there seemed to be relatively little secondary literature to draw upon. Of course there was magisterial work by Christopher Dyer, Marjorie McIntosh, and Paul Slack, but none of it quite did what I wanted to do in my paper. Building up an overall picture, however provisional, proved very hard.

If I were writing now, I would feel on far more solid ground. There is much new work with which I would have to engage. And yet the debate about the evolving place of the English parish in the history of welfare over the late medieval/early modern divide continues, which is heartening because it means that the questions with which I was grappling are still worthwhile. The principal reference must be Marjorie McIntosh's crowning monograph *Poor Relief in England 1350–1600* (Cambridge: Cambridge University Press, 2012), supplemented by her study of one extraordinarily comprehensive Tudor urban relief system, *Poor Relief and Community in Hadleigh, Suffolk 1547–1600* (Hatfield: University of Hertfordshire Press, 2013). Drawing on her unrivalled knowledge of churchwarden's accounts and many other types of documentation, McIntosh sees the decisive period for the transition from haphazard medieval parochial relief to a tax-based regular system not in the 1598/1601 legislation but in the reign of Edward VI. The Old Poor Law was essentially a creation of the long 1550s. The decade saw a major discontinuity. What preceded it was, for McIntosh, unimpressive in scale and range. Her summary is sobering. It is based on churchwardens' accounts and some other documents from no fewer than 58 parishes that survive from the period 1404–1546:

> Nearly a quarter of these accounts said that the wardens distributed alms to needy individuals at some point. The assistance they gave, however, had often been bequeathed by other people and was in most cases occasional, unpredictable, and of low value . . . not intended to provide regular support. Only a few parishes appear to have collected money specifically for the poor or to have provided ongoing help.
>
> (*Poor Relief in England*, p. 96; see further pp. 100–112)

These few were not evenly spread. McIntosh can locate the large majority (58 per cent) of the most active parishes in this respect in East Anglia and the south-west (p. 112 and online Appendix 9: http://www.cambridge.org/files/7613/6680/3700/online_appendix_9.pdf, accessed 10 August 2018). Her supporting Appendix F (printed in the book) shows that in fact a little more than 'nearly a quarter', specifically 32 per cent (19 out of 58), of documented parishes had churchwardens active on behalf of the poor in the period 1404–1546. As McIntosh acknowledges, however, this figure takes no account of bequests and distributions at funerals and obits since it does not draw on the evidence of wills. And of course it cannot include transfers the wardens did not report – which, while probably not very substantial, are unlikely to have been nil.

Now all this goes well beyond my impressionistic survey in its methodological rigour and its evidential base. But it is not inconsistent with my 'quarter-full glass'. Moreover, it is more restrictive than I was in defining what is to count as parochial relief, and it does not touch on the topic of healing, except very indirectly through the twelve almshouses known to McIntosh that were run by medieval parishes (p. 111 n. 80).

Apart from McIntosh's work, if I were writing now the scholarship which would require the most frequent reference has come from Christopher Dyer. Subsequent to the works I was able to cite, Dyer has published two highly pertinent articles: the first is 'Did the Rich Really Help the Poor in Medieval England?' delivered to the XXVI Semana de los Estudios Medievales, *Ricos y pobres: opulencia y desarraigo en el occidente medieval*, Estela, 2009 (Pamplona: Gobierno de Navarra, 2010), pp. 307–322, of which the author kindly sent me an offprint of the English text. (A text in Spanish can be found online at http://revistascientificas.filo.uba.ar/index.php/analesHAMM/article/view/2597, accessed 25 April 2018.) This was, secondly, much expanded into 'Poverty and its Relief in Late Medieval England', *Past and Present* 216 (August 2012), 41–78. Partly because Dyer makes much fuller use of wills than does McIntosh, he assigns a correspondingly greater role in poor relief to churchwardens than she would. He sees the village and parish combined as an important locus of material provision to the needy. And he depicts the later Middle Ages as a period of creative experimentation in the forms of such provision. These were sometimes based on unofficial quasi-rates. They were not necessarily haphazard and short-term, and they prepared the way for the key Tudor legislation. I think Dyer's wide-ranging expertise tends to confirm (and of course go well beyond) both what I wrote about the parish and my wider sketch of later medieval welfare.

To close, I shall simply note four other works which I wish had been available to me when writing:

Anne M. Scott (ed.), *Experiences of Poverty in Late Medieval and Early Modern England* (Farnham: Ashgate, 2012), including a further discussion by Dyer and a valuable study by the late Philippa C. Maddern of survival strategies of single mothers and their children.

Anne M. Scott (ed.), *Experiences of Charity 1250–1650* (Farnham: Ashgate, 2015), with pertinent contributions by Maddern again, Sharon Farmer, Neil S. Rushton, and Nicholas Dean Brodie.

G. W. Bernard, *The Late Medieval English Church: Vitality and Vulnerability before the Break with Rome* (New Haven, CT: Yale University Press, 2012), especially on episcopal piety and hospitality.

Gervase Rosser, *The Art of Solidarity in the Middle Ages: Guilds in England, 1250–1550* (Oxford: Oxford University Press, 2015).

14

MUSICAL SOLUTIONS[1]

Past and present in music therapy

I

'The present age is one of overproduction ... never has there been so much music-making and so little musical experience of a vital order.' Thus Constant Lambert, the composer. He was writing in 1934, in the classic *Music Ho! A Study of Music in Decline*.[2] The chapter is entitled 'The Appalling Popularity of Music'. It goes on to complain that, thanks to the 'gramophone', the 'wireless' and the loudspeaker, 'music of a sort is everywhere and at every time'. The result: total anaesthesia. If the BBC broadcast the Last Trump, Lambert expostulates, 'it is doubtful if it would interfere with the cry of "No Trumps" from the card table'.

> We have at present no idea of what havoc may be wrought in a few years' time by the combined effect of the noise of city life and the noise of city music – an actual atrophy of the aural nerves would seem to be indicated . . . We live in an age of tonal debauch where the blunting of the finer edge of pleasure leads only to a more hysterical and frenetic attempt to recapture it. It is obvious that second-rate mechanical music is the most suitable fare for those to whom musical experience is no more than a mere aural tickling, just as the prostitute provides the most suitable outlet for those to whom sexual experience is no more than the periodic removal of a recurring itch. The loud speaker is the street walker of music.[3]

Were he writing today, Lambert's metaphors would doubtless be even more florid. Music is omnipresent, and – worse – mechanized to an extent that he could scarcely have envisaged. Only within certain fundamentalist Muslim states is there any escaping its dictatorship over the acoustic environment, its unvarying and literally inhuman rhythm. The agents of infiltration now include the 'mini-system' and the cell phone. Much of their output is, however, ignored, left as background. The responses evoked by that which really is listened to, however 'profound' they may be, are fleeting. In a relatively

273

tiny market for recorded classical music, 'crossovers', tenor megastars, or concert warhorses predominate, while for the minority there is huge variety that encourages a detached promiscuity among collectors, a pseudo-culture of far vaster proportions than Malraux's 'museum without walls'.[4] To quote George Steiner, a more measured, but no less disheartened, critic of aural culture than Lambert:

> If we choose, we can put on Opus 131 while eating the breakfast cereal. We can play the *St. Matthew Passion* any hour of the day or week . . . the effects are ambiguous: there can be an unprecedented intimacy, but also a devaluation . . . A Muzak of the sublime envelops us.[5]

And with the mechanical beat and harmonic banality of most popular music, profundity, even of the fleeting kind furnished by the latest technology, is seldom in question. Not only can music be so readily meaningless, an addiction to decibels and metrical bass; it can be positively damaging, to the ear when brought too close to loudspeakers, to society when the sound falls directly on the inner ear from the headphone, perhaps to the whole intellect.[6]

Some experiments can be adduced which seem to illustrate that potential for damage, at a very basic, cellular level. But they also point towards an alternative, and less bleak, way of summing up our aural culture. Despite all the evidence that a greater quantity of music is more utterly ephemeral and trivialized in our time than ever before, attention can, increasingly, also be called to havens of serious and profound response that relieve the global landscape of rock and its offspring.

It is not just a question of a minority for whom listening to classical music is life itself. Picture the following. Six human cell cultures are aligned *in vitro*. Five are of tumour cells – malignant glioma, breast adenocarcinoma, colon adenocarcinoma, skin malignant melanoma and lung carcinoma; the remaining one is of normal dermal fibroblasts. The cultures are placed in separate humidified incubators. One incubator contains a water-resistant hi-fi speaker connected to a portable stereo system. The control incubator has no such musical attachment. Each culture is tested in triplicate for an average of four experiments. Music plays from cassette tapes from 5.00 p.m. to 9.00 a.m. continuously for ten days at a constant volume. One type of music consists of 'primordial sounds' – Sama Veda from the 'Maharishi Ayur-Veda system of natural health care'; the other is 'Back in Black' by the rock band AC/DC. Compared with no music at all, primordial sound significantly decreases the average growth across cell lines. In the presence of hard rock, however, growth of cells, though inconsistent, tends significantly to increase. 'We conclude,' write the authors of the research paper just summarized, 'that sound has an effect on the growth of neoplastic and normal human cells in vitro.'[7] But the possible newspaper headlines can be imagined: hard rock gives you cancer; Ayurvedic sound cures cancer. How can this happen?

Cells and intracellular structures apparently vibrate dynamically. These vibrations may play a role in the cell's self-regulation, affecting its shape, motility, and signal transduction. They can be changed by both growth factors and carcinogenesis. Incoming vibrations, such as sound waves, are perhaps transferred from the peripheral membrane to the nucleus and DNA. Sama Veda has a preponderance of low frequency tones and a regular slow rhythm, which may, by some means yet to be determined, restore the DNA to its own normal low-frequency vibrations. 'Back in Black', on the other hand, includes more high-frequency tones than the 'primordial sound' and its tempo and rhythm are alike irregular. It literally sets up the wrong vibrations.

The experiments and hypotheses I have been reporting are those of three members of the Department of Pathology, College of Medicine, Ohio State University. Their work was supported by the Lancaster Foundation, Bethesda, Maryland, and also by the Maharishi Ayur-Veda Foundation of America. There are three reasons for selecting their paper as an opening example in this collaborative historical enquiry into music's healing potential.[8]

First, it can stand as an extreme instance of how seriously the powers of music are nowadays being taken – a *ne plus ultra* of musical therapy to set against the provocatively glum panorama with which I prefaced it. For cancer, along with AIDS, is the most terrifying modern disease. And in this example, we are being told that music – without benefit of psychosomatic mechanism, cultural expectation, placebo effect and so on – is apparently capable of retarding the growth of cancer cells, at least *in vitro*.

Second, the paper represents the ambiguous status of musical therapeutics today. The research project could hardly be described as mainstream. It comes from the world of complementary medicine. It appears in the relatively new journal *Alternative Therapies in Clinical Practice*. And its purpose, one senses, is more to endorse than to test the 'system of natural health care known as Maharishi Ayur-Veda, which . . . utilizes "primordial" sounds as one of its techniques for restoring health'.[9] On the other hand, the authors can reasonably assert that they are not alone in their finding that sound or music can have a significant and positive impact on living organisms:[10]

A study conducted in India showed that experimental plants exposed to sound waves in the form of Nadeshwaram music showed more vigorous growth . . . In the US, Hicks demonstrated that corn receiving broadcast of a continuous low note had an increased yield . . . Retallack conducted a study in which plants showed a positive reaction when exposed to Ravi Shankar or Bach, growing toward the speaker, while a second group of plants exhibited a negative reaction to acid rock, growing away from the speaker and showing a random growth pattern.[11]

As such research comes to seem less marginal, the finding that plants or cell cultures have better musical taste than people will presumably lose its shock value. Meanwhile, its proponents can point to others involved in music therapy whose standing is less ambiguous than their own: professional music therapists and those researching music's psycho-physiological effects.

A third reason for using this paper is that it opens up a historical perspective. Besides a sweeping appeal to congenial research by others, it looks to the past for legitimation. It looks to the non-European past above all, to Ayurvedic healing in ancient India; but also to the medical antiquity of the Persians and Hebrews; and additionally to the classical tradition in Europe, a tradition which runs from the Greeks to the Renaissance and on into the nineteenth century.[12] Present-day enquiry is presented as continuous with the efforts of these much earlier cultures. The relationship of music to medicine is portrayed as almost always having been close. An analogy is implicitly drawn with traditional ways in which the regularity of music (harmonic or rhythmic) has been thought to alleviate irregularity or imbalance (dissonance) in the mind or body. To such traditions there has been only one interruption: 'the technological explosion of allopathic medicine in the 20th century'.[13]

To sum up so far: the findings of the research paper which I have been relaying are of ambiguous stature as normal science; they occupy an extreme position on the spectrum of musical possibilities, at the opposite end from the trivializing of so much contemporary music. Nonetheless, they open up a surprising range of therapeutic territories. These territories can be labelled – not altogether objectively – the 'heterodox', the 'professional', and the 'historical'. The professional is mainstream music therapy in Europe and America; the heterodox represents a variety of non-mainstream currents; history is the domain to which they both variously appeal for precedent or legitimacy. I shall spend the rest of this chapter looking at each in turn, to sketch what continuities and discontinuities have been discerned within and between them – and with how much justification. I shall thus be moving from the present back into the past.

II

The heterodox shows itself in a variety of forms and has been given a variety of more or less pejorative labels: New Age, para-scientific, esoteric, and so on. Animating many of these is an appeal to some non- (or perhaps omni-) denominational spirituality. Certainly there is a common aspiration to proclaim musical response as something more than a passing pleasure,

a temporary psychological and somatic reconfiguration. 'While I'm singing my soul is beautiful,' muses Luciano Pavarotti, drawing on the analogy
between personal and cosmic order which we shall encounter many more
times in what follows.

> It's not ego, like some think. It's therapy – for me and the audience.
> People who listen to music want to be happy in this stupid life today
> when everyone has taken to drugs . . . There have been periods in life
> when religion was important . . . The god of today is negative gossip.[14]

Until the tenor megastar changes all that, presumably. There are rock
equivalents, equally ready to substitute their health-restoring art for contemporary negativity. In the companion volume to one that this chapter
introduces, Linda Austern places The Smashing Pumpkins' album, *Mellon
Collie and the Infinite Sadness*, in a tradition of musical auto-therapy that
descends from Robert Burton.[15] Those seeking a less muscular therapy than
Messrs Pumpkins' or Pavarotti's find ready encouragement in CD catalogues and websites. 'David Naegele creates [in his CD *Temple in the Forest*]
a tranquil meditative environment . . . evoking an overwhelming feeling of
renewal and well-being.' One disc of music by Stephen Rhodes, based on
'mesmerising patterns of hypnotic harmony', is simply entitled *Music for
Healing*. Another, *Inner Peace*, is confidently promoted as 'stress-busting'.
    In this musical cauldron, Gregorian chant can meet New Age, pseudo-
orientalism or earth magic to promote spiritual journeying, or, more accu-
rately, its sales rhetoric. Debussy, Schubert, Aretha Franklin, and Crosby,
Stills, Nash and Young, are all recommended impartially as vehicles of
healing.[16] Played while in your bath, a track entitled 'Echoes of Ages', on
a CD called *Bliss*, will induce perfect relaxation.[17] The appeal to the past
may be a little more specific. Sung narratives of miraculous healing in the
Cantigas de Santa Maria compiled for the thirteenth-century King Alfonso
the Wise are recommended on a CD cover (SK 62263) as a cure for the evils
of modernity.[18] The School of Music Thanatology at the 'Chalice of Repose Project' within the St Patrick Hospital, Missoula, Missouri, advertises
a 'clinical practice that prescribes music [live voice and harp] to tend to
the needs of the dying. The school draws its inspiration from 11th-century
French monastic medicine.'[19] This is doubtless a serious and professional
form of palliative medicine. Its historical sense is a little weaker, though: in
medieval monastic ritual for the dying, it was the anointing of the sick which
was quasi-medicinal; the accompanying liturgy was directed to God.[20] In
dealing with this whole topic, it can be hard to know what to take seriously.
During 1998, BBC Radio 3 broadcast the assertion of an organist that we
each have a special tone which resonates with the whole being and promotes
health if sung or hummed for a long time – an old idea that 'goes back to the
walls of Jericho'. Only the date of the broadcast – 1st April – distinguished

this from many a programme extolling the mantra, or for that matter from another Radio 3 talk, this time about the monochord, a strung healing table of a kind that doubtless has equally venerable antecedents.

For all the apparent indifference generated by the mechanization of music in the second half of the twentieth century, there is clearly widespread heterodox interest in music's healing capacity, whether the music is part of complementary or New Age therapies, the vehicle of auto-therapy in the private world of the headphones, or something more mainstream. Here are two examples of that interest.

The first has been remarked with surprising infrequency in discussions of music therapy. It is the response to *Awakenings*. This was Oliver Sacks's famous account of the 'semi-survivors' of the sleeping sickness epidemic of the 1920s, patients very often immobilized into post-encephalitic Parkinsonism until revivified in various ways over four decades later by the 'miracle drug' L-DOPA. Fascination with their history is such that the book has run through several editions and its contents have inspired plays, documentaries, and a feature film.[21] In the book, as in some of its reincarnations, 'music has been the profoundest non-chemical medication for our patients'.[22] Music roused the akinetic to normal movement and calmed the excited – for the duration of its playing.[23] A musician patient, who knew all Chopin by heart, had merely to be told an opus number to play the music over to herself in her mind.[24] Most, of course, needed mechanical assistance:

> One minute would see Miss D. compressed, clenched, and blocked, or jerking, ticcing, and jabbering – like a sort of human bomb; the next, with the sound of music from a wireless or gramophone, the complete disappearance of all these . . . and their replacement by a blissful ease and flow of movement . . . It was necessary that the music be *legato*; *staccato* music (and especially percussion bands) sometimes had a bizarre effect . . .[25]

A more recent sign of popular preoccupation with such phenomena were the thousands of letters received by Paul Robertson,[26] the presenter of a Channel 4 series broadcast in May 1996, 'Music and the Mind', which was accompanied by a booklet of the same title. The resonances with a broader culture of musical therapy were unmistakable. After the opening exploration of the neurology of musical response, the second programme was called 'Healing and Harmony'. Not merely was the familiar equation of bodily and musical order repeated; the brain in particular was seen as 'musicalized'. To quote the booklet of the series: 'we use beautifully tuned systems of the brain to integrate a whole mass of complex information . . . So durable is the musical system that it often survives when other systems fail.'[27] (Hence music as, if nothing else, a therapy of last resort.) The human being is even presented as 'a kind of symphonic composition'. The similarity urged by philosophers of antiquity,[28] and which is likely in more recent times to be taken as metaphorical, becomes literal once again.

> The ancient belief that a 'harmonious' condition generates health and happiness, whilst a discordant state of mind and body encourages sickness and unease, has become part of the language of healers . . . heart-disease patients when making music are less able to coordinate and empathise with the rhythms of other music makers. But what is cause and what is effect? *Is disease damaging musicality, or is damaged musicality – being 'out of tune' – making people ill?*[29]

That recalls one of Oliver Sacks's informants, who referred to herself as being 'unmusicked' by Parkinsonism.[30] The larger point, however, is this: although Sacks and Robertson between them can sum up a widespread lay concern with music's healing properties, the reception of their work also illustrates how interest extends to more professional, clinical endeavours. Sacks [who died in 2015] was after all, a professor of neurology in New York. And Robertson's programme and booklet introduce us to the projects of two other specialists, both at work in Germany: Ralph Spintge, who runs a pain clinic and has compiled a database of the effects of music on 90,000 or more patients; and David Aldridge, Professor for Clinical Research Methods at the Institute for Music Therapy at the University of Witten Herdecke, whose research involves devising ways to analyse and assess what is actually going on in successful music therapy. It is Aldridge who wants us to see human life as a composition. 'Music is . . . isomorphic with the process of living'.[31] At Spintge's clinic, music of their choice is available to all patients, not just to distract them but, Spintge is convinced, to speed their recovery. Specially composed music is also played before, after, and even during operations:

> Fifteen minutes of soothing music lulls the patient into such a state of well-being that only 50 per cent of recommended doses of sedatives and anaesthetic drugs are needed to perform otherwise very painful operations. Indeed, some procedures are now undertaken without any anaesthetic . . . More invigorating music then alerts the patients' systems so they can actively respond to the surgeon. Once this is complete the music then takes the patient back into a relaxed state for recovery.[32]

III

As with cell cultures in the laboratory (with which we began), so with entire human beings; and as for the heterodox, the first of my three categories, so for the second, the professional: rhythm seems to be the key. 'Pieces [of music] composed to create specific physiological change . . . are designed to lock into the innate neurophysiological and biological rhythms that underlie the vital functions of the body.'[33]

Chronic pain and perioperative stress are but two of the areas presumably susceptible to this sort of analysis and in which music is today used as therapy. The full range defies brief summary, least of all by a non-specialist.[34] Suffice it to say that it embraces music played *to* patients (or clients); music both live and recorded, composed or improvised, conducted, sung or played *by* patients. The patients come individually or in groups, and on occasion their families are involved. They may be mentally or physically ill or disabled. Their ages span the prenatal (in some tentative experiments) at one extreme, and the comatose, the very elderly, and the terminally ill at the other. The music is sometimes ancillary, as in the operating theatre; sometimes it complements other therapies; sometimes it is the primary form of therapy. So it may be associated with every kind of technique from the most invasive to the mildest palliative. The physical settings in which music is used vary from the operating theatre and hospital ward to the specialized clinic or school, the day-centre, the charity, the home – or the prison.[35] A sonic spectrum might be envisaged running from the highest tinkling metallic percussion to the vibro-acoustic bed or chair, the speakers set into which play tones with a frequency of 40 Hz.[36]

Problems for which the low tones of vibro-acoustic therapy have been found efficacious include severe physical disability, rheumatoid conditions, muscle spasm, pulmonary disorders, and cerebral palsy. The list of problems or clinical contexts for which music therapy more generally has been pronounced helpful would of course be much longer. To offer no more than an alphabetical sample: asthma, AIDS, aphasia, autism, bereavement, cancer, deafness, dental problems, depression, dementia, eating disorders, emotional disturbance, epilepsy, inflammatory bowel disease, kidney failure, schizophrenia, multiple sclerosis, sexual abuse.

The profession whose work has brought all this to increasing public attention is now substantial in scale and nearly global in scope. There are hundreds of music therapists in Britain, proportionately many more in the United States. The World Federation of Music Therapy draws members from some twenty countries [2018 figures], including Ghana, Poland, and South Africa. (Only the Russian Federation and the Muslim Middle East seem unrepresented.)[37] There is clearly massive investment in the future of this profession. Meanwhile, the quantity of germane research papers increases ever more rapidly, to an extent that must simultaneously exhilarate and depress those therapists trying to keep abreast of it. The merest surfing of web databases such as the USA National Library of Medicine's 'PubMed' shows the range of titles in biomedical journals: '"Brain music" in the treatment of patients with insomnia'; 'Enhancement of spatio-temporal reasoning after a Mozart listening condition in Alzheimer's disease' (a variation on the educational use of background music which has become known as 'the Mozart effect');[38] 'The effect of constant baroque music on premature infants'; 'Music therapy: facilitating behavioural and psychological change in people with stroke'.[39] Success everywhere: few seem willing – or are allowed – to report that music made little or no difference in their particular cases, or worse, that it was positively damaging,[40] a music-therapeutic version of iatrogenic disease.[41]

The alluring article titles and their triumphalist tone prompt, then, the general question of what music therapists actually do with all this training and research. Their discipline's nature and purpose have proved remarkably hard to specify. The music produced (or reproduced) may decrease hormone levels, diminish stress, enhance immune functions, and reduce muscle tension, heart rate and blood pressure; but it may also be directed at less measurable goals such as self-expression or bolder socialization. The World Federation of Music Therapy's official definition is [1997] correspondingly open-ended:

> Music Therapy is the use of music and/or musical elements (sound, rhythm, melody, and harmony) by a qualified music therapist, with a client or group, in a process designed to facilitate and promote *communication, relationships, learning, mobilisation, expression, organisation and other relevant therapeutic objectives,* in order to meet physical, emotional, mental, social and cognitive needs. Music Therapy aims to develop potentials and/or restore functions of the individual so that he or she can achieve better intra- and interpersonal integration and, consequently, a better quality of life through prevention, rehabilitation, or treatment.[42]

Reference to curing is noticeably missing; the italicized aims are broad and increasingly vague; treatment comes last and is, it seems, connected only indirectly to the music. The therapy may be no more (though also no less) than an objectification of the problem, a form of diagnosis.[43] Criteria of success will be as elusive as definitions. The children with learning disabilities who might be taken as the emblematic clients of music therapists in the Anglo-American world are not so much being treated as communicated with. The music is both symbol and vehicle of the wider transaction between therapist and client, a transaction that seems to embrace both disease and cure, and indeed frustrates any attempt to separate them.

By way of illustration, consider Sophie.[44] At four months of age she was found to have difficulties with her fine and coarse motor control (she could not crawl or pull herself up to stand). Although her hearing was normal, she also failed to speak. She played alone, seemingly immune to distraction. No organic causes could be traced for any of this. In her first session with a music therapist, she was very anxious and played a small bell and chime bar almost inaudibly. By the fifth session, however, she was playing a drum in rhythms loosely related to those of the therapist's improvisation. Her parents began to find her freer and more sociable in daily life: she spoke in a babble but could remember words and was keen to communicate. In the remaining therapy sessions her improvisational skills developed considerably. Concurrently, her awareness of her surroundings and her independence of action increased in proportion.

When there are case histories like that to reckon with, it is entirely comprehensible that Leslie Bunt, an eminent and experienced music therapist, should write: 'we are at the stage when the "Does it work?" question seems rather meaningless given the complex interaction of so many variables involved in any piece of therapeutic work.'[45] How can the personal contribution of the therapist be distinguished from that of the music, or indeed from other kinds of 'treatment' which the musical one may complement, such as art therapy? Recall Yeats's 'how can we know the dancer from the dance?' ('Among schoolchildren'). Is such a distinction appropriate? How can the outcomes of therapy be categorized and assessed in ways that give weight to parental instincts as much as to clinical calibrations, to the psychosomatic as much as to the organic – above all, to the evolving *meaning*, for both therapist and client, of the problems being addressed?

It is easy to see why therapists resort to metaphor when trying to capture the elusive essence of their art: to the notion, for instance, that life is a musical composition, to which the actual music of the therapist is 'entrained' (attuned) so that subsequent adjustments of the music can bring with them analogous changes in the patient.[46] It is also easy to see why the aesthetics of Susanne Langer, for whom music was *par excellence* a symbolic analogue of the inner life, survive in the writings of music therapists when they have been rejected by most philosophers of art (for their Cartesian separation of the inner world from outward behaviour, their unanalysable concept of an emotion's logical structure, and the circularity implied in asserting that emotions can be described in musical terms).[47]

IV

'Each music therapy group becomes a miniature society.'[48] And yet it is precisely the social dimension that seems to be relatively neglected in the case histories of professional music therapists. Which is surprising, because it is from the wider social arena that some of the ailments and disabilities encountered by music therapists derive their significance, and it is in the wider social arena that all the outcomes of treatment must eventually be manifest. One body of writing which might assist and even inspire the music therapists – and put some perspective on their difficulties with definition and evaluation – is thus the social anthropology of music and healing, to which, still under the 'professional' heading, I shall devote the present section of the chapter. From this discipline, in reports mainly from sub-Saharan Africa but also, notably, from Sri Lanka and South-East Asia,[49] can be found examples of healing practice, 'professionalism' of a very different kind, that is stimulatingly alien. None of the usual distinctions seems to apply. In northern Malawi, for instance:

> *Vimbuza* – a multivocal term, a complex of meanings and references – encompasses a class of spirits, the illnesses they cause, and the music and dance used to treat the illnesses. As spirit, *vimbuza* is the numinous energy of foreign peoples and wild animals; as illness, it is both a spirit affliction and an initiatory sickness; as musical experience, it is a mode of trance. For patients possessed by *vimbuza* spirits, trance dancing is a cooling therapy; for adepts, it is the means for transforming a disease into a vocation; and for healers, it is the source of an energizing heat that fuels the divination trance.[50]

In such a world, sufferers become healers; both, at certain specified moments, become part of more complex transactions involving larger groups; singing, drumming and instrumental melody, words, dancing and imagery alike contribute to some all-encompassing ritual. The living and the ancestors, the human world and that of spirits may all be involved. As in some American or European music therapy, the music can be the diagnosis as well as the therapy; it can also be the disease itself.[51]

The afflictions addressed by rituals of this kind would not necessarily count as illnesses in Western biomedical terms. A classic example comes from the healing cult of the Congo basin made famous by John Janzen in *Lemba, 1650–1930: A Drum of Affliction in Africa and the New World*. As in other such cults, *Lemba* showed itself in the individual in physical symptoms such as abdominal pain and difficulty with breathing. It was, however, distinguished from those cults by its social exclusivity. It struck the elite households of the north bank of the Congo: chiefs, judges, traders. What the affliction was – what the *Lemba* drum and its associated magical medicines and bracelets were being deployed against – remained unclear. Janzen could not tell until (to quote one of his commentators),

> casually, he superimposed a map of the provenance of *Lemba* texts and artefacts on to one of the long-distance trade routes. They matched . . . the *Lemba* cult provided a way of calming conflicts of interest between the naturally competitive and divisive activity of trade and the social order of lower Zaire . . . *Lemba* protected their health from the disease of capitalism.[52]

Here, 'socio-somatic' seems a more appropriate category than psychosomatic. 'What is recognized as illness . . . is a model of the disorder rather than the disorder itself', a model constructed in and on the body.[53] Even so, some of the ways in which spirit-caused afflictions are resolved by indigenous healers, African or Asian, show points of contact with Western therapy. The music is highly personal – improvised and variable – personal to both the patient and the healer.[54] Whether spirits are invoked or not, the objective may well be the entrainment (metaphorically) of sick body and healing sound.

> Melodies rise, fall, cut straight across, or wind sinuously . . . What Temiars [of the Malaysian rain forest] describe as the disorientation of illness is counterbalanced by the sense of being 'located' on paths inscribed in song . . . vocalizations embody sonic action: 'blowing' cools the patient; 'sucking' helps extract the illness agent, bringing it to the patient's body surface, so it can be drawn out into the medium's hand, or swept away with a leaf whisk.[55]

The pity is all the greater, then, that music therapists and social anthropologists have, in recent decades, been writing largely in ignorance of one another. It was not always thus, as we shall see in a moment. And among music therapists, it is of course possible to find occasional reference to John Blacking, one of the pioneers of ethnomusicology, or to generalized notions of shamanism.[56] Yet there are no obvious signs that the major detailed ethnographies of healing cults – such as Janzen's *Ngoma*, Roseman's *Healing Sounds from the Malaysian Rainforest*, or Friedson's *Dancing Prophets* – have had much impact on the ways in which music therapists conceive their role.[57] In fairness, it should be added that those works are all relatively recent, and that sustained ethnographic interest of their type is hardly much older. Evans-Pritchard's classic account of Azande magic, first published as long ago as 1937, embraced the witch doctors' séance during which divinatory 'medicines' (magical trees and herbs) were activated by drumming, singing, and dancing.[58] Yet his was an isolated example. Even Victor Turner's highly influential discussions of Ndembu healing rituals published in the 1960s, notably his *The Drums of Affliction*, actually had little detail to offer about drumming, or indeed about the healing functions of music generally.[59] Not that anthropologists now have reason to feel superior when knowledge of cognate disciplines is in question. In 1996 Friedson could still write of the place of music in biomedicine in terms of muzak piped into doctors' waiting rooms – as if music therapy did not exist.[60]

The worlds of 'western' music therapy and 'traditional' musical healing are hardly far removed from one another in geographical terms. In Greek Macedonia, illness-generating social conflicts are both expressed and healed in the songs that accompany the fire-walking of possessed Anastenarides.[61] Spirit cults involving music can be found among expatriate communities in northern Europe, for example the Creole migrants from Surinam in an Amsterdam suburb.[62] Music therapy is already well represented in South Africa and will presumably spread to other parts of the continent, where its practitioners will find that biomedicine and indigenous therapies have already established a division of labour in the treatment of local ills. It will be fascinating to see how the two traditions of musical therapeutics interpenetrate.

No more need be said here about the ethnography of musical healing. The topic deserves much more sustained treatment, but it starts to receive that in contributions to Penelope Gouk's volume, *Musical Healing in Cultural Contexts* (by several authors discussed here, among others). One feature common to music therapists and musical healers is, however, worth noting now: the invocation of history. Both esteem ancestors more than contemporaries.

V

To views of the past, then; the last of the three headings that I proposed above.

> In the time of the Prophet Adam, Eve was sick [. . .] Adam looked for medicine; he looked and looked but couldn't find any [. . .] he asked the *bomoh* [Malay healer], 'Do you have any medicine to treat Eve?' This is what [. . .] the *bomoh* said: 'I have medicine for everything!' He brought over a *gebana* (hand drum); he had a *rehab* (spike fiddle). Adam asked what those things were. 'This is a bowl for medicine,' he said, pointing to the *gebana*. 'This is a medicinal herb', he said, pointing to the *rehab*. Then he treated his patient – he played. After he played, Eve was cured of her sickness.[63]

The shaman informant even went on to say that the original act of musical healing was Gabriel's reintegration, at God's behest, of Adam, after the infusion of divine breath had broken his body into little pieces. Music therapists and those engaged in related research may not look quite so far back for antecedents; sometimes a nineteenth-century precursor is venerable enough. But they do, as we have already seen, advert to early civilizations of the Mediterranean, the Middle East, and India. Having mentioned ancient Greeks, Egyptians, and Hebrews in the opening chapter of his account of contemporary music therapy, Leslie Bunt concludes by offering us, as the discipline's 'emblem', no less a figure than Orpheus.[64] In this he is to some extent following the example of Juliette Alvin. In what remains the classic short introduction to music therapy, Alvin too connects Orpheus with present-day concerns and ways of talking about musical performance, and, conversely, she relates the effects of a music box on an autistic child to something deep in mankind's biological past.[65] In a chapter which functions as a general survey of music in healing, she embeds, within a *tour de force* of potted medical history, a narrative of music in therapy that runs from 'primitive man' through Pythagoras, Cassiodorus, Bernard of Clairvaux, and Robert Burton,[66] to the physicians of the early modern age who were the first to write specific treatises on music's healing power.

285

Throughout, there is a presumption of continuity. It is made explicit at a later stage of Alvin's book: she prefaces her survey of the modern practice of music therapy – which occupies only the last 63 pages of a 163-page text – with a brief account of tarantism, the healing cult studied at some length in *Music as Medicine*.[67] The account is entitled 'The Continuous Thread'.[68] Elsewhere the presumption is implicit, but hardly less obvious. The figures named or quoted are (for her) more than remote precursors – they are colleagues, doing the same thing, with essentially the same means, as today's therapists. An account by Richard Brocklesby, Dr Johnson's physician, of the slow recovery of a pathologically grief-stricken Scottish patient is presented virtually as a case history in the modern clinical sense.[69] More tellingly, the substantial historical part of Alvin's book culminates in paired accounts of the biblical David playing on his lyre to relieve Saul of his 'evil spirit' [I Sam. 16: 14–23] and the castrato Farinelli (subject of a feature film) singing to lift the melancholic Spanish King Philip V. These not only suggest that comparisons between the two kings' cases can be made across the intervening millennia; they place as much emphasis on the evolving personal relationship between the two depressives and their singing therapists as on the uses of music in their respective treatments. 'Each of the approaches we have described is valid today; every music therapist uses them more or less consciously.' That is Alvin's general conclusion to her retrospect.[70]

The past is called upon to validate the present, to show that apparently novel approaches have in fact been tried for centuries. Alvin was one of the pioneers of the modern music therapy profession in Britain.[71] She gave so much space to history in her introduction to the subject presumably because music therapy was then still young and vulnerable to criticism: it needed an impressive pedigree. Newer textbooks, such as Leslie Bunt's, can be correspondingly briefer and more selective in their historical backgrounds because their profession is more securely established.[72] Nonetheless, authors of such works continue to rely on what, until postmodernity corroded it, could be felt as the cohesion and durability of the Hellenic- and Judaeo-Christian tradition. These authors take it as axiomatic that the past can be interpreted in much the same light as can the present – that David, or Pythagoras, can be seen as more or less a founding father of music therapy. If there has been any great interruption, any break in the continuity of musical thought and practice across the ages, then it would (for them) be quite a recent one. As those who treated cancer cells with Ayurveda put it, 'the technological explosion of allopathic medicine in the 20th century obscured the traditionally close relationship between music and medicine'.[73] Biomedicine – technologically triumphalist, dehumanizing, viewing the patient as a machine with broken parts rather than as a person for whom illness has meaning – was almost bound to undervalue the psychological or interpersonal dimension of healing.[74] Now, however, a more sensitive, holistic conception of medicine is firmly back in fashion – no longer simply the preserve of 'alternative' practitioners.[75] Music therapy can (it is implicitly contended) return from the margins to the centre and reclaim its inheritance.

VI

Grant for the moment that such an inheritance really exists. How are music therapists to feel its invigorating touch? The footnotes to the historical backdrops painted, on differing scales, by Alvin and Bunt inevitably refer mostly to a few secondary works, and their re-presentation of them is more a series of detached vignettes than connected historical writing. Bunt leans on Alvin, and both derive most of their evidence from an anthology of re-printed articles published in New York as long ago as 1948.[76] *Music and Medicine*, edited by Dorothy M. Schullian and Max Schoen, has endured as the major resource in English for those wanting something more than scattered anecdotes. Their collection, comprising articles already published as chapters in books or papers in musicological or medical journals, remains therefore in some ways the best available model for the present collection. In it, the findings of musicologists and medical historians march with those of social anthropologists and therapists, in a way that they have seldom, if ever, done since. The chapters essay a history of music therapy from the earliest times to the twentieth century (including a discussion of tarantism by one of the fathers of modern medical history, Henry Sigerist). And they show everywhere a familiarity with the primary sources that is still unusual in this particular field.

The context in which that project was conceived was the wartime use of music as a palliative in military hospitals and factories, the rapid expansion of the universities, and the first steps towards the establishment of professional training in music therapy. It is a context analysed by Penelope Gouk in the companion volume to this one and needs no elaboration here. What diminishes the value of the Schullian–Schoen collection over fifty years on, and suggests the need for its replacement, is precisely the depth to which it bears the stamp of its time. An opening discussion of 'Music and Medicine among Primitive Peoples' appears very much as a foil to that 'civilized' tradition, while a later contribution, by the composer Howard Hanson, pronounces the novelty of Boogie Woogie to be a harmful aural drug.[77] Such preconceptions distort the history presented. And that history has many gaps in it (most obviously the Middle Ages and the nineteenth century). Nonetheless the overall message is, predictably, one of continuity – from Pythagoras right through to the first professional music therapists, for whose calling the book was evidently to serve as manifesto. It is a continuity which is grounded in the achievements of 'dead European males' (or their texts) and which depends on Western 'art music' as the main therapeutic vehicle – both of which manifestations of 'elitism' make it automatically unpalatable in many quarters today.

In some ways the most solidly valuable part of the Schullian and Schoen anthology was the bibliography that Schullian contributed, including historical discussions reaching back to seventeenth- and eighteenth-century evidence.[78] Since 1948 a certain amount has been written on the topic in English, though none of it widely influential or combining breadth and scholarship.[79] Musicologists have had little of a historical kind to add; medical historians have done no better. It is perhaps symptomatic that the brief entry for 'music therapy' in *The New Grove Dictionary of Music and Musicians* confines itself to modern practices and omits Schullian and Schoen from its bibliography (although it does include a few historical texts). And no discussion of the topic is to be found in that otherwise authoritative and up-to-date conspectus, *The Companion Encyclopedia of the History of Medicine*.[80]

Meanwhile, however, the question of continuity seemed to have been settled elsewhere – on a scale, and at a scholarly level, that admitted no further doubt. In 1977, W. F. Kümmel published a revised version of his Habilitationsschrift, *Musik und Medizin: Ihre Wechselbeziehungen in Theorie und Praxis von 800 bis 1800*.[81] A densely learned text of over 400 pages, written in German and difficult to obtain, could not be expected to have much impact on Anglophone historians of medicine, still less on music therapists. The book is seldom cited and, one suspects, more often cited than read. Its sheer density has probably deterred proper evaluation. For that reason, and because it makes the strongest case yet for the continuity and significance of musical healing in the pre-modern past, I shall devote my final two sections to it.

VII

Kümmel quotes or paraphrases texts from right across the period indicated by his subtitle, in a profusion which attests massive reading in Latin and a range of vernaculars, among tomes of music theory, medicine, philosophy, theology and literature. Music, as it emerges here, was of profound importance in the Western medical tradition – and in the Middle Ages too, not just in antiquity and modern times as Foucault among others had argued ('since the Renaissance, music had regained all those therapeutic virtues antiquity had attributed to it.').[82] Theorists and practitioners of all kinds, from all the major European countries, and in almost every century, recommended listening or performing as a means of preventing or alleviating ill health.

'Every healing', as Novalis would say, 'is a musical solution.' 'Music heals the sick' had been the still more succinct conclusion of the music theorist Tinctoris, writing at the end of the Middle Ages but looking back to their dawn, and to the great encyclopaedist of that time, Isidore of Seville.[83] 'Throughout Spain,' the physician Rodericus a Castro wrote in 1614, 'whenever anyone falls seriously ill, it is usual to summon musicians'.[84] No mere collection of general assertions, the book's thematic chapters expound the history of music as a perceived remedy for: phrenitis, mania, melancholia, fever, pain, insomnia, plague, that mysterious virus 'the English Sweat',[85] lethargy, apoplexy, catalepsy, consumption, and epilepsy. To take a fairly extreme example that can be set beside our opening one of cancer cells: in the early sixteenth century the German religious reformer Ulrich von Hutten urged listening to singers and instrumentalists for those undergoing treatment (with a decoction of guaiac wood) for syphilis, a disease with which he was himself terminally afflicted.[86] The complete list of conditions thought to be musically treatable resembles the scope of modern music therapy in its diversity, embracing both mental and physical ailments, chronic conditions, and rapidly lethal epidemics. To it, moreover, we must add, first, those places or occasions in which music was thought to be helpful in an auxiliary capacity – in the bath and the hospital, and after having been bled; second, the capacities of music as preventive medicine: in pregnancy, early childhood, and old age, and as a factor in generally beneficial self-regulation.

The sheer volume and thoroughness of Kümmel's documentation seems to brook no contrary argument. Nor need such arguments be searched out in the present chapter. The task preliminary to that, which *should*, however, be undertaken here, is to gain some overall perspective on the hundreds of citations that Kümmel adduces in favour of the ubiquity and continuity of music in pre-modern therapeutics. Just how widespread and significant were the practices reported? What sort of continuity is being represented?

First, it is important to register that Kümmel has a far broader purview than music therapy. His title is *Music and Medicine*, and he is concerned with the whole spectrum of ways in which they may have interacted.[87] So he includes discussions of the 'music' of the pulse – a means of description and diagnosis which becomes a therapeutic technique in itself only towards the end of the long period surveyed in his book, when it was proposed that the pulse's rhythm might be altered by an actual musical counterpart.[88] Kümmel also pays considerable attention to the idea of music as a model of the human frame (*musica humana*), which, as we shall see, animates much discussion of music therapy, but for the sake of completeness is again pursued in his book as a subject in its own right. And he makes space for sections on music in child care, which often seems to have involved no more than the philosophy of lullabies; on *Tafelmusik*, to accompany eating and improve digestion; and on the recreational uses of music at spas – none of which topics is indisputably central to the history of musical healing. Subtract some of this material from the evidence submitted, and its mass seems a little less daunting and incontrovertible.

A second feature to note is that the range of sources pressed into service can undermine the author's thesis about the importance of musical medicine. Literature, philosophy, and music theory play at least as great a part in sustaining the case for ubiquity and continuity as do medical texts. While all equally part of the European intellectual tradition, they do not necessarily show that music was important in medicine. Indeed, the very abundance of non-medical evidence hints at an alternative argument which recurs in several chapters [in *Music as Medicine*]: that music therapy has often been more theorized than practised, has been of greater interest to philosophers than to physicians. Certainly Kümmel has comparatively little evidence of a practical kind to present. Case books or other detailed medical records are admittedly hard to come by until we have reached some way into the modern period. And Kümmel does include some extracts from *consilia* (letters of advice published by eminent physicians) and some individual case histories, mostly royal.[89] Nonetheless, it has to be said that there is far less evidence of music's actual use in therapy than might be expected. The medical sources make up only a part of the whole; and they are overwhelmingly prescriptive in character: they tell us more about ideals than about actuality.

The impression of ubiquity and continuity in musical healing is initially strengthened but then, on closer reading, called into question by Kümmel's manner of presenting his material. He organizes it thematically, which enhances our sense of the enormous range of medical tasks to which music has been applied. But that organization also has its disadvantages. Quotations as it were flash past, so that we can be moved from antiquity to the early nineteenth century within a matter of paragraphs. Evidence of all kinds jostles together without its authors being fully identified, their writings being characterized, or the immediate contexts of their assertions about therapy being set out. Disagreements about musical healing – its capacities and its limitations – get relatively little attention. Instances of music as a first resort are 'lumped' together with instances of it as a last one.[90] Moreover, evidence must be repeated under each of the disease headings to which it pertains, which can create the suspicion that the single march past of a huge army is actually the effect of a smaller number of soldiers coming round again and again.

VIII

The soldiers proclaim, essentially, a composite of some fundamentals of ancient medicine and one fundamental of ancient musical theory.[91] Let us step back from reviewing Kümmel and examine these a little further. The musical idea is that each mode or rhythm or type of music has its specific ethos, which can induce a specific response in the hearer. The medical ideas are threefold. First, there is in a sense only one disorder or disease: an imbalance of the four humours (blood, phlegm, yellow bile, black bile) that are the basic ingredients of the body.[92] Second, therefore, 'mental illness' as modern medicine conceives it is somatic in origin. On the other hand, third, the mind can hinder or generate ill health. This medicine is not entirely physicalist: the psychosomatic traffic is two-way. These various strands of thought remained distinct, and expressions of them often fragmented, in ancient writers such as Galen, the great physician of Roman imperial times and, like Hippocrates, one of the presiding geniuses of the European medical tradition. It was the Arabic scholars of the Islamic Middle East from the ninth century onward – the heirs of ancient Greek medical learning by way of translations – who synthesized the strands and thereby provided the framework within which the uses of music in therapy could be conceptualized.

The briefest exposition can be found in the work known to Western medicine as the *Isagoge* [*Introduction*] of Johannitius (Hunain ibn Ishaq), an Arabic synopsis so convenient that, in Latin translation, it was widely diffused across medieval Europe. This text distinguishes between the 'naturals' (chiefly the four elements, qualities such as hot or moist, and the four humours), the 'contra-naturals' (disease, its causes and 'sequels'), and the 'non-naturals'. The last are the pertinent ones here; they are the determinants of health. They include air and the environment, eating and drinking, exercise and baths, sleep, coitus, and the 'passions of the soul'.[93] Johannitius writes:

> Sundry affections of the mind produce an effect within the body, such as those which bring the natural heat from the interior of the body to the outer parts or the surface of the skin. Sometimes this happens suddenly, as with anger; sometimes gently and slowly, as with delight and joy . . . some affections disturb the natural energy both internal and external, as, for instance, with grief.[94]

Those sentences represent the conceptual gateway through which music comes into medicine – under the heading of 'delight and joy'. Music – of the appropriate ethos – can manipulate the accidents of the soul, mitigating those which cause disease, strengthening those which prevent it. That is why Gentile da Foligno, lecturer in the medical faculty at Perugia, advised all at risk of catching the Black Death of 1348 to avoid sadness, rage, and solitude because these upset the bodily complexion and encouraged disease. In the same vein, he counselled seeking joy and delight by means of 'melodies, songs, stories, and other similar pleasures'.[95] In the chapters that follow, as to some extent in earlier examples here, we encounter other grander formulations of how music 'works' medically – notably that which sees *musica instrumentalis* (actually including vocal music) as literally harmonizing *musica humana*, the disordered (that is, unhealthy) human frame, with the musical order of the cosmos, *musica mundana*. But the application of the non-naturals is an underlying constant of learned medicine so long as that medicine continues to subscribe to the tenets of ancient, and medieval Arabic, thought.

Take the example of melancholy. Its treatment across the two and a half millennia that separate Hippocrates and modern times has usefully been chronicled by Stanley W. Jackson (in a book written seemingly in ignorance

291

of Kümmel's). 'Much in the way of therapeutic advice', Jackson concludes, 'was based on classical concerns with *the regimen* . . . It often seemed as though the prescriber had run down a checklist of the six non-naturals.'[96] To that extent, it might be mere personal predisposition that an individual physician explicitly recommended music rather than one of the other possible ways of cheering the patient. And yet, with respect to melancholy at any rate, some changes of fashion are detectable across the centuries. Most of the ancient Roman authorities – Celsus, Soranus, Aretaeus of Cappadocia, Galen, Galen's late antique epigones – include no discussion of music in their recommendations for treatment.[97] Predictably, it is the Arabic scholars, notably Ishaq ibn 'Imran, who first consider it, and whose advice passed to the West in Latin translation.

> The physician must counteract melancholics' suspicions, mitigate their anger and grant them what they used to like . . . they should use reasoned and pleasant discourse . . . with diverse music and sweet-smelling, clear and delicate wine.[98]

Similarly mixed remedies reappear in some, but not all, of the major medieval texts. Following Constantine the African, translator of Ishaq, the medieval authority Bartholomaeus Anglicus (Bartholomew the Englishman) wrote that melancholics must be 'gladded with instruments of music and some deal be occupied'; in the 1530s Thomas Elyot counselled avoidance of anger, study or solitude, 'and rejoice thee with melody, or else be alway in such company, as best may content thee'.[99] The repetitions continue through the writing of Robert Burton and into the eighteenth century – and then music is apparently dropped. None of the major eighteenth- and nineteenth-century figures reviewed by Jackson specifically recommends it.[100]

If, with these examples in mind, we now return to the many other instances of musical therapeutics assembled by Kümmel, it becomes apparent that 'song' was frequently prescribed in the same breath as wine or women (the doctors are all male, their implied patients mainly so). That is, the physicians Kümmel cites are suggesting not music therapy so much as a more general 'soul' therapy, protecting health by lifting spirits. Music is only one of several obvious resources, a possibility always in the background but not inevitably the technique of choice, its explicit recommendation perhaps sometimes being arbitrary. A jolly story might serve equally well.[101] Most educated physicians did, however, know at least a little music theory, which might have inclined them to single it out. Music has never in its own right been a part of formal medical curricula in schools or universities. But it did enter the armoury of the learned because the study of the liberal arts was, until the eighteenth century if not later, nearly always a prerequisite of reading for a medical degree. And the primary arts text on music, as we shall see, was Boethius' treatise with its anecdotes of marvellous musical healings.[102]

The intellectual tradition just described lasts, as Kümmel's title shows, for a millennium, from the Arab synthesis of ingredients bequeathed by classical antiquity to the demise of humoral pathology in the early nineteenth century.[103] Within that long span, the beliefs anciently established remained valid, a few sceptical pronouncements apart. As an explanatory framework and a justification of music and other 'non-natural' diversions, they endured changing conceptions of human physiology (chemical, mechanistic, vitalist, neurological, and so on). That is why we shall find in subsequent chapters [of *Music as Medicine*] – and can already detect in both Kümmel's pages and recent music therapy textbooks – a limited number of anecdotes being endlessly recycled: of David or Pythagoras, or Farinelli. That is why Tinctoris, writing in the fifteenth century, leans on Isidore, writing in the seventh, who in his turn professes to have found instruction in still older vignettes.[104] The old nostrums remained for the most part unquestioned. Yet by the time the famous music critic Eduard Hanslick, scourge of Wagner and perfect Brahmsian, came to publish his tract *Vom Musikalisch-Schönen* [*On the Musically Beautiful*] in 1854, the tradition had dissolved. Hanslick can presume a certain ignorance in his readers in a way that would have been hazardous even half a century earlier.

> It may not be known to many music lovers [he writes] that we possess an extensive literature concerning the bodily effects of music and their medical applications. Rich in interesting curiosities but untrustworthy in observation and unscientific in explanation, most of these musico-medical writings seek to raise up some very complex and incidental property of music to the status of sovereign remedy.[105]

Hanslick quotes with obvious contempt the physician Peter Lichtenthal, whose *Der Musikalische Arzt* (1807) lists gout, sciatica, epilepsy, catalepsy, pestilence, delirium, convulsions, the jitters, nymphomania, and stupidity as among the disorders amenable to musical treatment. 'It is a bit of a problem', he concludes, 'that up to now no doctor has ever been known to send his typhus patients to Meyerbeer's [opera] *The Prophet* or to reach for a horn instead of a lancet.'[106] Perhaps Hanslick was himself more of a prophet than he knew. And the later nineteenth century was certainly not lacking in music therapy. But the framework was different by then; the non-naturals and the medical system that they represented had been left behind. Lichtenthal was among their last European advocates.

Kümmel's mass of evidence on this tradition that ends in the 1800s need not therefore be quite as overwhelming as it may first appear. To summarize: it includes some subjects not obviously central to the topic of musical therapeutics, and numerous texts that do not bear directly on medical practice. Many of the discussions of music mentioned are tralatician in nature: they repeat ancient commonplaces. The evidence is homogenized a little by being treated thematically and without sufficient respect for context. Above all, the medical tradition of the non-naturals – which does indeed last for the millennium embraced by the book's title – puts forward music as just one remedy among a range of useful diversions: it announces music's broad potential, but not always much more than that.

How far was that potential actually realized? Kümmel's work offers one answer – which may be too sanguine. Other studies that traverse some of his territory yield a very different picture. An authoritative history of epilepsy, for example, does not seem to find it worthwhile to mention any of the authors Kümmel musters in his pages on the musical treatment of the condition, and reveals no reference to music among the dietary recommendations it does adduce.[107] New studies of the history of gout and syphilis, similarly, have nothing of substance on musical treatment.[108] With the relatively few exceptions noted in the following pages, it seems that recent historical scholarship, whether consciously or not, has declined to endorse Kümmel's optimistic gloss on the evidence.

Clearly the matter requires further investigation. Some of that is undertaken here in *Music as Medicine*. Other aspects must be left to later occasions: [in *Music as Medicine*] we cannot match Kümmel's breadth of scope. The role of music in magic is one topic, perhaps peripheral to music therapy, that would repay more than sporadic notice. In magical incantations is it *prima la musica, dopo le parole* – or the other way round?[109] Which aspect of the magician's performance has been thought primarily efficacious? A related question might be asked of religious liturgy, on which we have already touched in the context of rites for the dying.[110] How, for example, should the singing of a Mass explicitly for the relief of fever, sung in honour of that ailment's patron saint, be understood to benefit sufferers? Is the saint's health-bringing intercession with the Deity thought to be in any sense dependent on the music of the Mass?[111] A slightly different example: at the graveside, is the singing of a ritual lament in any sense therapeutic?[112] These and like questions take us out from music therapy conceived as a part of learned medicine into a wider cultural world that seems to require a historical equivalent of the ethnography quoted earlier.

As part of such wider investigations, some attention should also be paid to the areas or the evidence in which we might expect to find music therapy but do not: the writings of that great composer-physician of the twelfth century, Abbess Hildegard of Bingen, for instance; of those Renaissance polymaths Girolamo Cardano, who discoursed on both music and medicine but not simultaneously, and Michael Maier, whose emblem book *Atalanta fugiens* (1617) keeps separate its fugues and its images of healing; or of Richard Napier, the English cleric and astrological physician, who in the early decades of the seventeenth century treated over 2,000 patients with mental disorders and whose casebooks are priceless evidence of early modern medicine.[113] Loud silences of that kind must alter our notion of the 'contours' of musical healing in the past. Not every cure is a musical solution.

Kümmel's work stimulates considerations such as these. Above all, it raises yet again the task of weighing continuity against discontinuity. Kümmel is careful to exclude the phrase 'music therapy' from his title and to distance the activities of the physicians he describes from those of modern music therapists.[114] For him the decline of humoral pathology marks a caesura in musical therapeutics. Before that, he contends, musical medicine was different – but it was continuous. Other writers, as we have seen several times now, are less scrupulous in the way they divide up the past, but are no less ready to accept a vision of continuity. For them, the past can readily be reclaimed by the present. There may be an intervening obstacle: usually the era of biomedicine's unquestioned dominance. Once that obstacle is conceptually vaulted over, however, the rest of history becomes available, *en bloc*, to endorse the claims and practices of today.

For such easy recourse, the present collection [*Music as Medicine*] hopes to substitute a less anachronistic historical panorama – one marked by change and disagreement as much as by smooth traditionalism, in which the absences figure alongside the presences. Some of the cultures discussed here have no concept of music that corresponds to ours; and their ideas of medicine and its capacity to heal rest on alien principles. The improvisations of today's music therapists – children of John Cage and Karlheinz Stockhausen – would have been shunned as cacophony only a few decades ago. Medieval physicians, trained to run through the non-naturals as part of preventive medicine, needed only to recommend music: they did not have to perform it themselves, and their involvement would usually have been extremely shallow by comparison with the intense interaction between patient and client that characterizes today's music therapy sessions.[115]

Modern music therapy needs a history from which it may derive a sense of its own particularity. That history must not, however, be written in Whiggish, teleological spirit. Medical history, for its part, needs music therapy – needs, that is, to include it in its master narrative of the past – but in just measure, a golden mean between excess and deficiency that should be the hallmark of scholarship as well as the ideal state of the body.

Notes

1 'Jede Kranckheit ist ein musicalisches Problem – die Heilung eine *musicalische Auflösung*' ('Every illness is a musical problem, its cure a musical solution'): Novalis, *Schriften*, vol. III, ed. R. Samuel et al. (Stuttgart, 1960), p. 310, no. 386.
2 London, 1934; 3rd edn 1966, p. 200.
3 Ibid. pp. 201, 204–205.
4 A. Malraux, *Museum Without Walls*, English trans. (London, 1967).
5 G. Steiner, *In Bluebeard's Castle: Some Notes Towards the Redefinition of Culture* (London, 1971), p. 90.

6 R. Scruton, *The Aesthetics of Music* (Oxford, 1997), pp. 496ff. [and see now for historical context James Kennaway, *Bad Vibrations: The History of the Idea of Music as Cause of Disease* (Farnham, 2012)].

7 H. M. Sharma, E. M. Kauffman and R. E. Stephens, 'Effect of Different Sounds on Growth of Human Cancer Cell Lines in Vitro', *Alternative Therapies in Clinical Practice*, 3.4 (1996), pp. 25–32 at 25.

8 P. Gouk (ed.), *Musical Healing in Cultural Contexts* (Aldershot, 2000) should be seen as complementary to the present volume [P. Horden (ed.), *Music as Medicine: The History of Music Therapy since Antiquity* (Aldershot, 2000)], being mainly anthropological in approach, in contrast to our historical thrust.

9 Sharma et al., 'Effect', p. 26.

10 Ibid. p. 25.

11 Sharma et al., 'Effect', cite: T. C. N. Singh and A. Gnanam, 'Studies on the Effect of Sound Waves of Nadeshwaram on the Growth and Yield of Paddy', *Journal of Annamalai University*, 16 (1975), pp. 78–99; C. B. Hicks, 'Growing Corn to Music', *Popular Mechanics*, 119 (1963), pp. 118–121; D. Retallack, *The Sound of Music and Plants* (Santa Monica, CA, 1973), pp. 20–33. See also P. Tompkins and C. Bird, *The Secret Life of Plants* (New York, 1973), pp. 145–162.

12 Sharma et al., 'Effect', pp. 25, 29–30.

13 Ibid. p. 29.

14 *Radio Times*, 11–17 July 1998.

15 '"No Pill's Gonna Cure My Ill": Gender, Erotic Melancholy, and Traditions of Musical Healing in the Modern West', in Gouk, *Musical Healing*, pp. 113–136. See also her chapter in Horden, *Music as Medicine*, 'Musical Treatments for Lovesickness: The Early Modern Heritage' (pp. 213–45).

16 E. Miles, *Tune Your Brain: Using Music to Manage Your Mind, Body and Mood* (http://www.tuneyourbrain.com.13 [no longer accessible]).

17 Britannia Music Company Catalogues, 1998–99. Compare 'New Spirit', a CD and book club that offers titles such as *The Tao of Music: Using Music to Change your Life*.

18 SK 62263. The compiler, Aegidius of Zamora, accepted in ch. 2 of his *Ars musica* the standard ancient topoi about musical healing; but that is another matter.

19 See http://www.stpatrick-hospital.org/chalice/musicthan.html [no longer accessible].

20 See F. Paxton, *Christianizing Death: The Creation of a Ritual Process in Early Medieval Europe* (Ithaca, NY, 1990), included in the 'Chalice of Repose' list of books for sale.

21 First published 1973, 4th edn, 1990: references are to the Picador paperback. See pp. xxi–xxiii for the textual history, 367–386 for the *Nachleben* of stage and screen.

22 Sacks, *Awakenings*, p. xiii.

23 Ibid. pp. 17, 125, 160, 270.

24 Ibid. p. 330.

25 Ibid. p. 60.

26 [The late] Paul Robertson, personal information. [See now Robertson's moving *Soundscapes: A Musician's Journey through Life and Death* (London, 2016).]

27 P. Robertson, *Music and the Mind* (London, 1996), p. 24.

28 Martin West, 'Music Therapy in Antiquity', in Horden, *Music as Medicine*, pp. 51–68.

29 Robertson, *Music and the Mind*, p. 25, italics added.

30 Sacks, *Awakenings*, p. 60 n. 45.

31 *Music Therapy Research and Practice in Medicine: From Out of the Silence* (London, 1996), p. 51.

32 Robertson, *Music and the Mind*, p. 27.
33 Ibid. p. 27.
34 Among a large literature, I have leaned most heavily on two monographs: L. Bunt, *Music Therapy: An Art Beyond Words* (London, 1994) [now in a 2nd edn with the same title, London, 2015, co-authored with Brynjulf Stige]; Aldridge, *Music Therapy Research and Practice in Medicine*. Among collections of articles, the most useful have proved to be: R. Spintge and R. Droh (eds) *MusicMedicine*, International Society for Music in Medicine, IV. International MusicMedicine Symposium ... 1989 (St Louis, MO, 1992); M. Heal and T. Wigram (eds), *Music Therapy in Health and Education* (London, 1993); T. Wigram, B. Saperston and R. West (eds), *The Art and Science of Music Therapy: A Handbook* (Chur, 1995); D. Aldridge (ed.), *Music Therapy in Palliative Care* (London, 1999). [I am also now grateful to Gary Ansdell, *How Music Helps in Music Therapy and Everyday Life* (Farnham, 2014). For a recent conspectus see e.g. N. S. Cohen, *Advanced Methods of Music Therapy Practice* (London, 2017); or O. S. Yinger, *Music Therapy: Research and Evidence-Based Practice* (St Louis, MO, 2018).]
35 Bunt, *Music Therapy*, p. 9.
36 Ibid. p. 55 [2nd edn, p. 62].
37 [See also Bunt, 2nd edn, p. 11; https://www.wfmt.info/ (last accessed 30 July 2018).]
38 C. F. Chabris et al., 'Prelude or Requiem for the "Mozart Effect"', *Nature*, 400 (26 Aug. 1999), pp. 826–828. Compare the journal *Psychology of Music*, 26 (1998), or *Musica Research Notes*, via http://www.musica.uci.edu/ [last accessed 28 July 2018].
39 [Search http://www.ncbi.nlm.nih.gov/PubMed/ (last accessed 30 July 2018) for the latest examples. Among journals see now *Voices: A World Forum for Music Therapy* (https://www.voices.no/index.php/voices, last accessed 30 July 2018, with Bunt, *Music Therapy*, 2nd edn, p. 25.]
40 Though compare L. Marchette et al., 'Pain Reduction during Neonatal Circumcision', in Spintge and Droh, *MusicMedicine*, pp. 131–136.
41 Bunt, *Music Therapy*, p. 30.
42 World Federation of Music Therapy, *Bulletin*, 1 (July 1997), italics added.
43 Aldridge, *Music Therapy Research*, pp. 181, 259.
44 I summarize Aldridge, *Music Therapy Research*, pp. 265–267. Bunt, *Music Therapy* includes many other case histories [in both editions].
45 Bunt, *Music Therapy*, p. 179 [apparently not reproduced in 2nd edn, but see esp. ch. 9 in that edition for more recent ruminations on what is involved. Also Ansdell, *How Music Helps*.].
46 C. D. Maranto, 'Applications of Music in Medicine', in Heal and Wigram, *Music Therapy in Health and Education*, p. 159.
47 See Bunt, *Music Therapy*, p. 73 [I should note in fairness that Lange is not present in the 2nd edn]; Aldridge, *Music Therapy Research*, pp. 161–162; J. Alvin, *Music Therapy*, first published 1966 (revised paperback, London, 1983), p. 92; S. Langer, *Philosophy in a New Key* (Cambridge, MA, 1942); *Feeling and Form: A Theory of Art* (London, 1953); Scruton, *The Aesthetics of Music*, pp. 147, 166–167. Langer's theories are discussed more fully in *The Philosophy of Music Education Review*, 1.1 (1993).
48 B. Hesser, 'The Power of Sound and Music in Therapy and Healing', in C. B. Kenny (ed.), *Listening, Playing, Creating: Essays on the Power of Sound* (Albany, NY, 1995), pp. 43–50 at 47.
49 J. M. Janzen, *Ngoma: Discourses of Healing in Central and Southern Africa* (Berkeley, CA, 1992); M. Roseman, *Healing Sounds from the Malaysian*

Rainforest: Temiar Music and Medicine (Berkeley, CA, 1991); B. Kapferer, *The Feast of the Sorcerer: Practices of Consciousness and Power* (Chicago, 1997), esp. pp. 115–120; R. Devisch, *Weaving the Threads of Life: The Khita Gyn-Eco-Logical Healing Cult among the Yaka* (Chicago, 1993). For older bibliography see S. M. Friedson, *Dancing Prophets: Musical Experience in Tumbuka Healing* (Chicago, 1996), pp. xii, 186 n. 3, but esp. R. Katz, *Boiling Energy: Community Healing among the Kalahari Kung* (Cambridge, MA, 1982). Note also F. Hurter, *Heilung und Musik in Afrika* (Frankfurt am Main, 1986).

50 Friedson, *Dancing Prophets*, p. 12. See also Janzen, *Ngoma*, ch. 1, e.g. p. 12.
51 Friedson, 'Dancing the Disease: Diagnostics and Therapeutics in Tumbuka Healing', in Gouk, *Musical Healing*, pp. 67–84.
52 G. Prins, 'But What Was the Disease? The Present State of Health and Healing in African Studies', *Past and Present*, 124 (1989), pp. 176–177. Compare Janzen, *Ngoma*, pp. 35–37.
53 M. Herzfeld, 'Closure as Cure: Tropes in the Exploration of Bodily and Social Disorder', *Current Anthropology*, 27 (1986), pp. 107–120.
54 E.g. Janzen, *Ngoma*, p. 143. See also Janzen, 'Theories of Music in African Ngoma Healing', in Gouk, *Musical Healing*, pp. 46–66, esp. p. 59.
55 M. Roseman, '"Pure Products Go Crazy": Rainforest Healing in a Nation-State', in C. Laderman and M. Roseman (eds), *The Performance of Healing* (New York, 1996), p. 252. See also Roseman, *Healing Sounds*, ch. 4. Janzen, *Ngoma*, pp. 176–7, compares healing 'cults of affliction' to institutions such as Alcoholics Anonymous.
56 Bunt, *Music Therapy*, pp. 72–73, 185 [2nd edn, p. 79]. Compare Alvin, *Music Therapy*, pp. 9–10, 19, 23.
57 See M. Pavlicevic, *Music Therapy in Context: Music, Meaning and Relationship* (London, 1998), a book by a therapist working in South Africa which, despite its title, largely ignores a promising ethnographic context.
58 E. E. Evans-Pritchard, *Witchcraft, Oracles, and Magic among the Azande*, abridged edn (Oxford, 1976), pp. 72–77.
59 Friedson, *Dancing Prophets*, pp. xiii–xiv; V. W. Turner, *The Drums of Affliction: A Study of Religious Processes among the Ndembu of Zambia* (Oxford, 1968). See also Turner, *The Forest of Symbols: Aspects of Ndembu Ritual*, first published 1967 (Ithaca, NY, 1970), ch. 10: 'A Ndembu Doctor in Practice', pp. 385, 389.
60 Friedson, *Dancing Prophets*, p. xi. Gouk, *Musical Healing*, to which Friedson contributes (pp. 57–84), represents a conference at which music therapists and medical anthropologists were at last able to communicate.
61 L. M. Danforth, *Firewalking and Religious Healing: The Anastenaria of Greece and the American Firewalking Movement* (Princeton, NJ, 1989), pp. 103–122. See also n. 56 above.
62 I. van Wetering, 'Women as *Winti* Healers: Rationality and Contradiction in the Preservation of a Suriname Healing Tradition', in M. Gijswijt-Hofstra, H. Marland and H. de Waardt (eds), *Illness and Healing Alternatives in Western Europe* (London, 1997), pp. 243–261.
63 C. Laderman, 'The Poetics of Healing in Malay Shamanistic Performances', in Laderman and Roseman, *The Performance of Healing*, p. 116.
64 Bunt, *Music Therapy*, p. 187 [2nd edn, pp. 192–193, 213–215].
65 Alvin, *Music Therapy*, pp. 12, 16. See further H. M. Tyler, 'The Music Therapy Profession in Modern Britain', in Horden, *Music as Medicine*, pp. 375–393.
66 On Burton see P. Gouk, 'Music, Melancholy, and Medical Spirits in Early Modern Europe', in Horden, *Music as Medicine*, pp. 173–194.

67 *Music as Medicine*, pt IV, chapters by D. Gentilcore, P. León, K. Lüdtke.
68 Alvin, *Music Therapy*, ch. 4.
69 Ibid. p. 46, quoting R. Brocklesby, *Reflections on Ancient and Modern Musick, with the Application to the Cure of Diseases* (London, 1749), pp. 34–35. [On Brocklesby see now P. Gouk, 'An Enlightenment Proposal for Music Therapy: Richard Brocklesby on Music, Spirit, and the Passions', in E. Altenmüller, S. Finger and F. Boller (eds), *Music, Neurology, and Neuroscience: Evolution, The Musical Brain, Medical Conditions, and Therapies* (Amsterdam, 2015), pp. 159–185.]
70 Alvin, *Music Therapy*, p. 58, drawing on I Sam. 16, 18, 19, 24. On Farinelli see now P. Barbier, *Farinelli: le castrat des lumières* (Paris, 1994), pp. 111ff. Contrast J. Godwin, *Harmonies of Heaven and Earth: The Spiritual Dimension of Music from Antiquity to the Avant-Garde* (London, 1987), p. 36, on how such anecdotes may be 'more a burden than an asset to the profession today': they exaggerate expectations.
71 Tyler, 'Music Therapy Profession in Modern Britain', pp. 381–386.
72 Bunt, *Music Therapy*, pp. 10–11. Compare W. B. Davis, K. E. Gfeller and M. H. Thaut, *An Introduction to Music Therapy: Theory and Practice* (Dubuque, IA, 1992), pp. 16–37 ('Music Therapy: An Historical Perspective').
73 Sharma et al., 'Effect', p. 29.
74 M. Foucault, *The Birth of the Clinic* (London, 1973) is the classic narration of the disappearance, in the late eighteenth to nineteenth centuries, of the sick person from the clinician's gaze, to be replaced by a body with lesions. On the more recent, reactive, 'patient as person' movement, see briefly R. Porter, *The Greatest Benefit to Mankind* (London, 1997), p. 682.
75 Though compare B. J. Good, *Medicine, Rationality, and Experience: An Anthropological Perspective* (Cambridge, 1994), ch. 3: 'How Medicine Constructs its Objects'.
76 [Bunt's 2nd edn stresses discontinuity much more, and cites Horden, *Music as Medicine* and Gouk, *Musical Healing* in support of that stance.]
77 'Emotional Expression in Music', in Schullian and Schoen, *Music and Medicine*, pp. 244–265. Compare the opinion quite widespread in 1920s and 1930s America that jazz was evil and corrupting: A. P. Merriam, *The Anthropology of Music* (Evanston, IL, 1964), pp. 241–244. For full discussion, see P. Gouk, 'Sister Disciplines? *Music and Medicine* in Historical Perspective', in Gouk, *Musical Healing*, pp. 171–196. [And see now Kennaway, *Bad Vibrations*.]
78 Schullian and Schoen, *Music and Medicine*, pp. 407–471.
79 Carl Gregor, Herzog zu Mecklenburg, *Bibliographie einiger Grenzgebiete der Musikwissenschaft* (Baden-Baden, 1962) adds over a decade's worth of material.
80 W. F. Bynum and R. Porter (eds), 2 vols. (London, 1993). See also I. G. Berrios and R. Porter (eds), *A History of Clinical Psychiatry* (London, 1995), which mentions music with reference only to David and Saul (p. 414).
81 *Freiburger Beiträge zur Wissenschafts- und Universitätsgeschichte*, vol. II, Munich.
82 *Madness and Civilization: A History of Insanity in the Age of Reason*, paperback edn, abbreviated translation (London, 1971), p. 178.
83 Kümmel, *Musik und Medizin*, p. 223. New edn and trans. R. Strohm and J. D. Cullington, *On the Dignity and Effects of Music . . . Two Fifteenth-Century Treatises*, Institute of Advanced Musical Studies, King's College London, Study Texts 2 (1996), ch. 14 (112), pp. 57, 73, with 64 n. 49. Compare, in the same volume, Egidius Carlerius, 'Treatise on . . . Church Music', 87, pp. 28, 44: 'euphonious music has sometimes even cured severe illnesses.'
84 Kümmel, *Musik und Medizin*, p. 227, citing Rodericus a Castro, *Medicus Politicus, sive de Officiis Medico-Politicus Tractatus* (Hamburg, 1662), p. 276.

85 M. Taviner, G. Thwaites and V. Gant, 'The English Sweating Sickness, 1485–1551: A Viral Pulmonary Disease?', *Medical History*, 42 (1998), pp. 96–98.
86 Kümmel, *Musik und Medizin*, pp. 334–335; U. von Hutten, *De Guaiaci Medicina et Morbo Gallico Liber Unus* (Mainz, 1519). For context see now J. Arrizabalaga, J. Henderson and R. French, *The Great Pox: The French Disease in Renaissance Europe* (New Haven, CT, 1997), pp. 100–103.
87 Kümmel, *Musik und Medizin*, p. 13.
88 See C. R. S. Harris, *The Heart and the Vascular System in Ancient Greek Medicine* (Oxford, 1973), ch. 7; N. G. Siraisi, 'The Music of the Pulse in the Writings of Italian Academic Physicians (Fourteenth and Fifteenth Centuries)', *Speculum*, 50 (1975), pp. 689–710; S. Hafenreffer, *Monochordon symbolico-biomanticum . . .* (Ulm, 1640), an eccentric early modern treatise on pulse.
89 On *consilia*, see N. G. Siraisi, *Taddeo Alderotti and His Pupils: Two Generations of Italian Medical Learning* (Princeton, NJ, 1981), ch. 9; J. Agrimi and C. Crisciani, *Les 'Consilia' médicaux*, Typologie des Sources du Moyen Age, no. 69 (Turnhout, 1994).
90 E.g. Kümmel, *Musik und Medizin*, pp. 236, 301, 319, 360.
91 Ibid. ch. 4.
92 See N. G. Siraisi, *Medieval and Renaissance Medicine* (Chicago, 1990), pp. 101–106, for this and what follows.
93 For the non-naturals, see G. Olson, *Literature as Recreation in the Later Middle Ages* (Ithaca, NY, 1982), pp. 40–44; L. García-Ballester, 'On the Origin of the "Six Non-Natural Things" in Galen', in G. Harig and J. Harig-Kollesch (eds), *Galen und die Hellenistische Erbe* (Wiesbaden, 1993), pp. 105–115.
94 Trans. E. Grant, *Sourcebook of Medieval Science* (Cambridge, MA, 1974), pp. 708–709.
95 J. Arrizabalaga, 'Facing the Black Death: Perceptions and Reactions of University Medical Practitioners', in L. García-Ballester et al. (eds), *Practical Medicine from Salerno to the Black Death* (Cambridge, 1994), p. 280. See also A. Wear, 'Fear, Anxiety and the Plague in Early Modern England', in J. R. Hinnells and R. Porter (eds), *Religion, Health and Suffering* (London, 1999), p. 355, for a seventeenth-century parallel; more generally Olson, *Literature as Recreation*, ch. 5.
96 S. W. Jackson, *Melancholia and Depression: From Hippocratic Times to Modern Times* (New Haven, CT, 1986), pp. 392–393. See also the contributions to Horden, *Music as Medicine*, by P. Gouk and L. Austern.
97 Jackson, *Melancholia*, ch. II.2; compare Kümmel, *Musik und Medizin*, pp. 290–291.
98 Trans. in R. Klibansky, E. Panofsky and F. Saxl, *Saturn and Melancholy* (London, 1964), p. 85, with Jackson, *Melancholia*, p. 59.
99 Ibid. pp. 64, 82. Further, P. Jones, P. Gouk, L. Austern in Horden, *Music as Medicine*.
100 Although he can produce a few references to it in writings of lesser figures: Jackson, *Melancholia*, pp. 300–304.
101 Olson, *Literature as Recreation*, ch. 2, esp. pp. 55–64.
102 Siraisi, *Medieval and Early Renaissance Medicine*, pp. 65–68; Kümmel, *Musik und Medizin*, pp. 70–71.
103 See L. J. Rather, 'Systematic Medical Treatises from the Ninth to the Nineteenth Century: The Unchanging Scope and Structure of Academic Medicine in the West', *Clio Medica*, 11 (1976), pp. 289–305.
104 Isidore, *Etymologiae*, IV.13.

105 Hanslick, *On the Musically Beautiful*, trans. G. Payzant (Indianapolis, 1986), p. 51. Contrast C. Burney, *A General History of Music*, 2nd edn (London, 1789, repr. New York, 1957): the opening 'Dissertation on the Music of the Ancients', section 10, dutifully, if sceptically, repeats the usual anecdotes.

106 Hanslick, *On the Musically Beautiful*, pp. 52–53. On Lichtenthal, see further C. Kramer, 'Music as Cause and Cure of Illness in Nineteenth-Century Europe', in Horden, *Music as Medicine*, pp. 338–352.

107 O. Temkin, *The Falling Sickness: A History of Epilepsy from the Greeks to the Beginnings of Modern Neurology*, 2nd edn (Baltimore, MD, 1971), pp. 66ff., 102ff., 232ff., 291ff. Compare Kümmel, *Musik und Medizin*, pp. 376–377 (not citing this work).

108 R. Porter and G. S. Rousseau, *Gout: The Patrician Malady* (New Haven, CT, 1998); Arrizabalaga et al., *The Great Pox*.

109 As in Richard Strauss's opera *Capriccio*. See West, 'Music Therapy in Antiquity', and his *Ancient Greek Music* (Oxford, 1992), p. 32. Contrast J. Combarieu, *La musique et la magie* (Paris, 1909), an attempt, in the grand manner, to derive the whole of music from magical incantation.

110 See C. Rawcliffe, 'Medicine for the Soul: The Medieval English Hospital and the Quest for Spiritual Health', in Hinnells and Porter, *Religion, Health and Suffering*, pp. 316–338.

111 F. S. Paxton, 'Liturgy and Healing in an Early Medieval Saint's Cult: The Mass *in honore Sancti Sigismundi* for the Cure of Fevers', *Traditio*, 49 (1994), pp. 23–43. Compare H. Sigerist, 'The Story of Tarantism', in Schullian and Schoen, *Music and Medicine*, pp. 96–98.

112 G. Holst-Warhaft, *Dangerous Voices: Women's Laments and Greek Literature* (London, 1992), p. 73.

113 B. Newman (ed.), *Voice of the Living Light: Hildegard of Bingen and her World* (Berkeley, CA, 1998); N. G. Siraisi, *The Clock and the Mirror: Girolamo Cardano and Renaissance Medicine* (Princeton, NJ, 1997), esp. p. 122; H. de Jong, *Michael Maier's Atalanta Fugiens*, Janus supplement 8 (Leiden, 1969), with F. Yates, *The Rosicrucian Enlightenment* (London, 1972), pp. 70–91; M. MacDonald, *Mystical Bedlam: Madness, Anxiety, and Healing in Seventeenth-Century England* (Cambridge, 1981).

114 Kümmel, *Musik und Medizin*, p. 412.

115 H. Tyler, 'Music Therapy', in T. Ford (ed.), *The Musician's Handbook*, 3rd edn (London, 1996), p. 92.

15

PARACELSUS

Renaissance music therapy and its alternative

I

The creative revival of interest in classical antiquity that we – like those who brought it about – call a Renaissance or rebirth was a movement that came at differing times and in differing forms in the visual arts, in letters, in philosophy, in music, and in medicine.[1] But so far as the history of music as therapy is concerned, one development was crucial. This development is what gives the subject its Renaissance, a period that differs from the preceding Middle Ages (which are, of course, 'middle' only because Renaissance scholars saw them as an intermediate embarrassment between antiquity and its rebirth). It distinguishes the fifteenth, sixteenth, and early seventeenth centuries[2] as an era when musical therapeutics attained a philosophical centrality, a cultural resonance, among educated Europeans greater than it has enjoyed at any time before or since – and greater than it seems likely to enjoy in the future, at least until the 'New Age' truly dawns.

The development in question was the re-establishment in European thought of an integrated vision of music which embraced both ethos and cosmos.[3] Music could have salutary effects on human beings because of its astrological significance as a mirror of the universe's 'deep structure'. Two currents within theorizing about music, the 'ethical' and the 'astrological', had come together in the Pythagorean–Platonic tradition in antiquity but had never been fully integrated. Correspondences between planets, signs of the zodiac, musical tones, elements, and bodily humours had then been systematically elaborated by Islamic scholars. But this integration could not influence European thought because the most pertinent texts had not been translated into Latin. If Plato is the key figure for us in antiquity, then Aristotle, with his scepticism about the music of the spheres, supplants him in the Middle Ages. Music is therapeutic in that period because of its power to moderate the 'accidents of the soul', not (or not usually) because it replicates the harmony of the cosmos within the human frame. Without being unduly schematic, we could see this as the triumph of Aristotle. The Renaissance in music therapy is the rebirth of Platonism in the mid-fifteenth century and its absorption into the larger framework of natural magic. This is not the magic of the village enchanter. It is a magic that is fundamental to a thoroughly articulated and, given its premises, highly rational world-view, which is better called 'occult philosophy'.[4]

The sources of that philosophy are various, but they certainly include Arabic texts (eventually accessible to interested Christian scholars), as well as the Jewish numerological mysticism of the Kabbalah. There are several early figures whose writings exemplify the Platonist revival.[5] Yet by far the most influential of them was the physician-philosopher-musician Marsilio Ficino (1433–1499).[6] The inspired songs of the 'second Orpheus' were intended, 'through fitting [musical] tones to the stars', to 'banish vexations of both soul and body', not just to provide diversion in discomfort. Ficino looked to newly recovered texts from both classical and late antiquity for a therapy that was far more ambitious in conception than anything detectable in medieval evidence. His work provided the starting point for many subsequent discussions – not particularly among theorists of music and medicine (as we might now style them) so much as in the writings of 'occult philosophers'. Physicians and musicologists reproduce ancient commonplaces, biblical and Pythagorean, about the power of music. (See, for instance, the *Istitutione harmoniche* [1558], bk 1, ch. 2, of Gioseffo Zarlino [1517–1590], so often taken as the paradigmatic text of early modern music therapy.)[7] Under this heading, nothing substantially new is added. The occult philosophers, by contrast, innovate by the subtlety and thoroughness with which they reinvent Pythagorean cosmology. And they are important not just in their own right but also for their profound yet equivocal connections with what can still (albeit controversially) be called the Scientific Revolution, as well as with the religious reformations of the early modern period, both Catholic and Protestant.[8]

Superimposed on the conception of music as regulator of the 'non-naturals' (a conception with a more or less continuous life from antiquity to the start of the nineteenth century), Ficino's astrological model, once publicized, proved comparably durable, lasting to the close of the eighteenth century, when explanations of musical healing were couched in mechanical or neurological terms that Ficino would not have recognized. Yet, as in antiquity so in the period of its rebirth, music therapy is apparently of far more widespread interest among philosophers than among physicians. Angela Voss can cite one example of an apparently successful Ficinian cure.[9] But, on the whole, early modern university-educated doctors were no more prone to 'dispense' music than were their medieval predecessors – or rather, they have covered their traces if they did, because scholars of the period seem to have no collections of case histories of music therapy at their disposal. A handful of anecdotes apart, music therapy flourishes most obviously – and perhaps to an unprecedented degree – in the realm of 'high culture'. The ideas in question are not, however, to be seen as mere metaphor:[10]

Historians . . . who depict a sixteenth- and seventeenth-century 'trivialization' of ideas of cosmic harmony into fiction or 'decorative metaphor and mere turns of wit' do not fully appreciate the staying power of this discourse. Their histories cannot account for the dispersion of the general idea of cosmic harmony across the conceptual and practical landscape . . . of magic and astrology, courtly ritual and pageantry, and writings by [diverse] authors . . . Faced with such persistence and pervasiveness, we should heed Haar's admonition 'to be cautious about labelling as metaphor only what was for so long believed in so earnestly'.

II

Such cosmology did not supply the only way in which musical therapeutics could be conceptualized during the sixteenth and seventeenth centuries. That is, the Platonic model did not entirely achieve 'market dominance'. A rather more eccentric one derives from the writings of the man whose medicine offered, for a long time, the only potent alternative to the Galenic humoralism upon which Renaissance Platonists predicated their understanding of *musica humana*. That man is Paracelsus.[11]

Theophrastus Philippus Aureolus Bombastus von Hohenheim (1493–1541) adopted the name Paracelsus, not (as is sometimes thought) in qualified homage to the first-century Roman medical authority Celsus, but as a Latinization of his 'surname', Hohenheim.[12] Little known in his own lifetime, Paracelsus' writings were widely diffused across Europe in numerous editions from around 1560 onwards. For the four humours of Hippocratic–Galenic tradition, Paracelsian medicine substituted salt, sulphur, and mercury as the primary substances. To the humoral imbalance as the systemic cause of disease, it preferred a quasi-ontological conception in which each disease was a distinct entity with a specific cause external to the patient. Against the allopathic medicine of the Galenists (countering humoral excess or deficiency with its opposite) it substituted a type of homoeopathy derived from the similarity of medicament and disease.

Admittedly, Paracelsus' belief in the detailed correspondence between body and cosmos (microcosm and macrocosm) and the role of spiritual essences in his physiology place him in broadly the same company as the occult philosophers; and his acceptance that beliefs were potentially pathogenic can be reconciled with the medieval conception of the accidents of the soul.[13] Nonetheless, there is little in the fundamentals of his thinking that should obviously have predisposed him to find curative virtue in music. His religious radicalism made him generally hostile to liturgy and ritual incantation.[14] His contempt for ancient wisdom, together with the alchemical basis of his therapeutics, seem to leave no opportunities for soothing sound.[15]

It is the more surprising, then, to find in Paracelsus' early treatise, *De religione perpetua* [*On the perennial religion*], the contention – rare or even perhaps unique in his massive literary output – that 'music is a cure for those troubled by melancholy and morbid imagination [*Fantasey*]', and that 'on the same account music drives away the spirits used by witches, by malefactors, and in sorcery'.[16] The context is a discussion of the benefits that accrue to a doctor armed with the 'religion of medicine', a doctor of upright character and genuine spirituality. Such a doctor will appreciate that a beneficent God has provided – and provided locally – all the appropriate remedies for local ills. Paracelsus' 'doctrine of signatures', according to which the remedy resembles the ailment, is intelligible by the light of nature; it requires no university learning. And just as in a garden there grow the plants that the physician needs, so there are kinds of music that will be efficacious against particular forms of insanity: listening to music resembles lunacy in that both involve the mind.

This is a music therapy which of course has some affinities with those of medieval Aristotelians and Renaissance Platonists, despite their general refusal to countenance the possibility that music could directly affect demons. Moreover, as later generations of Paracelsians syncretized their master's medicine with the Galenic mainstream, so the affinities would be magnified.[17] Yet at this early stage, in the master's own hands, it was, and remains, uncomfortably distinct.

Notes

1 [This paper is extracted from 'Commentary on Part III', in P. Horden (ed.), *Music as Medicine: The History of Music Therapy since Antiquity* (Aldershot, 2000), pp. 147–153.] For music see e.g. L. L. Perkins, *Music in the Age of the Renaissance* (New York, 1999). For philosophy, B. P. Copenhaver and C. B. Schmitt, *Renaissance Philosophy* (Oxford, 1992); further, C. B. Schmitt, Q. Skinner and J. Kraye (eds), *The Cambridge History of Renaissance Philosophy* (Cambridge, 1988). Medicine: N. Siraisi, *Avicenna in Renaissance Italy* (Princeton, NJ, 1987); A. Wear, R. K. French and I. M. Lonie (eds), *The Medical Renaissance of the Sixteenth Century* (Cambridge, 1985). This short note could not have been written without the unstinting assistance of Ian Maclean and Charles Webster.

2 For present purposes, it is not important to distinguish the Renaissance from a supposedly succeeding Baroque age.

3 For what follows see further Horden, *Music as Medicine*, especially the contributions of M. West, A. Shiloah, C. Page and P. M. Jones, and my own 'Commentaries' on Parts I and II.

4 As by Heinrich Cornelius Agrippa, cited by P. Gouk, 'Music, Melancholy, and Medical Spirits in Early Modern Thought', in *Music as Medicine*, p. 174. For context see G. Tomlinson, *Music in Renaissance Magic: Toward a Historiography of Others* (Chicago, 1993), ch. 3, with the review essay by P. Gouk, *Early Music History*, 13 (1994), pp. 291–306. Also P. G. Maxwell-Stuart (ed. and trans.), *The Occult in Early Modern Europe: A Documentary History* (Houndmills, 1999); B. Vickers (ed.), *Occult and Scientific Mentalities in the Renaissance* (Cambridge, 1984).

[R. Chiu, *Plague and Music in the Renaissance* (Cambridge, 2017), draws on *Music as Medicine* under the heading of music therapy.]

5 Tomlinson, *Music in Renaissance Magic*, pp. 77ff.

6 A. Voss, 'Marsilio Ficino, the Second Orpheus', in *Music as Medicine*, pp. 154–172; [A. Voss, '*Orpheus redivivus*: The Musical Magic of Marsilio Ficino', in M. J. B. Allen, V. Rees and M. Davies (eds), *Marsilio Ficino: His Theology, His Philosophy, His Legacy* (Leiden, 2002), pp. 227–241, esp. 239–240; J. Prins, *Echoes of an Invisible World: Marsilio Ficino and Francesco Patrizi on Cosmic Order and Music Theory* (Leiden, 2015), esp. pp. 186–208.]

7 Trans. in O. Strunk (ed.), rev. L. Treitler, *Source Readings in Music History* (New York, 1998), and discussed briefly by P. Gouk, 'Sister Disciplines? *Music and Medicine* in Historical Perspective', in Gouk (ed.), *Musical Healing in Cultural Contexts* (Aldershot, 2000), pp. 190–191. For a medical parallel, Epifanio Ferdinando, *Centum historiae seu observationes et casus medici* (Venice, 1621), pp. 266–268, 321. Peter Lauremberg, *Laurus Delphica seu consilium quo describitur methodus perfacilis ad medicinam* (Leiden, 1621), p. 31, supports his plea for musical knowledge in a physician with reminiscences of auto-therapy in his youth.

8 C. Webster, *From Paracelsus to Newton: Magic and the Making of Modern Science* (Cambridge, 1982); Vickers, *Occult and Scientific Mentalities*; D. C. Lindberg and R. S. Westman (eds), *Reappraisals of the Scientific Revolution* (Cambridge, 1990).

9 Voss, 'Marsilio Ficino', p. 162.

10 Tomlinson, *Music in Renaissance Magic*, p. 98, citing J. Haar, '*Musica mundana*: Variations on a Pythagorean Theme' (PhD thesis, Harvard University, 1960), p. 444.

11 H. R. Trevor-Roper, 'The Paracelsian Movement', in his *Renaissance Essays* (London, 1985), pp. 149–199; O. P. Grell (ed.), *Paracelsus: The Man and His Reputation, His Ideas and Their Transformation* (Leiden, 1998).

12 [See now C. Webster, *Paracelsus: Medicine, Magic and Mission at the End of Time* (New Haven, CT, 2008).]

13 H. Schott, '"Invisible Diseases" – Imagination and Magnetism: Paracelsus and the Consequences', in Grell, *Paracelsus*, pp. 315–316.

14 C. Webster, 'Paracelsus Confronts the Saints: Miracles, Healing and the Secularization of Magic', *Social History of Medicine*, 8 (1995), pp. 403–421.

15 Contrast A. Hayum, *The Isenheim Altarpiece* (Princeton, NJ, 1989), p. 46, who takes Paracelsus as, uncontroversially, a music therapist.

16 Leiden University, Codex Vossianus Chymicus 25, ff. 511–512a, ed. K. Sudhoff, *Versuch einer Kritik der Echtheit der Paracelsischen Schriften*, pt 2.1 (Berlin, 1898), no. 89, p. 419, trans. Charles Webster (personal communication, for which I am deeply grateful).

17 [See now P. Gouk, 'Harmony, Health and Healing: Music's Role in Early Modern Paracelsian Thought', in M. Pelling and S. Mandelbrote (eds), *The Practice of Reform in Health, Medicine and Science, 1500–2000: Essays for Charles Webster* (Aldershot, 2005), pp. 23–42, esp. pp. 29–30.]

POSTSCRIPT
Music therapy in Rabelais

No discussion, however brief, of the history of music therapy, or at least of representations of music therapy, in the Renaissance should have omitted the best vignette of all. It comes from the *Gargantua and Pantagruel* of François Rabelais (c.1483–1553), those massive, exuberant, ribald, satirical (Pythonesque?) 'chronicles' of the giant Gargantua and his son Pantagruel. A graduate of the famed medical school of Montpellier, who took his doctorate there in 1537, Rabelais was profoundly learned in medicine, as is well known. His love of music is also well known. Yet nothing in his career or his writings quite prepares us for the depiction of musical medicine in *Pantagruel* Book 5, chs 19–20. The problem with Book 5 is that it was published over a decade after Rabelais' death and scholars contest its authenticity. Some notes on music therapy could have survived among Rabelais' papers and been incorporated into a pseudonymous Book 5, perhaps by Jean Turquet de Mayerne. Whether that happened or not matters less here than the Rabelaisian spirit of the passage in question.

Pantagruel and his company are on a voyage, island hopping, starting with 'L'Isle sonnante' (Ringing Island). In a section of the book markedly alchemical in tone, they arrive at the Kingdom of Quintessence, called 'Entelechy', meaning 'coming into being'. The captain of the guard conveys them to the palace of the Queen. Although now 1,800 years old, she is still young and beautiful. The captain alludes to the power of English and French monarchs to 'touch' and thereby heal sufferers of the 'king's evil', scrofula; but he does that to show how Queen (or Dame) Quintessence surpasses them all in the range and immediacy of her cures, even without touching. She plays on an organ fashioned from medicinal plants: its pipes are made of sticks of cassia; its stops, of rhubarb; its keyboard, of scammony, and so on. Her officials, all of whom have obscure and pretentious titles (some of them alchemical) such as abstractors, spodizators and archasdarpenins, bring in the lepers.

> She played them a song, I know not what, and they were suddenly and completely cured. Then were brought in those who had been

poisoned. She played another song and they could stand up. Then the blind, the deaf [!], the mute, all likewise treated. This astounded us, rightly, and we fell to the ground, prostrating ourselves as if in ecstasy...

After dinner the officials explain that it is the Queen alone who does the impossible and cures the incurable; they deal with the rest. Pantagruel records that he saw cures of those afflicted with syphilis, dropsy, fever, and malaria; but these did not involve music.

The context of this episode is broadly clear. Alchemy is part of it: the Queen has after all learned to prolong life with the quintessence, sublimation of the philosopher's stone. She is a Renaissance neo-Platonic figure, from the world of Marsilio Ficino as relayed to Rabelais, or to his editor/continuator, by such writers as Cornelius Agrippa, referred to in the chapter above. Rabelais also knows, whether directly or indirectly, all the ancient anecdotes showing the therapeutic power of music, such as the one about Pythagoras healing both psychic and somatic afflictions by singing over the sick (Porphyry, *Life of Pythagoras*, 33). As a learned physician he is familiar with medicinal plants: Pantagruel had been cured of his stomach pains and constipation by taking huge quantities of scammony, cassia and rhubarb (*Pantagruel* ch. 22 = *Gargantua and Pantagruel* book 2, ch. 33). And he is aware of contemporary debates about why music may no longer have the curative power that it did in antiquity, and about whether, through sympathy, the material that the instrument is made of has anything to do with the effects of playing it. After Rabelais' death, but before the publication of Book 5, in 1564, Giovanni Battista della Porta, physician and polymath (?1535–1615) published in Naples the first of two versions of his *Magia Naturalis* (1558) in which he recommended healing with music played on the flute made from the medicinal plant appropriate to the disease.

This is still some way from the Queen's vegetable organ. Our Rabelaisian author seems to have invented that. Is he laughing? Is the Queen being used to mock the pretensions of Renaissance music therapists and all those who claimed to have certain and universal remedies? Perhaps only up to a point. The Queen is a dignified figure, even though we might be expected to chuckle as she greets her guests with extravagant wordiness – 'the scintillating probity in the circumference of your minds makes me certain of the virtue hidden within the belly of your spirits', and so on. If the tone is satirical, it is still remarkable that the protagonist is a woman. Women do not otherwise figure much in the annals of music therapy before the twentieth century (see pp. 315–16 below). The passage needs further exploration and specialist commentary, not least by those better versed than I am in the Renaissance *querelle des femmes* about the nature and status of women.

Bibliographical note

The text of Rabelais I used is the more or less standard edition, by Mireille Huchon, *Oeuvres complètes* (Paris: Gallimard, 1994). Translations are my own, but I consulted both the venerable one by W. F. Smith (London: Alexander P. Watt, 1893) and the latest and most authoritative one in the Penguin Classics series by M. A. Screech (London: Penguin, 2006). The passage in Book 5 was noticed briefly by W. F. Kümmel, *Musik und Medizin: Ihre Wechselbeziehungen in Theorie und Praxis von 800 bis 1800* (Freiburg: Karl Alber, 1977), pp. 234–235 (on which see Chapter 14 in this volume). Since then it has not, so far as I know, been considered by historians of music therapy. Nor has it been much discussed by Rabelais scholars beyond some annotation in editions of the text. The crucial publication is *Études rabelaisiennes*, vol. 40, ed. Franco Giacone, dedicated to the controversial *Cinquiesme livre* (Geneva: Droz, 2001). This includes a very helpful review of the arguments for and against authenticity by Richard Cooper (pp. 9–22), a general view of 'noise and music' in the fifth book as a whole by Olivier Millet (pp. 251–264), and a brief but detailed placing of the organ-playing Queen within the longer history of ideas of musical healing by Madeleine Lazard (pp. 243–50).

On music see Nan Cook Carpenter, *Rabelais and Music* (Chapel Hill: University of North Carolina Press, 1954), who defends the authenticity of Book 5 on the basis of its musicology. See more briefly her article in *Modern Language Quarterly*, 13 (1952), 299–304; also Frank Dobbins, *Music in Renaissance Lyons* (Oxford: Clarendon Press, 1992).

On della Porta see Rebecca Cypress, 'Giovanni Battista Della Porta's Experiments with Musical Instruments', *Journal of Musicological Research*, 35 (2016), 159–175.

On the 'royal touch', beyond the classic, Marc Bloch, *The Royal Touch: Sacred Monarchy and Scrofula in England and France*, first published 1924 (English translation, London: Routledge & Kegan Paul, 1973), see now Stephen Brogan, *The Royal Touch in Early Modern England: Politics, Medicine and Sin* (Woodbridge: Boydell, 2015).

I am grateful to Richard Cooper and Ian Maclean for expert advice.

16

ASPECTS OF MUSIC THERAPY IN THE NINETEENTH AND TWENTIETH CENTURIES

Romanticism, the USA, Mesmerism, Theosophy

I

The modern period – let us say, since 1800 – is paradoxically the least well explored of all the phases of music therapy's varied history.[1]

One reason for that comparative neglect is contingent. Neither musicology nor medical historiography has, until recent decades, adopted the broad cultural (postmodern) remit which would allow such a seemingly peripheral topic more than a brief airing. There is, however, another reason that goes deeper. It is that the very terms of reference of a history of music therapy in the modern period are uncertain, the contours of the subject are fundamentally obscure. Unlike antiquity, the later Middle Ages, or the Renaissance, this phase has no one clearly dominant paradigm: rather, it falls between two paradigms. The first of these is the humoral system of medicine. By the beginning of the nineteenth century this had more or less collapsed. Some treatments derived from it still flourish today, of course; but in European learned medicine it has been defunct for around two centuries. The legacy of classical antiquity, particularly of Hippocrates and Galen, it had been under assault since the time of the Scientific Revolution; yet it long continued to provide a broad framework which could accommodate even new medical philosophies. In the eighteenth century, Richard Browne, Richard Brocklesby or Louis Roger are intent on providing contemporary ways of approaching old problems, problems with which Marsilio Ficino was familiar.[2] The second paradigm is constituted by the professionalization that has taken place since the Second World War. This supplies a basis for global comparisons, even though it brings with it the danger that 'first-world' music therapy will be privileged over 'traditional' forms of musical healing. Much remains to be explored, but here at least, in the postwar decades, we have some bearings.

And between the two paradigms? It is still not clear where we should look – not clear which figure or idea should be connected with which other; what the important currents of thought are, what the subsidiary.

II

How, then, to represent the nineteenth century? Not much of relevance is to be expected of the history of general medical practice. In the long period from the end of antiquity to around 1800, there is no evidence that music was often recommended by the run of practitioners, however profound its artistic and philosophical resonances. The period 1800–1900 does not, in the present state of research, appear obviously different. Where we might look for music therapy is, rather, in the two of the great new phenomena of the time – phenomena not unconnected – Romanticism and institutional psychiatry.

Romanticism is exceedingly hard to characterize, in music or any other domain, and virtually impossible to characterize briefly. At least it can be said that Romantic musical thought substitutes an emphasis on the power of individual expression for the aesthetics of the eighteenth century, which dwelt mostly on imitation or which held out the possibility of a rational codification of musical effects.[3] Romantic music supposedly arises from deep in the composer's psyche and dives deep into that of its listener. Composing it might seem to require something akin to Platonic divine madness.[4] Hearing it could be comparably deranging. The arch-Romantic Wagner envisaged that his *Tristan and Isolde*, unless too badly performed to have any real effect, would drive its audiences mad.[5] Romantic music also, metaphysically speaking, reaches 'higher' or 'further' than ever before – beyond the *musica mundana* of ancient and Renaissance Platonism. For its greatest philosopher, Schopenhauer, music was the only art form that went beyond 'representations' to the very Will itself, that force underlying all apprehensible reality.[6]

In Romantic hands, therefore, music ought to be potent. Yet it is an ambivalent potency. In the early Romantic era, music can be either cause or cure of a disorder. And that disorder, which in a sense the age invented, is insanity: a psychological breakdown which does not necessarily have an organic component and which is treatable by means of psychiatry, the other medical 'invention' of the late eighteenth century. Even before Wagner began to derange his audiences, Liszt the recital pianist could already be found inspiring hysteria in his (especially female) listeners – hysteria of the kind which we associate with Beatles concerts. But Liszt also visited a Paris asylum to play to an inmate.[7]

In many asylums music apparently became, if not a regular feature, then at least a surprisingly common one from the last decades of the eighteenth century onwards.[8] It might seem as if this represented a continuation of the Galenic emphasis on 'diet', the daily regimen which included among its objectives the moderation of the 'passions of the soul' through entertainment. But the context is different, and there is as much discontinuity as continuity. Galenic medicine sees mental illness as essentially somatic, though the passions of the soul may have a part to play in its onset. There had been a 'therapy of the word', a 'talking cure', in Western medicine since antiquity, but it was always limited in scope.[9] The eighteenth-century treatment of insanity, at least to begin with, is a treatment of a disorderly body. That century may not have been quite the 'disaster for the insane' once discerned in it;[10] there was no 'great confinement' in asylums, nor the over-reliance on whips and chains that some historians have supposed. Nevertheless, humanitarian treatment in the private mad houses which began to flourish in the eighteenth century was still based on an essentially somatic understanding of mental health. The 'moral management' (or 'moral therapy') that characterized avant-garde asylums of the latter part of the eighteenth century and the first half of the nineteenth derived from the axioms that psychology was preferable to restraint, and that mental illness was precisely that, a failure of reason to be countered by rational means.

Now music for explicitly curative rather than liturgical purposes had not been heard in hospitals (apart from some monastic ones) or in institutions for the insane since the early Middle Ages in the Near East.[11] But with the advent of 'moral' treatment towards 1800,[12] it took its place in the asylum under new theoretical auspices. Its presence may also have had much to do with the commercialization of leisure and of social life generally. Moral managers were not necessarily medically trained. They were trying to restore their mentally abnormal patients to 'bourgeois' normality, within which music, both heard and performed, held an increasingly important place.

III

There is a chapter to be written on the USA to set alongside the European material that has dominated the historiography of music therapy. The histories of American and British music therapists were closely intertwined in the earlier twentieth century.[13] To grasp the American background to that, the nineteenth-century background, we must turn, on one hand, to secondary works which provide the likely context but say nothing about music and, on the other hand, to basic studies of the specific literature of music therapy which say little about the context.[14] What follows, then, is a preliminary attempt to bring the two sides together.

The earliest known North American publications on music therapy date from the late eighteenth century; they sound conventional, even old-fashioned.[15] An article in the *Columbian Magazine* for February 1789, entitled 'Music Physically Considered', seems to reassert the Galenic axiom of the interdependence of mind and body and the force of the 'passions of the mind' on bodily health; and it does so expressly in the face of Cartesian dualism[16] and the 'hydraulic' and 'neurological' physiologies of Boerhaave and Cullen, which left little scope for music therapy.[17] The article also cites a case of music's being used to cure extreme depression in a dancer. A few years later, in 1796, a short notice appeared in the *New York Weekly*

Magazine for 10 August, recounting the case of an unnamed music teacher (first a dancer, now a musician, as if only the musical were receptive to music therapy) whose fever had been abated and eventually, after a fortnight, dispelled by command performances of music – 'without any other assistance than once bleeding the foot . . .'.

Such is the *ancien régime* in North American music therapy: somewhat flimsy, unoriginal productions. Medical dissertations written in the early 1800s show a transition to a different phase of thinking, even if they do not represent a huge advance in scholarship.[18] In a nineteen-page tract of 1804, *An Inaugural Essay on the Influence of Music in the Cure of Diseases*, Edwin Atlee paid homage to the Galenic notion that excessive grief could lead to physical illness, and once more included fevers among the conditions susceptible to musical treatment. Yet he also asserted, in keeping with European 'moral' therapy, that music alone could attack the causes of mania, which he regarded as 'the consequences of a delirious or mistaken idea', not a physiological aberration. And he concluded by relating three cases known to him personally in which hearing music had relieved mental distress: those of a melancholic, a hysteric, and a maniac.

In 1806 there appeared another, equally compact work in the same vein. Samuel Mathews's *On the Effects of Music in Curing and Palliating Diseases* is steeped in much earlier authors such as Giorgio Baglivi and is still invoking David's playing to Saul. Although he takes his historical anecdotes from Burney's *History of Music*,[19] Mathews also appears forward-looking in his suggestions. He excites modern music therapists by his anticipation of what they call the 'iso' principle ('we should be particular in having the notes accommodated to the patient's mind').[20] And he was the first to recommend in print that music therapy should become part of clinical practice in institutions.

The brevity of these two pieces, and the fact that they give as much space to classic texts as to actual case histories, does not suggest that their subject was a particularly lively one in early nineteenth-century America. The dissertations were published in Philadelphia, and had been produced in partial fulfilment of the graduation requirements of the medical faculty of the University of Pennsylvania. Mathews admitted to having written his piece in a mere ten days;[21] and both authors were perhaps casting around for an untried topic. Like Joseph Comstock, who in 1801 treated an apparent case of tarantism with music,[22] they were, however, pupils of Benjamin Rush. Both Atlee and Mathews cited Rush extensively in their works and Mathews credited Rush with a plan – thwarted by practical difficulties – to introduce music therapy into the Pennsylvania Hospital.[23]

Benjamin Rush (1746–1813), pupil of William Cullen in Edinburgh, signatory of the Declaration of Independence, father of American psychiatry, is often taken as the chief American proponent of moral therapy.[24] And moral therapy, as has already been suggested, is likely to include music. Rush had exclusive charge of the insane in the Pennsylvania Hospital from 1787. Yet it seems he had not, by 1806, managed to include music in his therapies. The truth is that Rush was not quite the great advocate of musical healing that his pupils, and some of his later historians, would wish us to see in him. What he did introduce to the Pennsylvania Hospital, in 1810, 'to assist in curing madness', was his celebrated 'tranquillizing chair':

> It binds and confines every part of the body . . . Its effects have been truly delightful to me. It acts as a sedative to the tongue and temper as well as to the blood vessels. In 24, 12, six, and in some cases four hours, the most refractory patients have been composed.[25]

That is from a letter by Rush to his son. Nowhere in his published correspondence does he discuss the possibilities of music therapy. His enthusiasm is all for treatments at the somatic rather than the psychological end of the spectrum: 'warm and cold baths', 'copious bleeding', 'low diet', and the like.[26] In keeping with that preference, Rush's last medical book, *Medical Inquiries and Observations upon Diseases of the Mind*, published in the year before his death, while admittedly mentioning music therapy several times, is each time very brief and often somewhat abstract. Where individual patients do merit mention, it is not Rush's prescriptions that they are following. For example: 'I attend a citizen of Philadelphia, occasionally, in paroxysms of [hypochondriasis], who informed me that he was cured of one of them by hearing the old hundred psalm tune sung in a country church.' Or again: 'music has been much commended in this state of madness [mania] . . . Dr. Cox mentions a striking instance of its power over the mind of a madman.'[27] It is always someone else who describes or prescribes the music. And Joseph Mason Cox, though claimed by historians as a 'moral' therapist, was also the first to develop a working model of yet another mechanical device for subduing the insane, the 'swinging machine'.[28] He was no more a friend of music therapy than was Rush, whose tone in the *Inquiries* perceptibly brightens when he turns from music back to more congenial strategies for the management of lunatics – such as the use of terror, or even of torture.[29]

If this is moral treatment, then its arrival in America might be thought a mixed blessing. One begins to understand why early writers on music therapy such as Atlee and Mathews seem to have had little practical experience to go on, and look back to Baglivi. Perhaps music was never very prominent in the American version of moral treatment. The York Retreat, the British exemplar of a musical asylum, was widely imitated in the USA, starting with the Friends' Asylum near Philadelphia in 1817. Yet Rush's work remained the primary textbook on the treatment of insanity, and was hardly the best advertisement for music's cause.[30]

That may be why the first clearly documented institutional use of music in the USA apparently occurred not in a hospital or asylum, but in a school for the blind – the Perkins School established in south Boston in 1832 by Samuel Gridley Howe. His wife, Julia, composed children's songs and wrote the words for the 'Battle Hymn of the Republic'. Hers was probably the influence that determined the addition of music to the curriculum. In the Perkins School, as later, in other schools for the blind and indeed for the deaf, the music was not particularly therapeutic in intent; it was more to offer the handicapped 'intellectual gratification'.[31] The point (then as now) was presumably to communicate with the handicapped, to integrate them, to compensate for their physical deficiency with modest artistic success.

Meanwhile, after the brief flurry of the early 1800s, medical periodicals and dissertations seem to have been silent on the subject of music therapy for some time. A clutch of articles in the *Musical Magazine* for 1840–1841 rehashed anecdotes from antiquity to the time of Farinelli, once more drawn overwhelmingly from Burney's *General History of Music*, and registering none of the practical applications recorded or envisaged in the earlier publications.[32] Little is detectable thereafter until the 1870s. In 1874, James Whittaker published in the *Cincinnati Clinic* a renewed assertion of the possibilities of music therapy in the treatment of, above all, mild mental disturbance. Then, in 1878, *The World*, a New York newspaper, reported a set of experiments on the reactions to professional music-making that were evinced by pauper 'lunatics' in the Blackwell's Island (now Roosevelt Island) asylum. This was the first time that government-sponsored music therapy had been seen in the United States.[33] After some further published rehashes of Burney, a paper of 1892 by G. A. Blumer, Chief Executive Officer of the Utica State Hospital in New York, once more explicitly aligned the use of music therapy with moral treatment – long after it had passed out of fashion in asylums. Blumer also hired immigrant musicians to perform to the patients in his hospital.[34] Finally, as the century closed, a prominent neurologist, James L. Corning, published in the *Medical Record* an article reporting the first controlled attempt to treat disease with music. Combining the auditory and visual stimulation of patients who were presomnolent, Corning hoped that the music would bypass the cognitive faculties that were becoming (literally) dormant and would penetrate the unconscious. Appropriate music – which for Corning meant Wagner and other Romantics – was to facilitate the transfer of pleasant emotions from presomnolency into waking hours, thus lifting his patients' depression.[35]

At this point the present note begins to dovetail with Tyler's chapter in *Music as Medicine*. Early twentieth-century American developments are tabulated by her, and more detail of them is also conveniently available elsewhere.[36] So it will be enough to conclude here by signalling the major contribution that women were then making, for the first time, it would seem, in the entire history of music therapy: women such as Eva Vescelius, who treated insomnia, fever and other ailments with 'musicotherapy' in New York during the early 1900s, Margaret Anderton, who believed that particular pieces could be assigned to specific ailments (Schubert for insomnia, Brahms waltzes and, improbably, Sousa marches for the terminally ill), Harriet Ayer Seymour, Esther Gatewood, and indeed others. It is a remarkable list, only partly to be explained by women's role in caring for veterans of the First World War.

IV

The other domain of the history of music therapy I now want briefly to de-lineate is harder to characterize. 'Music therapy and occultism', or 'Music therapy and the esoteric' (or 'the para-scientific'), might serve as a heading but immediately engenders prejudice; and it is at once vulnerable to the charge of lumping together a diversity of ideologies. Occultism might be defined as the belief that nature has properties not amenable to the senses, properties beyond, or contrary to, those postulated by science – which the adept can learn to manipulate.[37] Such a definition does small justice to the complex connections between occult and mainstream scientific thought, either during the Renaissance, in which most modern occult traditions originated, or during the nineteenth to early twentieth centuries, when occultism achieved almost as large a cultural significance. Rather than try to disentangle that complexity, however, I shall simply illustrate it, by describing two types of music therapy very much a part of the wider picture, and without which no broad survey of the subject could be complete: the Mesmeric and the Theosophical.

First, Mesmerism. A caption to an early representation of a Mesmerist seance provides a useful introduction:[38]

> M. Mesmer, doctor of medicine in the faculty of Vienna in Austria, is the sole inventor of animal magnetism. That method of curing a multitude of ills (among others, dropsy, paralysis, gout, scurvy, blindness, accidental deafness) consists in the application of a fluid or agent that M. Mesmer directs, at times with one of his fingers, at times with an iron rod that another applies at will, on those who have recourse to him . . . The sick, especially women, experience convulsions or crises that bring about their cure . . . In the ante-chamber, musicians play tunes to make the sick cheerful.

The techniques and associated apparatus (including a tub of 'magnetized' water) would evolve. But the essentials are all there in that early description. Franz Anton Mesmer (1734–1815) studied medicine in Vienna and was an accomplished amateur musician. Friend of Gluck, Haydn, and the Mozart family (the infant prodigy's *Singspiel*, *Bastien and Bastienne*, was supposedly first performed in Mesmer's garden theatre), Mesmer was also skilful on the glass harmonica. The method of treatment which he elaborated may seem like a forerunner of hypnotism and psychoanalysis (brainchild of another Viennese physician);[39] but it is actually best understood against a background of both Renaissance cosmology and Enlightenment science. Mesmer's thesis of 1766, 'De planetarum influxu', was on the familiar Renaissance topic of the influence of the stars on the human body. From Renaissance sources such as Paracelsus and Fludd (his many critics were quick to puncture claims to originality) but also from the some of the physics of his own age, Mesmer derived the notion of a single universal fluid, visible (like its subspecies, ferromagnetism and electricity) only in its effects. This animal fluid (from *anima*, soul) was the medium for the interaction of heavenly bodies with the earth and with animate objects – or to put it in older terminology, of *musica mundana* with *musica humana*. Just as there was in Mesmer's scheme of things only one humour rather than four, so there was only one illness: not a humoral imbalance but a disorderly configuration of magnetic forces within an individual body. This disorder could be counteracted by passing a magnet, or later just a capable hand, over the patient's initially entranced and then convulsed body.

Magnetic fluid could, moreover, supposedly be directed and strengthened by sound.[40] No specifically Mesmeric music survives, at least from the circle of Mesmer himself.[41] And Mesmer never fully articulated its role in his curative sessions. Yet music – sung, or played on the glass harmonica by Mesmer himself or on the piano by an assistant – seems to have been a regular and more than ancillary part of the whole elaborate ritual. So much is clear from the recollections of disciples, among them the poet-physician Justinus Kerner (1786–1862), who himself played the Jew's harp as part of his magnetizing of a famous nineteenth-century 'case', that of the woman whom he immortalized in print as the seeress of Prevorst.[42] The enormous scholarly literature that Mesmerism has generated says relatively little about its musical aspect. Yet that literature has shown what a potent, popular force Mesmerism became in late eighteenth- and nineteenth-century Europe, despite the denunciations of various medical authorities. So there is a type of music therapy here, the possible diffusion of which has been too little noticed. And it is perhaps different from most other European types in that it seeks to induce rather than to end abnormal functioning – to provoke a crisis.

Whether musical or not, a Mesmeric seance was a performance. That does not make it wholly remote from contemporary medical or scientific orthodoxy. We should remember that the ancient postulate of an invisible universal substance held an essential place in Newton's mechanics, and that it was not finally banished from physics until the Michelson–Morley experiment of 1887, or indeed until the debates of the early 1900s surrounding Einsteinian relativity.[43] Nor was Mesmeric therapy obviously a failure – by the standards of either the humoral medicine of its time or of its obvious later *comparandum*, psychoanalysis. The effects may have owed everything to psychodynamics and nothing to magnetism; but they were palpable enough and, in the case of at least some female patients, palpably sexual.[44] Mesmerism has been seen as marking the end of the Enlightenment. In the present context, it might equally be called the revival of the Renaissance or the beginnings of Romantic occultism. But under neither heading should it be thought of as culturally marginal.[45]

Much of its resonance can be detected in the musical world. The most famous example is of course Mozart's comic portrayal of Mesmerism in the first act finale of *Così fan tutte*, in which Despina magnetizes the supposedly arsenic-poisoned suitors.[46] Less well known is Schubert's attendance at a Mesmerist session in 1825. The treatment was directed by the painter Ludwig Schnorr von Carolsfeld, and Schubert participated in it by playing some of his newly composed dances so that their effect on the patient, Louise Mora, could be observed while she was in a trance.[47] Liszt was described as mesmerizing his listeners.[48] Wagner too, as composer-conductor, was credited in some quarters with similar powers. A caricature of 1868 shows notes raining down from his baton into the eyes and mouths of a stupefied audience. Another, which appeared in the *Revue trimestrielle* during 1864, explicitly portrays him and Berlioz as engaged in a battle of mutual mesmerizing, score in one hand, baton in the other. Berlioz is the loser: his eyes are closed and he slumps forward in his chair.[49]

Magnetism runs through nineteenth-century esotericism like the powerful unifying force it was claimed to be. It provides the context within which to approach a range of figures who continued the eighteenth-century tradition of conjecturing the physiology of musical healing – a tradition represented, for Britain, by Browne and Brocklesby, and for France by Roger.[50] In 1874 Antoine Joseph ('Hector') Chomet published the revised text of a lecture that he had been invited to give in Paris in 1846, *Effets et influences de la musique sur la santé et sur la maladie*. In this he postulated a quasi-Mesmerist 'sonorous fluid', to set beside those which respectively conducted heat, light, and electricity, and which would explain the physical and psychological effects of music far more satisfactorily than could the already available theories. Two years later, in 1868, Louis Adolphe Le Doulcet, the self-styled Marquis de Pontécoulant, published a tract which bears even more deeply the stamp of 'occultized' Mesmerism, *Les Phénomènes de la musique, ou l'influence du son sur les êtres animés*. This author also conjectured a sonorous fluid to link performer and patient. He had for example 'seen a subject put to sleep by simply touching a guitar that had previously been magnetized, the sonorous fluid being propagated by the vibration of the strings'.[51] Whether or not such figures occupy 'a watershed in the history of music therapy', as their most sympathetic yet scholarly modern commentator has it,[52] they here provide a transition from the Mesmeric world to that of modern organized occultism.

In 1875, Madame Blavatsky, along with Henry Steel Olcott, founded the Theosophical Society in New York.[53] In true Pythagorean style she averred that sound may be produced of such a nature that the Pyramid of Cheops would be raised in the air, or that a dying man, nay, one at his last breath, would be revived and filled with new energy and vigour.[54]

Yet musical therapeutics were never very prominent in her thinking. It was rather among second-generation Theosophists that such matters came to the fore. In 1909, for example, Edmond Bailly started publishing *La magie du son* in his own journal, and this was the first part of a project for a book to be entitled *Du merveilleux dans la musique et de la thérapeutique musicale*.[55] Far more influential among this generation, however, was Rudolf Steiner (1861–1925). In 1913, Steiner had founded Anthroposophy (or Spiritual Science), a 'breakaway movement' from Theosophy that, unlike its progenitor, has had a lasting educational, medical, and musicological impact in Steiner schools and hospitals.[56] Music imbues Steiner's whole mode of expression. There is 'eurhythmy', a conception of movement as visible song.[57] And there is a thoroughly musical conception of the inner life: Steiner looked forward to 'a time when a diseased condition of the soul will . . . be spoken of in musical terms, as one would speak, for instance, of a piano that was out of tune'.[58] This is reminiscent of Novalis's 'every illness is a musical problem, its cure a musical solution' [cited at the start of Chapter 14 above]. But Steiner's pronouncements on 'the astral body, which is a musician in every human being, and imitates the music of the cosmos' are more thoroughly neo-Platonic, and seem to be a restatement of the analogy between *musica mundana* and *musica humana* in terms of Victorian spiritualism.[59] Steiner also believed that each musical interval of the chromatic scale expresses a distinctive kind of experience – the minor second, one of movement and activity within the self, extraversion with the perfect fifth, and so on.[60] And it is through the manipulation of such features, presumably, that a therapist can alter the astral body and realign it with the cosmic harmony. The ambition is to treat the whole person in artistic and spiritual terms, seeing illness as an opportunity for positive change rather than a setback that should be reversed.

Steinerian practice overlaps with the modern Western music therapy.[61] It does so, first, through influencing the practice of Nordoff and Robbins, itself extremely influential; second, through Steiner institutions such as the Herdecke Hospital of the University of Wittenberg, where the music of 'natural instruments' such as lyre and recorder is piped to patients in an otherwise 'high-tech' hospital.[62] David Aldridge writes of the music therapy practised at Herdecke as not of the Anthroposophical type. Yet he reproduces a Steinerian table of the emotions with which specific intervals may be linked.[63] Pervasive connections between Steiner therapists and mainstream professionals have clearly endured.

A final question: what place should be given to composers in the recent history of music therapy? Are there modern equivalents to Schubert, Liszt, or Wagner as quasi-Mesmerists? Alexander Scriabin and Arnold Schoenberg were, to differing extents, Theosophical adepts. Schoenberg's esotericism emerges in such works as the incomplete oratorio *Die Jakobsleiter*, but he does not seem to have conceived his music with therapeutic intent.[64] Scriabin, by contrast, thought of himself as another Orpheus, and planned the ultimate therapy of total dissolution. His final work was to be the *Mysterium*, of which – mercifully – only a 'Prefatory Act' was sketched (and has been posthumously reconstructed, and recorded). The whole would have been performed over seven days. (Seven was the number of human races according to Madame Blavatsky.) Even the 'Prefatory Act' by itself – to which, with unwonted pragmatism, Scriabin eventually confined himself – was to take place in a specially built temple in India, with spectators seated in tiers according to their degree of spiritual advancement. There were to be costumed speakers, processions, parades; dancers as well as musicians would take part, each in their thousands. Pillars of incense would form part of the scenery. And all this was merely the prelude to the final mystery, in which everyone would be dissolved in ecstasy. 'A brand-new race of purified, purged, clarified and spiritually advanced men is born . . . to repeat this monster act all over again, but on a higher plane.'[65]

Other composers, since Scriabin, have also seen themselves as therapists of a sort. Answering Hölderlin's question, 'What are poets for in a barren age?', Michael Tippett for instance portrayed the composer as virtually healing society – and as doing so very traditionally by contraries: restoring harmony and balance in a way that would not have surprised leading Renaissance figures.[66] A related theme of Tippett's work, derived from Jung, was the need to know both one's 'shadow', or dark side of the personality, and one's 'light', so as to achieve wholeness. It was a theme that Tippett dramatized in almost all his operas, from *The Midsummer Marriage* to *New Year*, and, pre-eminently, in the oratorio *A Child of Our Time*; and by dramatizing it he could be said to have attempted to induce it in his audiences. This is not, however, a particularly esoteric project, for all Jung's interest in the occult. Cyril Scott (1879–1970), by contrast, professed himself inspired by the Mahatma Koot Hoomi, a 'Master' described by him as a reincarnation of Pythagoras and over 150 years old.[67] Scott was a Neoplatonist and occultist with decided views on how music has surreptitiously influenced the whole history of mankind. He wrote books on medicine, health, and cancer, and looked forward to a 'type of music calculated to heal'.[68]

The main inheritor of the mantle of Wagner and Scriabin – his *magnum opus* also a gargantuan seven-day multi-media work, the opera cycle *Licht* – was, however, Karlheinz Stockhausen [d. 2007]. Stockhausen believed himself to have come from another world, the star Sirius, and his thought was for decades deeply coloured by that of Sri Aurobindo and by that of *The Urantia Book* of the Urantia Brotherhood of Chicago, as well as by Jakob Böhme, Nostradamus, Madame Blavatsky, and Jakob Lorber. Of all major recent composers, it was Stockhausen who showed the greatest interest in professional music therapy, while all the time relating it to his occult cosmological concerns.[69] Clearly, he saw all his compositions as potentially therapeutic. One excerpt from a characteristic discourse can serve as conclusion.

> Music should above all be a *means* of maintaining the soul's link with the beyond [Stockhausen said in an interview of 1973] . . . Nowadays there is something new, music therapy, which is becoming more and more popular . . . We have no idea about what music therapy can do. Only now are we slowly starting to rediscover that . . . Rather strangely, therapists only start helping people with music when they are already afflicted. My music is often used for therapy. Unfortunately that only happens when people are hospitalised and already completely unbalanced. Only very few people *know* that *every single one of us* basically needs music as a means of self-healing.[70]

Notes

1 [This paper is extracted from 'Commentary on Part V', in P. Horden (ed.), *Music as Medicine: The History of Music Therapy since Antiquity* (Aldershot, 2000), pp. 315–337.] Carl Gregor, Herzog zu Mecklenburg, *Bibliographie einiger Grenzgebiete der Musikwissenschaft* (Baden-Baden, 1962), contains over 120 entries on music therapy and cognate topics published since 1800 and I would guess that few of them have been explored by historians.
2 See Chapter 15 above; P. Gouk, 'Music, Melancholy, and Medical Spirits in Early Modern Thought', in Horden, *Music as Medicine*, pp. 173–194; A. Voss, 'Marsilio Ficino, the Second Orpheus', in *Music as Medicine*, pp. 154–172.
3 For some primary texts see P. Le Huray and J. Day, *Music and Aesthetics in the Eighteenth and Early-Nineteenth Centuries* (Cambridge, 1981).
4 R. Klibansky, E. Panofsky and F. Saxl, *Saturn and Melancholy* (London, 1964), ch. 1.
5 *Richard Wagner an Mathilde Wesendonk: Tagebuchblätter und Briefe 1853–1871*, 5th edn (Berlin, 1904), no. 66 (1859), p. 123. [See now J. Kennaway, *Bad Vibrations: The History of the Idea of Music as Cause of Disease* (Farnham, 2012).]
6 A. Schopenhauer, *Die Welt als Wille und Vorstellung* [*The World as Will and Idea*] (Leipzig, 1819), and many subsequent editions and translations.
7 See C. Kramer, 'Music as Cause and Cure of Illness in Nineteenth-Century Europe', in Horden, *Music as Medicine*, pp. 342–343.
8 For this and what follows, among a large literature see J. Goldstein, 'Psychiatry', in W. Bynum and R. Porter (eds), *Companion Encyclopedia of the History of Medicine*, 2 vols (London, 1993), vol. II, pp. 1350–1372, with good general bibliography. For Britain see further: R. Porter, *Mind-Forg'd Manacles: A History of Madness in England from the Restoration to the Regency* (London, 1987); Porter, 'Madness and its Institutions', in A. Wear (ed.), *Medicine in Society* (Cambridge, 1992), pp. 227–301; A. Scull, *The Most Solitary of Afflictions: Madness and Society in Britain 1700–1900* (New Haven, CT, 1993); C. MacKenzie, *Psychiatry for the Rich: A History of Ticehurst Private Asylum, 1792–1917* (London, 1992), ch. 1. On the contrasting world of pauper asylums, see J. Melling and B. Forsythe (eds), *Insanity, Institutions and Society, 1800–1914* (London, 1999). [For further literature see now G. Eghigian (ed.), *The Routledge History of Madness and*

Mental Health (Abingdon, 2017); A. Korenjak, 'From Moral Treatment to Modern Music Therapy: On the History of Music Therapy in Vienna (c. 1820–1960)', *Nordic Journal of Music Therapy* (2018), DOI: 10.1080/08098131.2018.1467481.]

9 P. Lain Entralgo, *The Therapy of the Word in Classical Antiquity* (New Haven, CT, 1970).

10 M. McDonald, *Mystical Bedlam: Madness, Anxiety, and Healing in Seventeenth-Century England* (Cambridge, 1981), p. 230; see also his 'Lunatics and the State in Georgian England', *Social History of Medicine*, 2 (1989), pp. 299–300.

11 A. Shiloah, 'Jewish and Muslim Traditions of Music Therapy', in Horden, *Music as Medicine*, pp. 73–75. W. F. Kümmel, *Musik und Medizin: Ihre Wechselbeziehungen in Theorie und Praxis von 800 bis 1800* (Freiburg, 1977), pp. 260–263, notes the apparent exception of the hospital of S. Spirito in Sassia, not far from St Peter's, the most elaborate hospital in early modern Rome, but music there was played as an accompaniment to eating, an aid to digestion.

12 See Goldstein, 'Psychiatry', pp. 1352–1357, for a helpful outline sketch. Compare A. Scull, *Social Order/Mental Disorder: Anglo-American Psychiatry in Historical Perspective* (Berkeley, CA, 1989), ch. 4.

13 H. M. Tyler, 'The Music Therapy Profession in Modern Britain', in Horden, *Music as Medicine*, pp. 375–393.

14 Remarkably, no chapter of synthesis on the nineteenth century is to be found in D. M. Schullian and M. Schoen (eds), *Music and Medicine* (New York, 1948).

15 For detail on what follows see G. N. Heller, 'Ideas, Initiatives, and Implementations: Music Therapy in America, 1789–1848', *Journal of Music Therapy*, 24.1 (1987), pp. 35–46 at 35–38.

16 While also drawing on Descartes' *Les passions de l'âme* [*The Passions of the Soul*] (1649).

17 On Herman Boerhaave (1668–1738), see G. A. Lindeboom, *Herman Boerhaave: The Man and His Work* (London, 1968); Boerhaave's very occasional interest in music therapy is noted by Kümmel, *Musik und Medizin*, pp. 300, 356. For William Cullen (1710–1790), see A. Doig, J. P. S. Ferguson, I. A. Milne and R. Passmore (eds), *William Cullen and the Eighteenth Century Medical World* (Edinburgh, 1993). For Cullen's treatment of insanity, see his *First Lines of the Practice of Physic*, 4 vols, new edn (Edinburgh, 1786), vol. III, pp. 266ff.

18 W. B. Davis, K. E. Gfeller and M. H. Traut, *An Introduction to Music Therapy: Theory and Practice* (Dubuque, IA, 1992), p. 22; Heller, 'Ideas', pp. 38–39; W. B. Davis, 'Music Therapy in 19th Century America', *Journal of Music Therapy*, 24.2 (1987), pp. 76–87 at 77; E. T. Carlson and M. B. Simpson, 'Tarantism or Hysteria? An American Case of 1801', *Journal of the History of Medicine and Allied Sciences*, 26 (1971), p. 301.

19 For Baglivi, see D. Gentilcore, 'Ritualized Illness and Music Therapy: Views of Tarantism in the Kingdom of Naples', in Horden, *Music as Medicine*, p. 265. C. Burney, *A General History of Music*, 2nd edn (London, 1789, repr. New York, 1957), 'Dissertation on the Music of the Ancients', section 10.

20 Mathews, *On the Effects of Music*, p. 14, cited from Heller, 'Ideas', p. 40.

21 Davis, 'Music Therapy', p. 78.

22 Carlson and Simpson, 'Tarantism', p. 302.

23 Heller, 'Ideas', p. 40; Davis, 'Music Therapy', p. 78.

24 Goldstein, 'Psychiatry', p. 1357. Biographies of Rush include those by N. G. Goodman (Philadelphia, 1934), C. Binger (New York, 1966), and D. F. Hawke (Indianapolis, 1971).

25 *The Letters of Benjamin Rush*, ed. L. H. Butterfield, 2 vols (Princeton, NJ, 1951), vol. II, p. 1052.

26 Ibid. pp. 443, 763, 766–767, 769.
27 *Medical Inquiries and Observations upon Diseases of the Mind* (Philadelphia, 1812, facsimile edn, New York, 1962), pp. 122–123, 211, 228, 329, 355; quotations from pp. 123, 211.
28 J. M. Cox, *Practical Observations on Insanity* (London, 1806), pp. 140ff., with Scull, *Social Order/Mental Disorder*, pp. 71–73.
29 *Medical Inquiries and Observations*, pp. 11, 229. Contrast D. Ramsay, *An Eulogium upon Benjamin Rush MD* (Philadelphia, 1813), p. 47, who writes approvingly of Rush's never having needed to use chains or whips.
30 G. N. Grob, *The Mad Among Us: A History of the Care of America's Mentally Ill* (New York, 1994), ch. 2 and pp. 66–70; Scull, *Social Order/Mental Disorder*, ch. 5 ('The Discovery of the Asylum Revisited: Lunacy Reform in the New American Republic'); N. Dain, *Concepts of Insanity in the United States* (New Brunswick, NJ, 1964). For a Canadian instance of music therapy in the asylum, see S. E. D. Shortt, *Victorian Lunacy: Richard M. Bucke and the Practice of Late Nineteenth-Century Psychiatry* (Cambridge, 1986), pp. 133–134.
31 W. W. Turner and D. E. Bartlett, 'Music among the Deaf and Dumb', *American Annals of the Deaf and Dumb*, 2 (Oct. 1848), p. 6, cited by Heller, 'Ideas', pp. 41–42.
32 Heller, 'Ideas', pp. 43–4.
33 Davis, 'Music Therapy', pp. 79–81.
34 Blumer, 'Music in its Relation to Insanity', *American Journal of Insanity*, 50 (1891–92), pp. 350–364, cited by Davis, 'Music Therapy', pp. 81–94.
35 J. L. Corning, 'The Use of Musical Vibrations Before and During Sleep . . .', *Medical Record*, 14 (1899), pp. 79–86, cited by Davis, 'Music Therapy', pp. 85–86.
36 H. M. Tyler, 'The Music Therapy Profession in Modern Britain', in Horden, *Music as Medicine*, pp. 375–393; Davis et al., *An Introduction to Music Therapy*, pp. 26–30.
37 R. Galbraith, 'Explaining Modern Occultism', in H. Kerr and C. L. Crow (eds), *The Occult in America: New Historical Perspectives* (Urbana, IL, 1983), pp. 15–19.
38 R. Darnton, *Mesmerism and the End of the Enlightenment in France* (Cambridge, MA, 1968), pp. 6–7.
39 See H. Ellenberger's classic *The Discovery of the Unconscious: The History and Evolution of Dynamic Psychiatry* (London, 1970), pp. 57ff., where Mesmer's work is presented as a turning point in the evolution of dynamic psychotherapy. Note also A. Crabtree, *From Mesmer to Freud* (New Haven, CT, 1993). For Mesmer's career, conflicts with the medical establishment, and larger impact, among a substantial recent literature see F. A. Pattie, *Mesmer and Animal Magnetism* (Hamilton, NY, 1994); A. Gauld, *A History of Hypnotism* (Cambridge, 1992).
40 E. Völkel, *Die spekulative Musiktherapie zur Zeit der Romantik: Ihre Traditionen und ihr Fortwirken* (Düsseldorf, 1979), pp. 118–134. L. Brockliss and C. Jones, *The Medical World of Early Modern France* (Oxford, 1997), p. 792.
41 Robert Darnton, personal communication.
42 *Die Seherin von Prevorst*, 2 vols (Stuttgart, 1829). See the abbreviated English translation by Mrs Crowe, *The Seeress of Prevorst* (London, 1845), p. 73. Völkel, *Die spekulative Musiktherapie*, pp. 126, 128–131; for Kerner, pp. 135–139. Ellenberger, *Discovery of the Unconscious*, pp. 79–81.
43 G. N. Cantor and M. J. S. Hodge (eds), *Conceptions of Ether: Studies in the History of Ether Theories, 1740–1900* (Cambridge, 1981).
44 Brockliss and Jones, *The Medical World of Early Modern France*, p. 789.
45 See T. James, *Dreams, Creativity, and Madness in Nineteenth-Century France* (Oxford, 1995), ch. 3. For the USA, see R. C. Fuller, *Mesmerism and the American*

Cure of Souls (Philadelphia, 1982) [and now E. Ogden, *Credulity: A Cultural History of US Mesmerism* (Chicago, 2018)].

46 Compare the portrayal of moral therapy in Paisiello's *Nina*: S. Castelvecchi, 'From *Nina* to *Nina*: Psychodrama, Absorption and Sentiment in the 1780s', *Cambridge Opera Journal*, 8.2 (1996), pp. 91–112 at 94.

47 L. Feurzeig, 'Heroines in Perversity: Marie Schmith, Animal Magnetism, and the Schubert Circle', *19th-Century Music*, 21.2 (1997), pp. 223–243. Compare H. Goldschmidt, 'Schubert und kein Ende', *Beiträge zur Musik Wissenschaft*, 25 (1983), p. 290. Feurzeig tries, unconvincingly, to show that Mesmerism permeated some of Schubert's songs: pp. 240–243.

48 Kramer, 'Music as Cause and Cure', pp. 341–342.

49 A. Winter, *Mesmerized: Powers of Mind in Victorian Britain* (Chicago, 1998), pp. 314–15.

50 Gouk, 'Music, Melancholy, and Medical Spirits in Early Modern Thought'. For what follows see also J. Godwin, *Music and the Occult: French Musical Philosophies 1750–1950* (Rochester, NY, 1995), pp. 141–142.

51 (Paris, 1868), p. 21.

52 Godwin, *Music and the Occult*, p. 142.

53 See P. Washington, *Madame Blavatsky's Baboon: Theosophy and the Emergence of the Western Guru* (London, 1993).

54 H. P. Blavatsky, *The Secret Doctrine*, 2 vols (London, 1888, and many subsequent editions), vol. I, p. 555 (addenda to bk 1, no. 10).

55 Godwin, *Music and the Occult*, p. 157.

56 R. Steiner, *Anthroposophy: An Introduction* (1950, trans. London, 1983), *The Nature of Anthroposophy* (New York, 1964), *The Essential Steiner*, ed. R. McDermot (San Francisco, CA, 1984).

57 R. Steiner, *Eurhythmy as Visible Music* (London, 1977).

58 *Essential Steiner*, p. 349.

59 Ibid. p. 348. Compare D. P. Walker, 'The Astral Body in Renaissance Medicine', *Journal of the Warburg and Courtauld Institutes*, 21 (1958), pp. 119–133.

60 A. von Lange, *Man, Music and Cosmos* (London, 1992).

61 K. E. Bruscia, *Improvisational Models of Music Therapy* (Springfield, IL, 1987), pp. 30–32.

62 Gary Ansdell, personal communication.

63 *Music Therapy Research and Practice in Medicine: From Out of the Silence* (London, 1996), pp. 8, 152.

64 [D. Schroeder, 'Arnold Schoenberg as Poet and Librettist: Dualism, Epiphany, and *Die Jakobsleiter*', in R. A. Berman and C. M. Cross (eds), *Political and Religious Ideas in the Works of Arnold Schoenberg* (New York, 2000), pp. 41–59.]

65 F. Bowers, *Scriabin*, 2nd rev. edn, 2 vols (New York, 1996), II, p. 254. See also B. de Schloezer, *Scriabin: Artist and Mystic* (Oxford, 1987), pp. 236ff., 260ff.

66 *Moving into Aquarius*, new edn (St Albans, 1974), p. 156 (and p. 100).

67 M. Trend, *The Musik Makers: The English Musical Renaissance from Elgar to Britten* (London, 1985), pp. 144–147 at 146.

68 C. Scott, *Doctors, Disease and Health* (London, 1938), *Medicine, Rational and Irrational* (London, 1946), *An Outline of Modern Occultism* (London, 1935), *Music: Its Secret Influence Throughout the Ages* (London, 1958), quotation from p. 200.

69 M. Kurtz, *Stockhausen: A Biography* (London, 1992), pp. 185, 188, 190, 196, 207.

70 *Towards a Cosmic Music: Texts by Karlheinz Stockhausen*, ed. T. Nevill (Shaftesbury, 1989), p. 58. See also J. Cott, *Stockhausen: Conversations with the Composer* (London, 1974), pp. 113–114, a discussion of the music therapy of chickens.

17

THE PREHISTORY OF INFANT SEXUALITY

I

One feature of the popular view of the sexual instinct is that it is absent in childhood and only awakens in the period of life described as puberty . . . It is true that in the literature of the subject one occasionally comes across remarks upon precocious sexual activity in small children – upon erections, masturbation and even activities resembling coitus. But these are always quoted only as exceptional events... So far as I know, not a single author has clearly recognized the regular existence of a sexual instinct in childhood; and in the writings that have become so numerous on the development of children, the chapter on 'Sexual Development' is usually omitted.

So wrote Sigmund Freud, opening the second of the *Three Essays on the Theory of Sexuality* of, originally, 1905 (Pelican edn, 1977: 88). To this, even in the first of the work's several editions, he added a confirmatory footnote:

The assertion made in the text has since struck me as being so bold that I have undertaken the task of testing its validity by looking through the literature once more. The outcome of this is that I have allowed my statement to stand unaltered. The scientific examination of both the physical and mental phenomena of sexuality in childhood is still in its earliest beginnings. (Freud 1977: 89 n. 1; for the different editions, see Van Haute and Westerink 2016)

We can of course trace the development of Freud's thinking during the years preceding the publication of those remarks in considerable detail – through his abandonment of the 'seduction theory', his elaboration of the Oedipus complex, and his still tentative ideas on childhood sexuality in the aetiology of neurosis that were aired in a paper of 1898 (Gay 1985: 58).

Yet Freud did not, of course, *discover* infant sexuality as a 'regular' and not just an 'exceptional' phenomenon. His own footnotes hint as much. Almost every element in his conception of the topic had to some extent been anticipated during the nineteenth century by the sexologists. It is enough to recall such names as Maudesley, Dessoir, and Krafft-Ebing, or Havelock Ellis and Albert Moll (Kern 1973: 121; Sulloway 1979: 278; Van Haute and Westerink 2016). They did not all regard signs of childhood sexuality as rare or pathological. To take earlier and perhaps less familiar examples: in the 1840s Pierre Jean Corneille Debreyne, a theologian-physician, insisted in his writings on the frequency of infantile masturbation (Ellenberger 1970: 295), and Adolf Patze, an otherwise obscure German physician, observed, in a footnote to a pamphlet on bordellos, that 'the sexual drive already manifests itself among little six-, four-, and even three-year-old children' (Gay 1985: 58; 1989: 144).

Beside the writings of these sexologists we can set evidence such as that of Strindberg's autobiographical novel *The Son of a Servant* (*Tjänstekvinnans son*, 1886). In this, he records his realization, at the age of twelve, that many eight- or nine-year olds regularly attempted intercourse in the woods on the way home from school (Kern 1973: 119). And, because Strindberg is hardly a dispassionate witness to his time, let us also note the chilling case of a seven-year-old girl in Cleveland, Ohio. In 1894, as the ultimate remedy for her supposed persistent masturbation, she was subjected to clitoridectomy (Gay 1984: 304; compare DeMause 1976: 390, 420).

It can hardly be said, then – although Freud came close to saying it – that the nineteenth century was entirely ignorant of what he, Freud, took to be the ways of young children. His contribution was not to 'discover' infantile sexuality, or even to assert its normality, but rather to define its purported stages – oral, anal, phallic – and to integrate these into a full developmental scheme (Kern 1973: 137; Sulloway 1980: 457).

For all that, whether we consider his ideas science or metaphor, we live (even now, still) in the age of Freud, and not, say, of Krafft-Ebing. That is one of two reasons why I begin with him. His spreading influence in the last century shows us what a mutation in the prevailing conception of childhood can look like; it shows how widespread yet discrete 'perceptions' of supposed sexuality in young children do not necessarily amount to the sort of collective acceptance which we might call 'cultural recognition'; and that can be useful.

Freud himself exemplifies the mutation on a personal scale. It took him some years to become reconciled to the implications of his presumed discovery. Even in the first edition of *The Interpretation of Dreams* (actually published in 1899) he could still – as had Rousseau – aver that childhood is 'innocent of sexual desires' (Pelican Freud, 1976: 37). If we remember how Freud maintained that view, in the face of what he himself had written since abandoning the seduction theory, we can perhaps better make sense of those much earlier figures who upheld childhood innocence despite what others at the time thought to be contrary evidence.

A second reason for beginning with Freud is that his comments about the sexology of his time could also be applied mutatis mutandis to modern historical discussion of this theme. There are isolated references but few syntheses. This may be partly because Freud so dominates our thinking that those nineteenth-century figures who anticipated him seem, by themselves, to constitute the obscure prehistory of the subject. Anything written or said before 1845 belongs to a scarcely imaginable early phase of that prehistory, its Jurassic period (Gay 1989: 144). And when pre-nineteenth-century evidence of childhood sexuality is brought into play, it is likely to treated as in some way special; it will be pressed into the service of a preconceived theory – as when Philippe Ariès (1973: chs 4, 5) drew on Héroard's record of the supposed promiscuity of the infant Louis XIII in his long-debated (and ultimately rejected) exposition of the discovery of childhood (Marvick 1976). We need greater chronological depth. To that extent the subject is, as Freud said, 'still in its earliest beginnings'.

The following is thus sketchy and serendipitous. It sidesteps the problem of defining the expression of sexuality by accepting only relatively unambiguous evidence of sexual behaviour *attributed* to children. In other words, in Freudian terms the topic is genital rather than oral or anal. There will be nothing on the history of – even for psychoanalysts – ambiguous activities such as thumb-sucking or potty training. Nor is what follows an attempt to recreate the actual behaviour or the emotions and drives of children in the past, or in other cultures: it is about adult ideas of children in their cultural contexts. Yet nor is it an exercise in uncovering child abuse or identifying potential abusers. The condemnations of what were presumed to be childhood expressions of sexuality might have been sharpened in particular cases by ugly motives – but that motivation is mostly lost to us and is in any case not my focus here.

II

Rather than begin at the beginning, let us go first to the early Middle Ages, and to a vivid yet relatively little-known and still less explicated text. I shall then work outwards from that, looking both earlier and later, and eventually try to reach some tentative conclusions about the phases into which the history of this subject might be divided.

The text on which I focus is just one subsection in the *Penitential of Cummean* (ed. Bieler 1963: 108–135). But I should first introduce the whole work and the genre to which it belongs. A penitential is a schedule of sins and their prescribed penances, drawn up for the convenience of confessors. It developed as a genre in the British and Irish churches from the sixth century (Meens 2014, a magisterial survey; see now also Abraham 2017: ch. 1). With the exception of what is known as the *Old Irish Penitential*, the *Penitential of Cummean* is the most comprehensive of the early texts from Ireland (Bieler 1963: 5; Meens 2014: 57–62). *Cummean* survives complete in only three manuscripts, of the ninth and tenth centuries (Körntgen 1993: 91–98; Meens 2014: 60 n. 105). Its author was most likely Cumineus (Cumianus), or Cummaine Fota, bishop of Clonfert, who according to the Annals of Ulster died in 662 (McNeill and Gamer 1938: 98). Therefore, the text falls within a century or so of the identifiable insular beginnings of the genre in Ireland (Charles-Edwards 1992: 78). The *Penitential of Cummean* is the first that we have to be organized according to John Cassian's fifth-century formulation of the eight capital sins (*Conferences* 5.2; see McNeill and Gamer 1938: 19; Bieler 1963: 246 n. 4).

In common with much of the early penitential material, Cummean has a great deal to say about sexual misdemeanours – a propensity that prompted the notorious horrified judgement of that great Bede scholar and Celticist Charles Plummer: 'it is hard to see how anyone could busy himself with such literature and not be the worse for it' (Plummer 1898, vol. I: clviii). Indeed, the interest displayed by the penitentials in the subtle taxonomy of sexual acts and aspirations is matched only by their concern with food and its various possible sources of contamination (Bieler 1963: 163, 177, 217). Cummian's section on fornication is the longest of his Cassianic eight. But the canons that are of concern here come in a later and subsidiary section headed 'The decrees of our fathers . . . on the playing (*ludi*) of boys' (Bieler 1963: 127).

To summarize: Boys talking alone and (thereby?) breaking the rules of the elders, three special fasts. Those who kiss simply (*oscula simpliciter facientes*), six fasts; licentiously (*inlecebrosum*), but without pollution (that is, from semen), eight; with pollution or embrace, ten (10.1–2, Bieler 1963: 126–127). These boys, as the next canon (3) indicates, are adolescents under 20. But then attention shifts to an earlier age, to (apparently) the pre-pubescent: '*minimi* imitating acts of fornication (*fornicationem imitantes*) and stimulating one another, but who are not defiled because of their immature age, twenty days penance; if frequently, forty' (10.4, Bieler 1963: 128–129, trans. modified). Bieler renders *minimi* as children. But the whole section concerns delinquent boys: girls are mentioned only as the objects of delinquency (canon 17). Alongside this canon on *minimi* should be set one that comes a few lines later (9): 'a small boy (*puer paruulus*) misused/abused (*oppressus*) by an older one (*maiore*), if he is ten years of age [or older?], shall fast for a week; if he consents, for twenty days'.

What should a proper commentary on these canons look like – beyond the preliminary suggestion that here may be a moment, a significant point, in the history of ascribed infant or (perhaps better) prepubescent sexuality, when someone claims to be identifying and attempting to discipline it? First, a general prefatory point. We can say nothing about the frequency with which matters of this kind presented themselves to seventh-century Celtic confessors – or indeed to any medieval confessors. But we can, I think, detect the spirit in which they were considered. There may be a degree of realism: imitation of mature sexual behaviour might be thought all too likely in the cramped and undivided sleeping conditions of many medieval households (Thacker 1992: 160). There is also a humanity, an understanding alertness to intention, in Cummean and others of his kind, and that humanity contradicts (if contradiction were needed) the ideas of Charles M. Radding (1978: 589), on the early medieval preoccupation with act rather than motive. Against Radding, and other commentators who suspect that these texts are mechanical and superficial – mere literary exercises – I would set Cummean 2.14: 'he who for a long time is lured in thought to commit fornication, and resists too half-heartedly (*tepidius*), shall do penance for one or two or more days according to the duration of the thought' (Bieler 1963: 114–115). Despite the tabulation and the tariffs, there is no emphasis on mere externalities here – which is as we should expect in a relationship of confessor to penitent characterized at the time as 'soul friendship' (Charles-Edwards 1992: 92). Perhaps that is the context in which we should interpret the unusual provision for the (probably) abused child who does not consent but is nonetheless penanced (Payer 1984: 42, 171 n.129).

Those are impressions about the 'spirit of the laws'. I turn to more specific points about the letter of the law. First, as we read the earlier penitential material, both Welsh and Irish, nothing prepares us for these canons. We become all too used to prescriptions for the remission of fornication, adultery, incest, sodomy, bestiality, masturbation, the kissing of virgins, abortion, and unsatisfied lust. But these nearly all concern adults. Cummean's prescription for *minimi* apparently comes out of nowhere. A late ninth-century Bobbio MS now in the Ambrosian Library represents a missing source of Cummean's Penitential (Bieler 1963: 6; Meens 2014: 8). But the canons of interest are not in this presumed source, the 'Ambrosian Penitential'; and that throws into even sharper relief the apparent novelty of Cummean's concern to discipline prepubescent sexuality.

Next, we must clearly ask about the ages of young males involved. It would surely be a mistake to expect too much precision in the wording (Payer 1984: 42). Medieval schemes of the ages of man are notoriously inconsistent. We are presented here with *minimi, pueri paruuli*, and *pueri*. Adulthood is seemingly not reached until well after the age of 20. A boy is small at around ten, and capable of punishable sin even when passive to an elder's advances. (And yet, disconcertingly, in a slightly later continental text, a *puer parvulus* can be 20: Meens 1994: 53–54). Can *minimi* be understood strictly as very small boys, significantly younger than ten, to some degree responding to the common medieval definition of *infantia*, derived from Isidore, as running from birth to seven (Isidore, *Origines* 11.2, with Metz 1976: 18)? Children who appear in the early penitentials are never called *infantes*; mostly they are labelled *pueri* (Meens 1994: 53). But we must not press too heavily on these clauses, for in them *pueritia* certainly extends later than the 14 we might expect; indeed, *infantia, pueritia,* and *adolescentia* as Isidore would define them have been run together (Shahar 1990: 22, 264–265), creating, as Rob Meens has put it, a 'long *pueritia*' (1994: 54 n. 3; see also Abraham 2017: ch. 2). It does, however, seem that boys younger than the fourteen or so years of age that were usually taken to mark the beginning of adolescence are involved here, even perhaps boys still in infancy. The tenor of the canons accords with the view later taken by a number of didactic authors that from seven onwards a child needs careful attention and training (Shahar 1990: 24). And there are closer comparisons that can be drawn with Cummian's reference to age ten – for example some later canonists' notion that a sub-stage within *pueritia* commenced half-way through it in the eleventh year (Shahar 1990: 24; Metz 1976: 19).

We also need to look for context in the history of the sacraments. It can be assumed that Cummean's boys would have been baptized. In slightly later continental penitentials, the penance for those who let their children die unbaptized rises sharply if the child is older than three: perhaps the maximum permissible age for baptism (Meens 1994: 59–60). We might further assume that the boys had been confirmed – although confirmation is, in terms of the surviving evidence, the most elusive of the early medieval sacraments (Blair and Sharpe 1992; Metz 1976: 60–61). What are the implications of this sacramental context for our understanding of the canons? The medieval western theology of the matter, deriving of course from Augustine, is in essence that children are born with original sin, which is washed away at baptism, and are then blameless for at least a few years until, around the age of seven, they develop a capacity for acquired or personal sin. Emphasize the original sin, the weakness of the young child's soul, and you have what Shahar has reasonably characterized as the negative medieval view of childhood. Emphasize the weakness of the infant's body – its incompleteness, dependence, vulnerability; recall also Isidore of Seville's etymology of *pueritia* (boyhood) from *puritas* (purity), and you have the positive image (Shahar 1990: 14–19, 45ff.). Which image is favoured will naturally depend on the rhetorical context: the early Middle Ages can hardly be expected to speak to us with one voice. The canon law of later centuries might place the age of discretion, and the capacity for betrothal, at seven (Metz 1976: 28, 65), and the boys seem to have passed beyond that. But we must remember that this is an early and not a high medieval text, that the age of the boys is far from clear, and that early medieval canon law on such matters was far from settled. We can presume that, among these *minimi*, the effects of baptism were wearing off. Yet the penance, of twenty days fasting, is hardly severe in comparison with the years of abstention that Cummean elsewhere prescribes. Twenty days is for instance the penance for minor theft by what we would call a young adult, for 'an evil word or glance' of a sexual nature, and for small boys who strike one another (1.13=10.11; 2.12; 10.21).

One way out of the thicket may have been provided by Peter Cramer in his monograph *Baptism and Change*. He writes of an ambiguity in early medieval thought on baptism, and contrasts a view of it as a 'once-for-all triumph' with the notion that it is, rather, 'an image, and an intense re-enactment, of the *continuously-repeated* [my emphasis] ethical journey from sin to repentance' (Cramer 1993: 116). I suggest we invoke the latter view to begin to interpret Cummean's canons. Such enquiries as he postulates are perhaps staging-posts on that journey. That is why it would be a mistake to expect to determine exactly what stage in their sacramental progress Cummean's boys were supposed to have reached.

Enough sacramental theology. The next question to ask is: what sort of boys are we dealing with; whose sexuality is being disciplined? Was the 'audience' for this part of the penitential a restricted one? Canon 17 refers to a 'boy coming from the world', as if into a monastery, as an oblate. It is tempting to associate the concern for pre-pubescent homosexuality with monasticism, because it is an expression of that anxiety about the proximity of monks to one another which goes back to the very beginnings of the monastic movement (Rousselle 1988: 148; Boswell 1981: 159, 183, 188). Cummean certainly addresses his penitential overwhelmingly to men and boys; females are rarely mentioned. He was presumably a monk as well as a bishop. And yet there is no compelling reason why the scope of the canons of concern here should have been strictly limited to monks and quasi-monastic 'lay clients' (Frantzen 1982: 29 n. 33; Meens 2014: 59–60), either when Cummean drew them up or in their later life. Elsewhere (e.g. 2.2, 17, 22) Cummean distinguishes penances for monks from those for clergy and laity. And in any case monasteries were not, in this place and period, the specialized and exclusive institutions that we might imagine (Sharpe 1992: 99, 101). Therefore, we should be chary of attributing a specifically monastic colour to the early Irish penitentials.

What sort of occasion should be envisaged for the perhaps delicate enquiry into, and confession of, imitated fornication? An evocative source, though imbued with too much optimism to be taken as reportage, is the eighth-century *Dialogue* of Egbert of York: during the twelve days before Christmas, he writes, not only the clergy in their *monasteriis* (minster churches) but also the laity with their wives and families (families defined by kinship or by co-residence) would resort to their confessors, and would wash themselves of carnal concupiscence by tears, community life, and almsgiving (Thacker 1992: 161).

But at what age were children able to confess and do penance in the early Middle Ages? In her book on childhood, Shulamith Shahar (1990: 25, 266; see also Metz 1976: 65) rightly reports that some theologians later held that a child was capable of sin and should therefore confess from the start of *pueritia* – that is, from seven onwards. In the sixth century, Pope Gregory the Great had identified the development of the capacity for post-baptismal sin with the beginnings of speech; indeed, he knew of a child who learned to blaspheme at the age of five (de Vogüé 1978–80: Dialogues IV.18, with Mounteer 187: 241). If speech brings sin, it might have been argued, it also facilitates confession, and the expiation of sin. In any case, confession, however 'private' in Cummean's time, was hardly a matter for the individual alone. We may envisage Cummean's *minimi* as talking quietly to their confessor in the *cubiculum sacerdotis* to which a continental *ordo confessionis* refers (Kottje 1987). Can we so easily envisage the preceding process as one involving just their consciences, and no familial or societal prods – or indeed hindrances, for this was perhaps one area (among many) in which a family might not want to cooperate with the Church's scrutiny of its venial sins, or might not reckon them sins at all?

III

To say that is to hint at a wider cultural background than I have so far embraced. What background is relevant? One could of course go back a long way and cast the net widely. Much has for instance been written about the passive homosexuality of very young boys in ancient times from classical Greece to the time of the later Roman empire (Rousselle 1988: 134; see now also Vickers and Nash Briggs 2007), about the abuse involved in ancient child abandonment and prostitution, and about very early – that is, prepubertal – marriage for girls (the last quite rare, it now seems: the mock wedding of an immature boy and seven-year-old girl in *The Satyricon*, 14.24–25, is far removed from the norm suggested by epitaphs) (Boswell 1981: 81).

These subjects clearly overlap my own; but at what points they do so is unclear, because the evidence for them mostly concerns the children far less than it does their elders. And when children are brought into the picture, questions of status and honour are usually far more important than those of pleasure and pain. In classical Greece, an honourable (adult) *erômenos*, according to Dover's classic yet still controversial account, 'does not seek or expect sensual pleasure from contact with a [boy] *erastês*' (1978: 103). Doubtless some *erômenoi* did, and in theory they were treated, Plutarch asserted, 'as the lowest of the low' (103 n. 87). In practice, as the pagan Libanius and Chrysostom claim to witness, from their divergent standpoints, in Antioch of the fourth century, children of ten or even seven were keenly corrupted (Laes 2011: 250–252; for wider scholarly context on 'Greek love' and pederasty, see Davidson 2007, esp. chs 4 and 5, and the overview of Lear 2014).

Overall, we can generalize that both the Greeks and the Romans upon whose writings we depend managed simultaneously to uphold the modesty of young children as a precious commodity and to condone frequent child abuse as we would now define it. They also, in part as validation of those abusive traditions, asserted that the prepubescent had sexual appetites of their own (Boswell 1981: 81). In comedies and satyr plays, boys were seen as sexual beings from an early age and addressed as *posthôn*, 'penis'. A fragment of Aeschylus even has the satyr Silenus propositioning the baby Perseus (Golden 2005: 48). In keeping with that attitude, Xenophon approves the practice of the Persians: 'we do not discuss sexual matters in front of very young boys; if lax discipline should give free rein to their passions, the young might indulge them to excess' (Golden 2005: 57, *Cyr.* 1.6.34).

I turn next to the Christian sources. It is the patristic material that supplies the most pertinent context for Cummean's canons. We cannot avoid Augustine. The striking passage does not come from the *Confessions*, in which Augustine unwittingly threw down the gauntlet to the psycho-historians. Nor does it come from one of the texts in the front line of Augustine's debates with Origen and Pelagius about original sin and the soul's origin. It is, rather, from the discussion of baptism in book 10 of the *Literal Commentary on Genesis* (XIII.23).

> We shall not deal with *pueri grandiusculi* to whom some [Pelagius? Caelestius?] are unwilling to attribute personal sins except from the age of fourteen when puberty begins. We would willingly admit this if there were no other sins than those that concern the genital organs. Who would dare to deny that theft, lying and perjury are not sins except those who want to commit them with impunity?' (Agaësse and Solignac 1972, vol. 2: 182–4)

No pre-pubescent sexuality there, though many other sins are.

It is the eastern Roman world that gives the sort of background I hoped to find in western sources. Sometime in the middle decades of the fourth century, Basil of Ancyra (Ankara) wrote a treatise on virginity as a guide for the female ascetics of his region. 'A man of recondite learning and singularly unruffled powers of observation', as Peter Brown puts it (1989: 267), also a former doctor, Basil claimed to know that there was really no such thing as sexual innocence, whatever one's youth or ascetic commitment: 'no young girl', he wrote, 'is so innocent as she reaches puberty as not to be aware to some degree of the nature of that person from whose side she was torn [Adam]) . . . In the unripeness of their limbs children are detected imitating copulation with men' (Migne, *Patrologia Graeca* 30.801BC; Brown 1989: 268; compare Gould 1994: 46).

IV

Basil had medical experience, and the girls about and for whom he was writing in that passage were approaching puberty. And that points toward an obvious line of enquiry that I have so far omitted: medical or scientific writings on adolescence.

Aristotle, or more likely pseudo-Aristotle, writing on *Physical Problems* (XXX.953b36, Golden 2005: 48 n.), had observed that boys enjoy rubbing their penises even before they have quite reached an age when they are able to ejaculate. The various medical traditions of antiquity and the Middle Ages evince a comparably restricted range of interest in prepubescent sexuality. That is, they look no further back in the life of the child than the period leading up to the first seminal discharge or to menarche. Puberty is not thought to have origins deep in infancy. Indeed, if the discussion needed to be extended in any direction, the medical writers would take it further on into adolescence because, in boys, the earliest discharges were often considered sterile (Eyben 1972). The case of women was of course more complicated because of debate on the function of female seed; but Soranus (*Gynaecology* I.33) writes of badly brought-up girls who arouse in themselves premature desires (trans. Temkin 1956: 31) and who may even conceive before menarche (Temkin 1956: 25; Rousselle 1988: 35).

According to Aristotle, boys first produced semen toward the end of the fourteenth year, but it remained sterile until the seventeenth or even the twenty-first year. For Galen, following Hippocrates, puberty came after the end of the fourteenth year or even one or two years later; and it lasted until the age of twenty-five. In the wake of Joan Cadden's excellent monograph, *Meanings of Sex Differences in the Middle Ages* (1993), medieval variations on this theme can easily be mustered. But it is to the *De animalibus* of Albertus Magnus that we turn for, as Cadden writes (1993: 146), 'the fullest medieval account of puberty'. Cummean dealt with boys who imitate intercourse but are too immature to pollute themselves. Albert recognized that sexual desire can awaken in both boys and girls before either can achieve emission. They then turn to masturbation, and 'pollutions' may arise before long (*De Animalibus* book 9, 1.1.6–7, quoted Cadden 1993: 146 n. 114).

Albert fancies that he can tell us what girls on the brink of maturity imagine when they are lustful, as well as what they do. Yet a humoral aetiology of sexual development, derived largely from Galen, sets firm parameters to Albert's thought and observation. His psychology of female adolescence is embedded in an account of physiological processes. The general notion inherited from antiquity that human development is a process of desiccation, and that adolescence is the transition from the predominance of blood to that of yellow bile, militated against the perception of precocious sexuality in children. To put it another way, the medical tradition gives us the preliminary to puberty, proto-pubescent sexuality we might call it, not the prepubescent kind.

V

Glancing at the medical-scientific view of puberty has brought us back from antiquity into the Middle Ages. In the last section of this paper, I am concerned to establish to what extent prepubescent sexuality continued to be recognized after Cummean. That way I can, after a fashion, work my way back toward Freud, with whom we began.

A canon such as Cummean's, once recorded, ought to have remained within the medieval confessor's repertoire. But it does not. To cut a long textual history short: the canons about child sexuality reappear, slightly modified, in the vernacular *Old Irish Penitential*, plausibly datable to the eighth century (2.28, immature boys and girls kissing; 2.30, little boys imitating fornication: ed. Gwynn 1915: 144; Bieler 1963: 264–265; Meens 2014: 62; Abraham 2017: 75–76).

In England, their reception is less obvious. That concerning a *parvulus* being abused by an older boy comes back in the penitential attributed to Bede (3.22,32, Payer 1984: 151). In the penitential attributed to Theodore, archbishop of Canterbury, there is a canon concerning a mother who imitates fornication with her little son (McNeill and Gamer 1938: 186.20), but only she is to do penance. Otherwise nothing in the insular tradition, it seems.

On the continent, meanwhile, the canons became more widely diffused, especially through the composite so-called *Excarpsus* of Cummean (2.15, Schmitz 1898: 610). But here significant textual variations start to appear. Some manuscripts drop the word 'imitation' and make the behaviour of the *minimi* real fornication, thereby, perhaps, shifting the focus from prepubescence to the more familiar ground of what I have called proto-pubescence. Various other penitentials of the Carolingian period include excerpts from or echoes of the Cummean canons (Schmitz 1898: 186, 330, 355). The Valicellian penitential of the later ninth century has a clause about the mutual pollution, manual or femoral, of ten-year olds, and this reappears in Regino of Prüm in the early tenth century. Then the trail thins and in effect peters out (Payer 1984; Lutterbach 1999: 108).

Perhaps it was obliterated. Some degree of conscious editing is almost certainly involved. Carolingian church reformers of the eighth to ninth centuries did not like the often contradictory penitential canons that had been imported from Ireland and had gained currency in Frankish manuscripts, although they did not dispense with the penitential as a genre (Meens 2014: 114–123). If continental texts such as the so-called St Gall penitential represent the unofficial, more chaotic side of the continental penitential tradition, then a collection such as that of Halitgar of Cambrai can count as reformed and official (111–112, 131–132). Halitgar incorporated some of Cummean's canons on *pueri* into his own. But he left out the one about imitated fornication. To judge simply by what is in the texts, concern for this kind of sin on the part of confessors seems to disappear before we reach the high Middle Ages. And if we look forward in time to the *summae confessorum*, the more systematic and sophisticated confessors' manuals produced from the twelfth century onwards, then we find much less of the same interest in the sexuality of the very young. In Alan of Lille, Bartholemew of Exeter, Thomas of Chobham, and their ilk, the sections on fornication are overwhelmingly preoccupied with the delinquency of adults (Payer 2009).

The change, if I am right about it, is easier to describe than to explain. One explanation might be couched in terms of the predominance of the positive view of childhood in the High Middle Ages. Or again, the more frequent confessions of adults, in the wake of the Fourth Lateran Council, may have left confessors little time or energy to worry about children's doings and need guidance on them from the *summae*. Indeed children may no longer have been expected to confess (Orme 2001: 215). Another explanation is that the early penitentials are monastic in character, and that their canons on boys reflect an especial concern with oblates; their function was later taken over by monastic rules. The *summae confessorum*, by contrast, concern the sins of the laity, and the sexual misdemeanours of lay children was felt to be of less importance. I have already given one reason for receiving this attractive hypothesis with caution. It is simply that the early penitentials are not narrowly and specifically monastic in colour. Another reason for rejecting it is that prepubescent sexuality as it were re-emerges in the literature of confession at the end of the Middle Ages. This has been seen as something entirely new. John Bossy, for instance, describes Gerson as a 'pathfinder' (1985: 49). Cummean had trodden the path before him.

The later medieval texts in which prepubescent sexuality comes to the fore are well known, and have been drawn together by Shulamith Shahar. In his *Instructions for Parish Priests*, John Myrc counselled against letting children over seven sleep together 'lest they between them breed the liking of that foul deed' (Shahar 1990: 101). The main figure of interest, though, is that great advocate of sympathetic enquiry into childhood sin – and scourge of masturbators – Jean Gerson. Boys, he observed, of ten begin to masturbate at the age of five, or even as young as three (Brundage 1987: 535; Shahar 1990: 176).

Since we have moved into the later Middle Ages, evidence other than that of penitentials and associated texts becomes more plentiful. But its tenor is not new. From pagan antiquity onward, there had been numerous warnings about the susceptibility of the very young. Doctor Bernard de Gordon, for instance, had asserted that the young child should be prevented from seeing adult pudenda and indecent acts (Demaitre 1977: 481; Shahar 1990: 19, 100). In his *Yconomica* of 1352, Konrad of Megenberg admonishes those who teach young girls to masturbate (Krüger 1973: 89). More vividly, the author of a set of miracles attributed to Giovanna of Signa (d. 1307) emphasizes the struggle of parents to inculcate a sense of shame in their female offspring.

A man named Duccio Aringhi . . . had a daughter named Laurentia, who as an infant had been taken out of her cradle by her mother. When the swaddling clothes had been removed, the girl always put her hands in her lower fontal area and near her groin [instead of behind her back as healthy girls would], indicating in her own body a quite unnatural vice. Much distressed by this, the father commended her to the blessed Giovanna, vowing that if she should be freed [from this vice] he would take her to the saint's tomb with candle worth five *solidi*. (Trans. Goodich 1994: 495, adapted.)

Yet more extreme is the early fifteenth-century Dominican Giovanni Dominici, condemned to haunt the pages of the *Journal of Psychohistory*. In his opinion, the child's modesty should ideally be protected from the age of three. From that age on, he should not see naked adults, he should wear a nightshirt reaching below the knee, he should not be hugged, kissed, or petted, he should not share a bed with siblings (Shahar 1990: 101).

I hope I shall not be charged with impiety if, in this somewhat context, suggestive of child abuse as well as child sexuality, I now introduce some Christian iconography. Leo Steinberg in his highly controversial *The Sexuality of Christ in Renaissance Art and in Modern Oblivion* (1995) drew attention to the large body of Renaissance devotional imagery in which the genitalia of the infant or the dead Christ 'receive such demonstrative emphasis that one must recognize an "*ostentatio genitalium*" [Steinberg's coinage] comparable to the *canonic ostentatio vulnerum*' (1996: 1). Steinberg argues that, if there is such an *ostentatio genitalium*, it must be interpreted above all in terms of the theology of the Incarnation. There is something more than descriptive naturalism in those pictures in which the Christ child's member appears to be erect. Granted – but the naturalism may be there in the background, iconographically speaking, to the theology. We have already come across infantile erection and masturbation. And I could, earlier, have recalled the tradition running from the medical writings of antiquity to Fallopio and beyond (Rousselle 1988; Steinberg 1996: 117) of encouraging parents and nurses to manipulate their boys' penises, like other parts of their bodies, into an acceptable size and shape. It would, quite generally, be convenient to associate this imagery with the renewed emphasis on prepubescent sexuality that seems to prevail in the texts I have just reviewed. The imagery certainly develops at the 'right' time, the later fourteenth century, during which the Christ child is first depicted naked or only partially covered. But that change has many causes, theological and artistic, that have nothing to do with sex. So the association, if it be allowed at all, can only be a loose one.

Such looseness seems, as I try to sum it up this whole project, inevitably to characterize the history of childhood sexuality. I have no grand conclusion about how much of the evidence I have reviewed arises from adult projection, how much from relatively unprejudiced observation. Nor can I be at all confident that I have avoided confusing change in the nature and quantity of the evidence with broader historical change. I have proposed that Cummean's penitential may signal a 'moment' of some kind in the perception and mild discipline of such sexuality, a change in the degree of cultural recognition accorded to it. I would like to be able to identify other such moments, because I think that a history divided into phases in this way makes more sense of the recalcitrant texts than one conceived in terms of, for example, repression simply increasing across the centuries, period by period. (That, incidentally, is why this has been a paper free, until now, of Foucault. His best remarks on the Middle Ages, not in the *History of Sexuality*, but in lectures of the 1970s at the Collège de France, still do not go very deep; and his criticism of the 'danger of child sexuality' and plea for decriminalizing the relations between adults and minors, in a debate of 1978, reads very uncomfortably today (Foucault 2003: 170–176; 1988: 271–285).)

One of these other moments perhaps lurks somewhere in the later Middle Ages. Another, with which I began, is marked by the writings of Freud in the years around 1900. And it may be that still another has occurred more recently. I said that we still live in the age of Freud. But if so, it is the Freud of the seduction theory rather than the Freud of the *Three Essays*. What Freud said about the writings on child development of his own time applies again to their textbook successors. Most of them leave childhood sexuality out. There has been little serious work since Kinsey. The cultural recognition forced on us by Freud has been tacitly withdrawn. We now once again assert the innocence of children and reserve our attention for abusive adults.

Acknowledgements

For comments and references that have much improved earlier versions of this paper, I am most grateful to Peter Biller, William MacLehose, Janet Nelson, Chris Wickham, and Joseph Ziegler, as well as to participants in seminars at which its preliminary forms were aired, in London and Oxford. Faults and inadequacies that stubbornly remain are of course all mine.

References

Abraham, E. V. (2017). *Anticipating Sin in Medieval Society: Childhood, Sexuality, and Violence in the Early Penitentials.* Amsterdam: Amsterdam University Press.

Agaësse, P. and Solignac, A. (ed. and trans.) (1972). *Oeuvres de Saint Augustin. La Genèse au sens littéral.* 2 vols. Bruges: Desclée de Brouwer.

Bieler, L. (ed.) (1963). *The Irish Penitentials.* Dublin: Dublin Institute for Advanced Studies.

Blair, J. and Sharpe, R. (eds) (1992). *Pastoral Care Before the Parish.* Leicester: Leicester University Press.

Bossy, J. (1985). *Christianity in the West, 1400–1700.* Oxford: Oxford University Press.

Boswell, J. (1981). *Christianity, Social Tolerance, and Homosexuality: Gay People in Western Europe from the Beginning of the Christian Era to the Fourteenth Century.* Chicago: University of Chicago Press.

Brown, P. (1989). *The Body and Society: Men, Women, and Sexual Renunciation in Early Christianity.* London: Faber and Faber.

Brundage, J. A. (1987). *Law, Sex and Christian Society in Medieval Europe.* Chicago: University of Chicago Press.

Cadden, J. (1993). *Meanings of Sex Difference in the Middle Ages: Medicine, Science, and Culture.* Cambridge: Cambridge University Press.

Charles-Edwards, T. (1992). The Pastoral Role of the Church in the Early Irish Laws. In J. Blair and R. Sharpe (eds), *Pastoral Care Before the Parish*, 63–80. Leicester: Leicester University Press.

Cramer, P. (1993). *Baptism and Change in the Early Middle Ages, c.200–c.1150.* Cambridge: Cambridge University Press.

Davidson, J. (2007). *The Greeks and Greek Love: A Radical Reappraisal of Homosexuality in Ancient Greece.* London: Weidenfeld and Nicolson.

de Vogüé, A. (ed. and trans.) (1978–80). *Grégoire le Grand. Dialogues.* 3 vols. Paris: Éditions du Cerf.

Demaitre, L. (1977). The Idea of Childhood and Child Care in the Medical Writings of the Middle Ages. *Journal of Psychohistory*, 4: 461–490.

DeMause, L. (ed.) (1976). *The History of Childhood.* London: Souvenir Press.

Dover, K. (1978). *Greek Homosexuality.* London: Duckworth.

Ellenberger, H. F. (1970). *The Discovery of The Unconscious: The History and Evolution of Dynamic Psychiatry.* London: Allen Lane.

Eyben, E. (1972). Antiquity's View of Puberty. *Latomus*, 31: 677–697.

Foucault, M., ed. L. D. Kritzman (1988). *Michel Foucault: Politics, Philosophy, Culture: Interviews and Other Writings 1977–1984.* New York: Routledge.

Foucault, M. (2003). *Abnormal: Lectures at the Collège de France 1974–1975.* London: Verso.

Frantzen, A. J. (1982). The Tradition of Penitentials in Anglo-Saxon England. *Anglo-Saxon England*, 11: 23–56.

Freud, S. (1976). *The Interpretation of Dreams.* Harmondsworth: Penguin.

Freud, S. (1977). *On Sexuality: Three Essays on the Theory of Sexuality and Other Works.* Harmondsworth: Penguin.

Gay, P. (1984). *The Bourgeois Experience: Victoria to Freud*, vol. I: *The Education of the Senses.* Oxford: Oxford University Press.

Gay, P. (1985). *Freud for Historians.* New York: Oxford University Press.

Gay, P. (1989). *Freud: A Life for Our Time.* London: Papermac.

Golden, M. (2015). *Children and Childhood in Classical Athens.* 2nd edn. Baltimore, MD: Johns Hopkins University Press.

Goodich, M. (1994). Sexuality, Family, and the Supernatural in the Fourteenth Century. *Journal of the History of Sexuality*, 4.4: 493–516.

Gould, G. (1992). Childhood in Eastern Patristic Thought: Some Problems of Theology and Theological Anthropology. *Studies in Church History*, 31: 39–52.

Gwynn, E. J. (1914). An Irish Penitential. *Ériu*, 7: 121–195.

Kern, S. (1973). Freud and the Discovery of Child Sexuality. *History of Childhood Quarterly*, 1.1: 117–141.

Körntgen, L. (1993). *Studien zu den Quellen der frühmittelalterlichen Bußbücher.* Sigmaringen: Jan Thorbecke.

Kottje, R. (1987). Busspraxis und Bussritus. *Segni e riti nella Chiesa altomedievale* (Settimane di Studio del Centro italiano di studi sull'alto medioevo, Spoleto), 42: 369–395.

Krüger, S. (ed.) (1973). *Konrad von Megenberg. Ökonomik (Buch I).* Stuttgart: Anton Hiersemann.

Laes, C. (2014). *Childhood in the Roman Empire: Outsiders Within.* Cambridge: Cambridge University Press.

Lear, A. (2013). Ancient Pederasty. In T. K. Hubbard (ed.), *A Companion to Greek and Roman Sexualities*, 106–131. Chichester: Wiley-Blackwell.

Lutterbach, H. (1999). *Sexualität im Mittelalter. Eine Kulturstudie anhand von Bussbüchern des 6. bis 12. Jahrhunderts.* Cologne: Böhlau.

Marvik, E. W. (1976). Nature versus Nurture: Patterns and Trends in Seventeenth-Century French Child-Rearing. In L. DeMause (ed.), *The History of Childhood*, 259–301. London: Souvenir Press.

McNeill, J. T. and Gamer, H. M. (1938). *Medieval Handbooks of Penance: A Translation of the Principal Libri Poenitentiales and Selections from Related Documents.* New York: Columbia University Press.

Meens, R. (1994). Children and Confession in the Early Middle Ages. *Studies in Church History* 31: 53–65.

Meens, R. (2014). *Penance in Medieval Europe 600–1200.* Cambridge: Cambridge University Press.

Metz, R. (1976). L'enfant dans le droit canonique medieval. *Recueils de la Société Jean Bodin*, 36.2: 9–96.

Mounteer, C. A. (1987), Roman Childhood 200 BC to AD 600. *Journal of Psychohistory*, 14: 233–254.

Orme, N. (2001). *Medieval Children.* New Haven, CT: Yale University Press.

Payer, P. J. (1984). *Sex and the Penitentials: The Development of a Sexual Code, 550–1150.* Toronto: University of Toronto Press.

Payer, P. J. (2009). *Sex and the New Medieval Literature of Confession, 1150–1300.* Toronto: Pontifical Institute of Mediaeval Studies.

Plummer, C. (1898). *Venerabilis Bedae opera historica.* 2 vols. Oxford: Clarendon Press.

Radding, C. M. (1978). The Evolution of Medieval Mentalities: A Cognitive-Structural Approach. *American Historical Review*, 83.3: 577–597.

Rousselle, A. (1988). *Porneia: On Desire and the Body in Antiquity*, trans. F. Pheasant. Oxford: Blackwell.

Schmitz, H. J. (1898). *Die Bussbücher und das kanonische Bussverfahren*, vol. II of *Die Bussbücher und die Bussdisciplin der Kirche.* Mainz: Franz Kirchheim.

Shahar, S. (1990). *Childhood in the Middle Ages.* London: Routledge.

Sharpe, R. (1992). Churches and Communities in Early Medieval Ireland: Towards a Pastoral Model. In J. Blair and R. Sharpe (eds), *Pastoral Care Before the Parish*, 81–109. Leicester: Leicester University Press.

Steinberg, T. (1996). *The Sexuality of Christ in Renaissance Art and in Modern Oblivion.* 2nd rev. edn. Chicago: University of Chicago Press.

Sulloway, P. (1980). *Freud: Biologist of the Mind.* London: Fontana.

Temkin, O. (trans.) (1956). *Soranus' Gynecology.* Baltimore, MD: Johns Hopkins University Press.

Thacker, A. (1992). Monks, Preaching and Pastoral Care in Early Anglo-Saxon England. In J. Blair and R. Sharpe (eds), *Pastoral Care Before the Parish*, 137–170. Leicester: Leicester University Press.

Van Haute, P. and Westerink, H. (2016). Sexuality and its Object in Freud's 1905 Edition of *Three Essays on the Theory of Sexuality. International Journal of Psychoanalysis*, 97: 563–589.

Vickers, M. and Nash Briggs, D. (2007). Juvenile Crime, Aggression and Abuse in Fifth-Century Athens: A Case Study. In G. Rousseau (ed.), *Children and Sexuality: From the Greeks to the Great War*, 41–69. Houndmills: Palgrave Macmillan.

18

THOUGHTS OF FREUD

I've always lived only in the *parterre* and basement of the building. You claim that with a change of viewpoint one is able to see an upper storey which houses such distinguished guests as religion, art, etc. You're not the only one who thinks that; most cultured specimens of *homo natura* believe it. In that you are conservative, I revolutionary. If I had another lifetime of work before me, I have no doubt that I could find room for these noble guests in my little subterranean house.
Freud, letter to Ludwig Binswanger, 1936.[1]

The monument of psychoanalysis must be traversed – not by-passed –like the fine thoroughfares of a very large city, across which we can play, dream, etc.: a fiction.
Roland Barthes, *The Pleasure of the Text.*[2]

The extra lifetime's work denied to Freud has been granted to his adherents. Some of those noble guests can now find accommodation in the psycho-analytic basement – through developments which Freud could hardly have foreseen. New psychoanalytic methods of literary criticism in America pro-vide one striking example of the devious and unexpected means by which his thought renews its claim to our attention. The history that explains these methods begins with Freud's early reputation outside Germany. Its middle chapters involve politics, philosophy, and art as well as psychoanalysis. And it ends – for the moment – in this:

Thomas flang his sword into a bush.
It's not fair! he exclaimed.
What's not fair?
Why do I feel so bad? he asked, looking round him in every direction, as if for an answer.
Are you ill?
I could use a suck of the breast, Thomas said.

Not in front of him.
They retired from the Dead Father's view, behind a proliferation of
Queen Anne's lace.

Donald Barthelme's novel *The Dead Father* obviously courts reference to
the Oedipus complex.[3] It is indeed a product of the Freudian age – when
the furtive ways of the unconscious are widely acknowledged, when the
jargon of psychoanalysis has become a lingua franca, and when Freud's
theories are an undisputed part of the novelist's potential subject matter.
Yet Barthelme's novel deliberately leaves us uncertain whether psychoanalysis is, as Barthes supposed, a plaything of the imagination or, as Freud
hoped, a revolutionary and all-embracing means of interpretation. That
uncertainty reflects its style. Like a French *nouveau roman* the novel is
self-conscious about its fictionality. It systematically undermines the reader's habitual attempt to enter a credible imaginary world. Its heavy-handed
allusions to Freud ironically 'resist' the analysis of either the author or his
characters.

The psychoanalyst-critic is not to be outdone, however. New perspectives
await exploration. The narrative's inner workings, rather than the ostensible
plot, become the focus of interest. The Dead Father of Barthelme's title is,
we note, a giant, dead 'only in a sense'. He is being dragged towards his grave
by Lilliputian progeny. He lusts after his daughters in a manner reminiscent
of Freud's discarded 'seduction theory'. But he is restrained by his otherwise
ineffectual son, who learns how to cope from 'A Manual for Sons', reproduced as part of the text. Just as it ironically engages with traditional means
of literary representation, so Barthelme's novel also confronts traditional
literary images of the father. And this is more than a matter of surface
allusion. It concerns the essence of the novel as an example of discourse.
Paternity is the clue to both structure and latent theme: to the very nature of
the language being used.

> The death of fathers: When a father dies, his fatherhood is returned
> to the All-Father, who is the sum of all dead fathers taken together
> … Fatherless now, you must deal with the memory of a father. Often
> that memory is more potent than the living presence of a father,
> is an inner voice commanding, haranguing, yes-ing and no-ing –
> a binary code, yes no yes no yes no yes no, governing your every,
> your slightest movement, mental or physical. At what point do you
> become yourself? Never, wholly, you are always partly him.[4]

That prompts a reading of the novel which Barthelme can anticipate but
not forestall – in the psychoanalytic terms, less of Freud himself than
of 'the French Freud', Jacques Lacan (1901–1981). It is not easy to give a
brief account of ideas whose author prided himself on a style that imitates

delirium. Suffice it to say that Lacan's radical psychoanalysis amounts to a rewriting of early Freud –*The Interpretation of Dreams, The Psychopathology of Everyday Life, Jokes and their Relation to the Unconscious* – in the light of post-structuralist theory of language. His analysis of infantile sexuality is couched in the vocabulary of signifier and signified that continental linguistics has learned from Saussure. The child's Oedipal encounter with the father marks its entry into 'the symbolic order' of culture, its constitution as a subject. A prior 'imaginary' mode of signification is exemplified by the child's unmediated desire to be what its mother desires (the 'phallus'): an inability, Lacan argues, to distinguish signifier from signified, word from object. This happy state gives way to the anxiety of post-structuralist discourse. In 'the symbolic order' words and objects never again coincide; the unity of the self is a precarious by-product of the yes-and-no of language.

> It is in the *name of the father* that we must recognize the support of
> the symbolic function which, from the dawn of history, has identi-
> fied his person with the figure of the law.[5]

The father's name, not the father himself. Only the signifier is ever present: the father himself is absent – dead 'in a sense', as Barthelme said. And desire has been pushed down into the unconscious, adding extra, concealed dimensions of meaning to the discourse which the name of the father initiates and authorizes. The unconscious, to quote Lacan's best-known utterance, is structured like a language. Its Freudian primary processes of condensation and displacement are reformulated in linguistic terms as metaphor and metonymy.

> There is in effect no signifying chain that does not have, as if at-
> tached to the punctuation of each of its units, a whole articulation of
> relevant contexts suspended 'vertically', as it were, from that point.[6]

The literary work can thus be anthropomorphized. The critic treats the text as an equivalent of unconscious discourse; he interprets the theme of the absent father as an allegory of the generation of covert meanings which repressed desire leaves beneath the surface. Lacan's analysis of Hamlet as being in 'a certain position of dependence upon the signifier' – that is, the phallus, of which Claudius is an incarnation – reveals the extent to which he has transformed Freudian theory.[7] The way is therefore open for a psychoanalytic approach not only to writers like Barthelme, but to Homer, Dickens or Faulkner as well, which seeks out the paternal signifier buried within the text.[8]

> The general action of the novel supposes that Esther's wise passivity,
> which establishes the positionality of the father in the new Bleak

House, also casts back over the voice of the other who tells the public story of the reign of the symbolic order. Esther's narrative lays down the law of signification that permits this larger element of *Bleak House* to be given meaning.[9]

That there should be critical interpretation of Dickens guided by a structuralist version of French psychoanalysis and published in America in the 1980s is one of those paradoxes with which any appraisal of Freud's continuing impact must come to terms. What is striking is not the mixture of insight and absurdity which characterizes the enterprise: it is that psychoanalytic criticism of this sort should be practised in America at all.

America had, of course, welcomed psychoanalysis from the beginning. Freud rightly described the ideas he brought on his visit there of 1909 as 'the plague'. The environment had to some extent been prepared by, among others, Ernest Jones, James Jackson Putnam and William James, who cited the Freud–Breuer *Studies on Hysteria* with enthusiasm in his *The Varieties of Religious Experience*. The disease spread rapidly. But it was reduced to a state of mild endemicity by the 'neo-Freudians', who took their cue from the schismatic Alfred Adler. They elaborated an ego psychology which, in both theory and therapy, gave far more weight to the individual's socialization than to the instinctual origins of behaviour. Theirs was an optimistic, perhaps complacent, rereading of Freud.[10] Lacan, for whom there was no such thing as an autonomous ego or a reality principle, criticized them with unconcealed venom.[11] In literary circles meanwhile, the type of psychoanalytic interpretation whose major exponents included Edmund Wilson, Kenneth Burke and Lionel Trilling had lost its vitality by the 1960s. Their theories inevitably remained peripheral to a literary culture largely dominated by the New Criticism. Only Harold Bloom's idiosyncratic account of poetic influence as the 'belated' poet's Oedipal confrontation with his 'strong' predecessors testified thereafter to the continuing possibility of a respected Freudian criticism.[12]

So it was an alien form of literary exegesis that came to be transplanted from France to America. But the surprise is not only in the transplantation: that has to be seen in the wider intellectual context of the wholesale expropriation by American universities, Yale especially, of post-structuralist theories associated with the name of Jacques Derrida.[13] What could not have been predicted was that there would be a French psychoanalysis worth adopting. Lacan's rise to pre-eminence – or notoriety – and the growth of a psychoanalytic culture around him owed a great deal, as Sherry Turkle has demonstrated, to the 'events' of 1968.[14] Lévi-Strauss's anthropology and structuralist linguistics had of course made their mark on French intellectual life well before then; and the schisms within the psychoanalytic establishment which would punctuate every stage of Lacan's career had already begun.[15] But until those decisive months of '68, combined hostility to Freud's thinking on the part of the Catholic Church, the Communist Party, the psychiatrists, the existentialists, and the prevailing 'bourgeois ideology', meant that there could be no such general enthusiasm for psychoanalysis in France as there had been in America. (Sartre's psychoanalytic biographies represent the zeal of the late convert.[16])

In the land of Bergson and Janet, psychoanalysis was looked on first as a German and then as an American inspiration – and thereafter to be distrusted. Freud's only real success with the French before the 1960s was among the Surrealists; and it was a qualified success.[17] That both Lacan and Lévi-Strauss should have frequented Surrealist circles in the early phase of their careers indicates the subsequent importance of this early link. Certainly, both were profoundly influenced by what they learned from the Surrealists. Lévi-Strauss has written in *Tristes tropiques* that psychoanalysis, Marxism and geology were what contributed most to his intellectual formation (each encouraging the search for structures hidden below the surface of things).[18] He has also, in true Surrealist fashion, said that his books write themselves. The obscurity of his style and mode of argument suggest that his anthropology has had more in common with both Surrealist writings and Lacan's delirious seminars (in which Surrealism was often mentioned) than differences of subject might lead us to suppose.[19] This community of interest would nonetheless have been insufficient by itself to shake the general antipathy to Freud's ideas.

1968 brought the catalyst of major change. Freud was no longer the preserve of Surrealists, their sympathizers, and a small number of analysts. Psychoanalytic slogans became rallying cries ('a policeman dwells in each of our heads, he must be killed'). The Sorbonne lecture hall, scene of protracted utopian debate, was rechristened *L'Amphithéâtre Che Guevara– Freud*. And like Marcuse, Reich and Foucault, Lacan was one of those elevated to the status which only the French seem capable of according their 'intellectuals'.[20] A new psychoanalytic ideology developed out of, and about, his ideas. In this ideology, the couch became what the cafe was to the existentialists. Lacan's *Écrits* was almost a coffee-table book, more venerated than read or understood. Schoolchildren wrote essays on 'psychoanalysis and the notion of the epistemological break'. And *Freud Explained to Children* (with illustrations) was a popular gift.

Not only were there more psychoanalysts than ever before in France; the very short sessions characteristic of Lacanians enabled them to analyse more patients each day than is possible for an orthodox Freudian. The patients arrived expecting to talk about the name of the father and the like, some even clutching *Écrits*. This vastly exacerbated the analyst's perennial problem of dealing with those who know too much for their own good, and who unconsciously create new forms of resistance out of psychoanalytic gleanings. And the outrageous, subversive quality of Lacan's thought is tamed into a set of nostrums much as Freud's own theories were domesticated by American ego psychology.

Renewed French interest in Freud (as mediated by Lacan) in the years around 1968 did, however, give rise to something more than another version of radical chic. A Lacanian approach to semiotics (the comparative investigation of signifiers) resulted in textual exegesis more varied, and usually more subtle, than a search for symbolic fathers.[21] The rapprochement with Marxism prefigured in the cult of Marcuse during '68 went beyond Marcuse's simplistic equation of psychic repression and political oppression – notably in some of Althusser's essays.[22] It also led to *Anti-Oedipus* by Gilles Deleuze and Felix Guattari, designed, in part, to harmonize Freud with Marx once and for all, and to show the interdependence of Oedipal conflict and capitalism.[23]

The immense popularity of this work in France since its publication in 1972 is a further sign of how well Freud had been integrated into that bewildering blend of political rhetoric, linguistics and metaphysics which has constituted so much of modern French philosophy. In the early 1950s Merleau-Ponty, the leading phenomenologist, had all but rejected Freud's theory of the unconscious as having no bearing on the phenomenologist's method of philosophy by introspection. Just over a decade later Paul Ricoeur would, to the disgust of the Lacanians with whom he had been closely associated, publish a phenomenological 'close reading' of Freud (Freud only, not Lacan). He there asserted Freud's absolute centrality to the business of philosophical interpretation.[24] Echoing Ricoeur's 'situating' of Freud in contemporary debate, Vincent Descombes summed up the change like this.

> In the recent evolution of philosophy in France we can trace the passage from the generation known after 1945 as that of the 'three H's' to the generation known since 1960 as that of the three 'masters of suspicion': the three H's being Hegel, Husserl and Heidegger, and the three masters of suspicion, Marx, Nietzsche and Freud.[25]

The usefulness of that triadic contrast perhaps led Descombes to underestimate the extent to which Heidegger's thought has survived the period of transition. But his main point stands. Those continental schools of philosophy that laid as much emphasis on the material, especially the political, circumstances of a philosophical utterance as on its conceptual validity naturally welcomed psychoanalysis to the philosophical ranks.[26] The common preoccupation of Nietzsche, Marx and Freud with the concealed origins and significance of human behaviour (in the will to power, in material interest, or in libido) is immediately relevant to a post-structuralist concern with the elusiveness of meaning. That is why, for example, Freud's work is frequently referred to by Derrida, still the most widely known and controversial of French philosophers. Freud, like Lacan, and indeed like many others, may be the victim of Derrida's deconstructive exegesis. Yet his thought is also exemplary for the philosophical exposure of the 'metaphysics of presence' which Derrida finds in western thought.

> That the present in general is not primal but, rather, reconstituted, that it is not the absolute, wholly living form which constitutes experience, that there is no purity of the living present – such is the theme, formidable for metaphysics, which Freud, in a conceptual scheme unequal to the thing itself, would have us pursue. This pursuit is doubtless the only one which is exhausted neither within metaphysics nor within science.[27]

* * *

In 1914, already reflecting on the history of the psychoanalytic movement, Freud predicted that 'the scene of the decisive struggle over psycho-analysis' would be the ancient centres of culture where the greatest resistance to his ideas had been displayed.[28] Even so, he might have been startled to learn of his popularity and intellectual standing in France – and of his appeal, through Lacan, to novelists and literary critics in America, for so long the land of ego psychology. Yet he would not have been surprised to find himself dubbed a master of suspicion, a Derridean – to use a phrase ripe for deconstruction – *avant la lettre*.[29]

The mastery was evinced, and the ultimate reputation for it assured, by a relatively small body of work. Had Freud published only *The Interpretation of Dreams*, the *Three Essays on the Theory of Sexuality*, and various supporting papers, he would have given Lacan and Derrida quite enough material with which to refashion him in their own image. His contribution to modern thought would hardly have been diminished. And others could have proceeded to extend his systematic impieties (as Kenneth Burke once described them) beyond the realm of individual psychology with ample theoretical justification.

Indeed, one possible view of Freud seeks to protect him from his own and his disciples' extravagances. It sees his clinical work as the essence of his achievement: that communion of one unconscious with another which constitutes the analysis of the neurotic. It has little time for the wanton speculation about the unconscious significance of cultural phenomena that was characteristic of the first generation of pupils, such as Rank or Ferenczi (for whom all containers were womb-like and all swords penial). And it reminds us that Freud's ventures of this kind, whether on Leonardo or Moses, literature or society, were often tentatively conceived, reluctantly published, and readily disavowed. (As Freud said to Abram Kardiner of *Totem and Taboo*, 'don't take that seriously – I made that up on a rainy Sunday afternoon'.[30])

Not only have such diversions been extraordinarily influential; they actually lie at the very heart of Freud's thinking – whatever he may have said about them. They are as central to the psychoanalytic project as clinical observation; and they followed ineluctably from what Freud was observing and thinking. It was he, not Jung or any of the other early followers, who liberated psychoanalysis from the regime of consultancy. The omnicompetence he claimed for his technique of explanation was inherent in the nature of psychoanalysis as a general theory of the mind and as the science of the unconscious.

Historically, the point is easily documented. There are no wholly separate periods in Freud's work, apart from his long pre-psychoanalytic involvement with neurophysiology (and historians have seen even that as deeply pertinent to the genesis of his most significant ideas).[31] There was, admittedly, in the 1920s a return to the psychology of the ego, a subject which Freud can be seen to have neglected since the (posthumously-published) *Project for a Scientific Psychology* of 1895. And Freud himself wrote in his *Autobiographical Study* that his scientific career had been a long detour away from his original interest in problems of human culture – to which, newly armed with the theory of the death instinct from *Beyond the Pleasure Principle*, he returned at the end of the '20s in *The Future of an Illusion* and in *Civilization and its Discontents*.

But these are shifts of emphasis, not fresh departures. As the lists of Freud's writings by subject matter included in the Standard Edition reveal at a glance, the psychoanalysis of the arts and of anthropological topics like myth and religion interested him from the beginning.[32] The behaviour of 'savage tribes in antiquity' was first discussed, not in *Totem and Taboo* but (albeit briefly) in a pre-psychoanalytic essay on hysterical paralysis which Freud probably began to write in 1886.[33]

The reflections on the Oedipus complex in Sophocles and Shakespeare in *The Interpretation of Dreams*[34] are, like so many other aspects of Freud's thought, fully anticipated in a letter to Wilhelm Fliess of the late 1890s written during Freud's self-analysis. And it is notable that he should immediately turn for confirmation of a very personal discovery to works of literature.

> One single thought of general value has been revealed to me. I have found, in my own case too, falling in love with the mother and jealousy of the father, and I now regard it as a universal event of early childhood, even if not so early as in children who have been made hysterical . . . If that is so, we can understand the riveting power of *Oedipus Rex*, in spite of all the objections raised by reason against

its presupposition of destiny . . . A fleeting idea has passed through my head of whether the same thing may not lie at the bottom of *Hamlet* as well.[35]

With Freud, fleeting ideas had a habit of becoming certainties. The creative élan with which he at once turned his hand to the interpretation of whatever facet of social life engaged him is amply demonstrated in other letters to Fliess:

> The idea of bringing in the witches is gaining strength, and I think it hits the mark. Details are beginning to crowd in. Their 'flying' is explained; the broomstick they ride on is probably the great Lord Penis. Their secret gatherings, with dancing and other amusements, can be seen any day in the streets where children play... The story of the Devil, the vocabulary of popular swear-words, the songs and habits of the nursery – all these are now gaining significance for me . . . In connection with the dancing in witches' confessions, remember the dance-epidemics in the Middle Ages . . . I have an idea shaping in my mind that in the perversions, of which hysteria is the negative, we may have before us a residue of a primaeval sexual cult which, in the Semitic East (Moloch, Astarte), was once more, perhaps still is, a religion . . .[36]

Art, history, folklore, anthropology, comparative religion: Freud's vast reading supplied material in abundance.[37] Psychoanalysis was not first evolved and then applied. Its application contributed greatly to its evolution. For this reason, and also because of the paucity of case histories with which they were familiar, Freud's disciples who met regularly – and under his strict personal supervision – at the Vienna Psychoanalytical Society ranged as widely as he did during the movement's early years.[38] Their first three recorded meetings, in October 1906, were taken up with Otto Rank's distillation of the incest motif from poetry and folklore. During the course of these, in interesting contrast to Sir Ernst Gombrich's exposition, father hatred was identified as a dominant motif in Schiller's work.[39] And Freud opined that incest was rare in Shakespeare because he adapted existing plots and his texts were therefore 'not really his own'. Those later subjected to analysis included Christ, Oedipus, Goethe, Kleist, Hoffmann and Dostoevsky. There was also talk of the 'psychic life of the nation', primitive agriculture, and 'the corset in custom and usage among the peoples of the world'.

The group's catholicity was to be echoed in the journal *Imago*, published between 1912 and 1941 and devoted to the non-medical applications of psychoanalysis. In its first issue Freud stressed the need to extend the scope of psychoanalysis to subjects as diverse as criminology, philology and ethics, as well as myth and religion. And in later years the journal included, among numerous other works from his pen, the essays ultimately collected as *Totem and Taboo* and *Moses and Monotheism*.

No one, indeed, was more catholic in analytical research than Freud. The economy and subtlety of his arguments are always betrayed by rapid summaries, which make them sound like the caricatures of interpretation to which Freud's disciples were generally so prone. But certain recurrent themes do emerge. Setting aside an interest in occultism (which Freud had in common with Jung to a greater extent than is often realized)[40] and in the use of analysis in legal proceedings,[41] there are five main themes in what might be summed up as his psychoanalysis of culture.[42]

One theme comprises Freud's successive polemical accounts of the instinctual elements in contemporary religious belief and practice. Early on, he drew a celebrated analogy between religious observance and obsessional neurosis.[43] In his book on Leonardo, God appeared as 'the exalted father'; he explained the cohesion of the Catholic Church in libidinal terms in *Group Psychology and the Analysis of the Ego*; trust in God was a substitute for paternal protection in *The Future of an Illusion*; religious sentiment was 'oceanic' – involving regression to a primitive stage of ego development – in *Civilization and its Discontents*.

A second theme, bound up in this analysis of religion as the 'neurotic' product of instinctual renunciation, is the interpretation of culture (or civilization) as ever-stronger repression – with the probability of corporate neurosis, rather than sublimation, increasing in proportion. 'We may well raise the question whether our "civilized" sexual morality is worth the sacrifice which it imposes on us,' Freud wrote in 1908.[44] And by the time of *Civilization and its Discontents* (1930) the conflict at the heart of culture had been rendered still more insoluble (and indeed confused in its theoretical presentation) by the inclusion of the death instinct. For in Freud's early formulations, civilization was a sacrifice of libidinal instinct for the sake of ego instinct, or self-preservation. But now:

> civilization is a process in the service of Eros, whose purpose is to combine single human individuals, and after that families, then races, peoples and nations, into one great unity, the unity of mankind. Why this has to happen, we do not know; the work of Eros is precisely this. These collections of men *are* to be libidinally bound to one another. Necessity alone, the advantages of work in common, will not hold them together. But man's natural aggressive instinct, the hostility of each against all and of all against each, opposes this programme of civilization. This aggressive instinct is the derivative and the main representative of the death instinct which we have found alongside of Eros and which shares world-dominion with it. And now, I think, the meaning of the evolution of civilization is no

longer obscure to us. It must present the struggle between Eros and Death, between the instinct of life and the instinct of destruction, as it works itself out in the human species.[45]

We have to interpret the subjects of Freud's biographical interest, the third theme in his writings, as figures in this dire secular drama. The most distinguished 'pathographies' are those of the creative artists whose works may be used to shed light on their neuroses (the book's title is, after all, *Leonardo da Vinci and a Memory of his Childhood*). But, despite differences in the evidence used, no significant distinction should be drawn between Freud's studies of Leonardo, Jensen, Goethe and Dostoevsky and his analyses of Woodrow Wilson or Dr Schreber.

The fourth theme in his work is the comparative analysis of material whose underlying similarity Freud had already asserted in letters to Fliess, where he set the Sophocles play alongside his own Oedipal memories and the history of witchcraft alongside children's games and symptoms of hysteria. It all began with *The Interpretation of Dreams*. 'Previously,' Freud later explained,

> psycho-analysis had only been concerned with solving pathological phenomena . . . But when it came to dreams, it was no longer dealing with a pathological symptom, but with a phenomenon of normal mental life which might occur in any healthy person. If dreams turned out to be constructed like symptoms, if their explanation required the same assumptions – the repression of impulses, substitutive formation, compromise-formation, the dividing of the conscious and the unconscious into various psychical systems – then psycho-analysis was no longer an auxiliary science in the field of psychopathology, it was rather the starting-point of a new and deeper science of the mind which would be equally indispensable for the understanding of the normal.[46]

This discovery is, for example, what underlies Freud's interest in the similarity between the purported antithetical meanings of words in ancient languages and the double meaning of certain elements in dreams; or his analysis of 'the theme of the three caskets' in myth, lore and Shakespearian drama; or his ethnography of the virginity taboo.[47]

It also, of course, underlies that amalgam of anthropology, history and theory of the neuroses that constitutes *Totem and Taboo*. But this work, together with its sequel on Moses, is best seen as representative of the fifth and last of the preoccupations which inform Freud's non-clinical writings: a search for origins. 'Another presentiment . . . tells me, as I knew already – though in fact I know nothing at all,' Freud had written to Fliess in May 1897, 'that I shall very soon discover the source of morality . . .'[48] In *Totem and Taboo* Freud triumphantly located the source not only of morality, but of religion, society and the incest taboo, in the aftermath of the aboriginal patricide. The book on Moses revealed the origins of monotheistic religion in the murder which re-enacted that of the primal father. And Freud elsewhere had a miscellany of like speculations to offer: on the acquisition of fire for example (a renunciation of homosexual eroticism), and on the origins of clothing (women, inspired by pubic hair, invented weaving to conceal their lack of a penis).[49]

These last two features of the evolution of Freud's thought – the comparative study of symptoms, dreams and myths, and the search for prehistoric origins – are both crucial to the psychoanalysis of culture. The broadening of explanatory scope from the aetiology of the neuroses to the origins of weaving depended upon a series of increasingly bold theoretical steps. The first was to generalize from the pathological to the normal in human affairs. The second was to dispense with the 'patient's' free associations and thus to make possible a historical and sociological psychoanalysis.[50] The third was to postulate that the interpretation of works of art, myths, folklore and primitive behaviour could all be interpreted in the same way as dreams, jokes, slips and symptoms; for all of them originated in universal 'archaic' processes of the mind such as condensation, displacement and symbolization.[51]

The argument supporting this postulate was, at heart, circular. Freud had used Sophocles's *Oedipus* to give shape and substance to the results of his self-analysis; but he then sought to demonstrate the play's latent content by referring to its universal power of awakening unconscious memories such as his own.[52] A further step was necessary: the extension from biology to psychology of Haeckel's biogenetic law.[53] If ontogeny recapitulates phylogeny, if the stages of individual development reflect those of humankind, then primitive man the myth-maker was genuinely childlike in psychological make-up. The final step – conceptually not chronologically – in this methodological progression was to adopt the Lamarckian theory that acquired characteristics could be genetically inherited. Freud's unswerving adherence to Lamarck's discredited theory (which he at one stage planned to reformulate in psychoanalytic terms)[54] has often been considered a minor aberration confined to the books on totemism and Moses and having no bearing on the rest of his achievement. Certainly, the most obvious use of the theory was in the explanation of a sense of guilt in monotheistic religion as a genetically inherited memory trace of murdering the primal father.

But Freud invoked it on numerous occasions, calling its incorporation into his ideas 'the coping-stone of psychoanalysis';[55] and it may also have coloured his hypotheses about infant sexuality.[56] Like so much else, Lamarckianism is prefigured in the Fliess correspondence, where Freud speculates on the hereditary transmission of acquired neuroses.[57] Its full deployment seems, however, to have been precipitated by his analysis of the

'Wolf Man', from which he could confirm the universality of the Oedipus complex as a 'hereditary schema' independent of individual experience.[58] And in the twenty-third *Introductory Lecture*, during a discussion of infantile fantasy, Freud had this to say:

> The only impression we gain is that these events of childhood are somehow demanded as a necessity, that they are among the essential elements of a neurosis. If they have occurred in reality, so much to the good; but if they have been withheld by reality, they are put together from hints and supplemented by phantasy. The outcome is the same, and up to the present we have not succeeded in pointing to any difference in the consequences, whether phantasy or reality has had the greater share in these events of childhood. Here we simply have once again one of the complemental relations that I have so often mentioned; moreover it is the strangest of all we have met with. Whence comes the need for these phantasies and the material for them? There can be no doubt that their sources lie in the instincts; but it has still to be explained why the same phantasies with the same content are created on every occasion. I am prepared with an answer which I know will seem daring to you . . . It seems to me quite possible that all things that are told to us to-day in analysis as phantasy . . .were once real occurrences in the primaeval times of the human family, and that children in their phantasies are simply filling in the gaps in individual truth with prehistoric truth. I have repeatedly been led to suspect that the psychology of the neuroses has stored up in it more of the antiquities of human development than any other source.[59]

Lamarckianism was not peripheral to his thought: it was absolutely central. 'The psychological peculiarities of families, races and nations, even in their attitude to analysis, allow of no other explanation.'[60]

Realizing the strength and pervasiveness of this conviction is more than a scholarly matter of accurate biography. It helps us judge between two possible versions of Freud – and we can therefore estimate whether the psychoanalysis of culture that others have performed in his name is a travesty or a continuation of what he set out to achieve.

Throughout his career Freud wavered in answering the questions that must constantly be rehearsed by those who grant psychoanalysis any credence at all. How much can psychoanalysis interpret and explain? At what point in human affairs do conscious and preconscious motives yield to unconscious ones? After hearing a paper on chess at a meeting of his infant Psychoanalytical Society, Freud remarked: 'this is the kind of paper that will bring psychoanalysis into disrepute. You cannot reduce everything to the Oedipus complex. Stop!'[61] There is the first of the two Freuds speaking.

For him, psychoanalysis was the science of the unconscious; it had as little to say about the 'normal' psychology of everyday life, the ego's encounter with the cultural environment, as chemistry had to say about biology.[62] 'Starting from unconscious perception,' he wrote in *An Outline of Psycho-Analysis*, his final summation, the ego

> has subjected to its influence ever larger regions and deeper strata of the id, and, in the persistence with which it maintains its dependence on the external world, it bears the indelible stamp of its origin (as it might be 'Made in Germany').[63]

Such was socialization – a process to be noted, not explained; but a process which was none the less of enormous significance for psychoanalysis. Freud always held that the possible aetiologies of neuroses should be seen as a 'complemental series' of endogenous and exogenous factors, with the two extremes of the spectrum of possible combinations seldom occurring.[64] Symptoms were, in his terminology, 'compromise formations' between unconscious and preconscious, caused by instinct but shaped by external circumstance.[65] Myths were, similarly, the distorted secular dreams of youthful humanity.[66] The unconscious meaning of works of art could be more or less obscure according to what sort of tradition nourished the 'individual talent' and how advanced (in terms of repression) was the culture which sustained the tradition; the Oedipal content of *Hamlet* was thus better hidden than that in Sophocles' play, as the Elizabethans were generally more neurotic than the Greeks.[67]

There is, then, according to this view of Freud, a great deal of 'normal' life in which psychoanalysis can and should take no interest. (Even Lacan seems to have recognized that.[68]) And there are a great many phenomena of which it can never produce a sufficient explanation.

The similarity between diabolical possession and hysteria which Freud – and Charcot before him – had already noticed in the 1880s[69] could, for example, no more lead to a full historical account of possession than obsessional neurosis could be a complete explanation of a particular religious observance. 'We need not be surprised to find,' Freud wrote in 'A seventeenth-century demonological neurosis' of 1923,

> that, whereas the neuroses of our unpsychological modern days take on a hypochondriacal aspect and appear disguised as organic illnesses, the neuroses of those early times appear in demonological trappings... The states of possession correspond to our neurosis ... In our eyes, the demons are bad and reprehensible wishes, derivatives of instinctual impulses that have been repudiated and repressed. We merely eliminate the projection of these mental entities into the external world which the middle ages carried out.[70]

Why such projections took one form rather than another is a question for history rather than for psychoanalysis. And the analogy of religion and neurosis turns out, on similar grounds, to be no more than that – an analogy.[71]

Freud's aesthetics can, after the same fashion, be interpreted as both circumspect and incomplete. We may take seriously his frequent disclaimers that psychoanalysis by itself provides a full understanding of a work of art's origins. Psychoanalysis really has nothing to say about the nature of artistic talent. (This is perhaps because Freud's theory of art did not keep pace with his developing views on the constructive power of the unconscious.[72]) It could be added that Freud adhered to an impoverished quasi-Aristotelian conception of aesthetic response; that he only dealt with artistic form as a 'fore-pleasure' which bribes the spectator to pay attention; and that he had little to say about how sublimation occurs.[73] Freud as the tentative aesthetician is perhaps encapsulated by reference, not to the Leonardo essay but to Rembrandt. Freud told Jones that Rembrandt was his favourite painter.[74] And the series of self-portraits is surely the greatest psychological document in the history of art. Yet Freud recognized its opacity to an analysis like those he offered of *Gradiva* or 'Moses'. He left the series alone.

The modest Freud had a more ambitious internal counterpart. It was the other Freud who, in his eightieth year, pronounced the agenda for psychoanalysis used above as an epigraph. This is the man in whose eyes 'the whole course of the history of civilization *is no more than* an account of the various methods adopted by mankind for "binding" their unsatisfied wishes'.[75] The reduction was made possible by postulating that the 'myth-work' and the 'art-work' (to invent Freudian terminology) were on the same spectrum of disguised wish-fulfilments as the joke-work and the dream-work. And Haeckel and Lamarck were enlisted so that what escaped analysis on the purely synchronic front could be caught by analysis on the historical front, and then restored to the contemporary picture as an inherited repression. Form and content, tradition and individual talent, symptom and neurosis: nothing escaped.

> A child who produces instinctual repressions spontaneously is thus merely repeating a part of the history of civilization. What is to-day an act of internal restraint was once an external one, imposed, perhaps, by the necessities of the moment; and, in the same way, what is now brought to bear upon every growing individual as an external demand of civilization may some day become an internal disposition to repression.[76]

All that psychoanalysis needed was patience.

* * *

'Thoughts of Freud, naturally.'[77] Such was Franz Kafka's reaction on reading over one of his own stories the night after he had finished writing it. Kafka has been called the Dante of the post-Freudian age. But what that age thinks of Freud – what it has made of his manifold legacy – defies even supremely creative epitomizing. The problem of determining what is to count as influence can hardly be solved *a priori* – something which literary criticism has apparently conceded in replacing 'influence' with 'intertextuality' or 'discourse' as an all-purpose linking term less redolent of personal encounter. Tracing Freud's impact on the humanities is not only a search for ideological paternity – who read whom – in all its Oedipal horror. It is also, more importantly, like Freud's own work an archaeology: the uncovering of obscure paradigms of thought. One could trace for example the rise and fall of psychohistory, from Freud's Leonardo to the psychogenetic theory of everything propounded by Lloyd DeMause;[78] the unexpected fortunes of Freud in the field of art history, typified in the application of Kleinian theory to architectural criticism by Adrian Stokes;[79] psychoanalysis in sociology, from Talcott Parsons to the Frankfurt School of Marxists, or in Anglo-American philosophy from Wittgenstein to Davidson.[80]

There is always more to be said. And this is not merely because each age and culture reinterprets orthodox psychoanalysis to suit its own purposes; it is mainly because psychoanalysis itself is being continually reformulated. The American 'psychoanalytic psychologist of the self' Heinz Kohut has for instance, like Freud and Lacan, held forth on Shakespeare, as well as on that most Freudian of modern writers, Thomas Mann. A new set of doctrines provides a new analysis of culture.[81]

Just as there is more to be said of Freud and his epigones, so there is more to be uncovered about those on whom they have depended.

Two problems arise. The first is that of Freud's own ambiguous place in the history of ideas. A good writer, Nietzsche proposed in *Human, All Too Human*, has not only his own mind but the minds of his friends as well. It is only since the publication of Ellenberger's massive work *The Discovery of the Unconscious* that we have grown used to disregarding the legend of Freud as an isolated hero battling for recognition in a hostile scientific environment.[82] Increasingly, the early development of psychoanalysis comes to seem like a creative synthesis of numerous existing scientific ideas – each of which may well have been as influential on modern culture as psychoanalysis itself. We must beware of attributing too much to Freud – or at least to Freud alone. And that caution should lead to an adequate recognition of the writers of all kinds whose thought psychoanalysis has embraced or unwittingly echoed. In a characteristic early essay Auden remarked that the whole of Freud's teaching may be found in *The Marriage of Heaven and Hell*.[83] If that goes too far, the underlying point is well made. The more we learn, say, about the impact of Schopenhauer or Nietzsche on Freud's century the more we find which we might otherwise have thought purely Freudian.[84] Freud's indebtedness to nineteenth-century German philosophy has become apparent only surprisingly recently.

For a related reason, the effort to plot the courses Freudianism has taken must also give due weight to the more general history of ideas. We have been taught by Philip Rieff to speak of 'the emergence of psychological man' (or woman). We have given him (or her) a name – and a set of attributes – but not a habitation. Naturally, a broad contrast can be drawn between psychological man and his communist counterpart – for whom, since Stalin and the Chinese Revolution, the prevailing psychiatry has normally been a punitive Pavlovianism. But the history of 'Freud's French Revolution' shows how much that simple contrast leaves unsaid about the specific conditions, intellectual and sociological, in which a genuine psychoanalytic culture arises.[85] The emergence of psychological man cannot be taken for granted.

Nor, of course, should his demise. From some perspectives, psychoanalysis might seem to have withered in the face of the plentiful empirical and philosophical onslaughts that have been directed against it.[86] But the possible weakness of the discipline itself does not necessarily invalidate all examples of its heuristic application; these too demand appraisal. Like Marxism, psychoanalysis is a monument we cannot erase. To compare Freud with other significant psychologists of our age – Jung, Piaget, Pavlov, Skinner, Eysenck, the Gestalt school – is to be struck once again by how much more Freud has had to offer. Throughout the English- and German-speaking worlds the psychoanalysis of culture is, admittedly, unfashionable. Consciously or not, most accounts of human behaviour rehearse Durkheim's methodological postulate: 'every time a social phenomenon is directly explained by a psychological phenomenon, we may rest assured that the explanation is false.'[87] To use psychoanalysis under these circumstances is always to make a special case; and that remains true even if it is the general form rather than the specific content of Freud's ideas that is pressed into service.[88] Yet psychoanalysis is never beyond resuscitation, whether as a useful fiction, the greatest of modern myths, or the queen of sciences. There may for all we know be further revolutions like that in France, and they may be founded on yet more surprising intellectual alliances. At best, Freud's is 'perhaps the most important body of work committed to paper in the twentieth century', a worthy successor to Darwin's. At worst, extending a comparison drawn by a trenchant critic, it may be like Homer's stories of Olympus – masterly but unscientific.[89] To be compared to Homer even in failure is no bad thing.

Notes

1 Quoted by Ronald W. Clark, *Freud: The Man and the Cause* (London, 1982), p. 497.
2 (London, 1976), p. 58.
3 (London, 1977). The quotation is from p. 10.

4 Barthelme, *The Dead Father*, p. 144.

5 Jacques Lacan, *Écrits: A Selection* (London, 1977), p. 67.

6 Ibid. p. 154.

7 Jacques Lacan, 'Desire and the Interpretation of Desire in Hamlet', *Yale French Studies*, 55–56 (1977), p. 11. Cf. his 'Seminar on "The Purloined Letter"', *Yale French Studies*, 48 (1972), a reading of Poe.

8 Cf. *The Fictional Father: Lacanian Readings of the Text*, ed. Robert Con Davis (Amherst, MA, 1981).

9 Thomas A. Hanzo, 'Paternity and Subject in *Bleak House*', in Davis, *The Fictional Father*, p. 43.

10 Cf. J. A. C. Brown, *Freud and the Post-Freudians* (London, 1961); Russell Jacoby, *Social Amnesia: A Critique of Contemporary Psychology from Adler to Laing* (Boston, 1975).

11 Cf. *Écrits*, pp. 6, 171.

12 Cf. Bloom's *The Anxiety of Influence* (London, 1973) and *Poetry and Repression* (New Haven, CT, 1976).

13 Cf. Christopher Norris, *Deconstruction: Theory and Practice* (London, 1982), ch. 6, for a useful brief survey of the phenomenon.

14 *Psychoanalytic Politics: Jacques Lacan and Freud's French Revolution* (London, 1979), to which I am generally indebted in what follows.

15 Cf. Catherine Clement, *The Lives and Legends of Jacques Lacan* (New York, 1983).

16 Richard Ellmann, 'Freud and Literary Biography', in P. Horden (ed.), *Freud and the Humanities* (London, 1985), pp. 58–74, at pp. 72–73.

17 S. Dresden, 'Psychoanalysis and Surrealism', in Horden, *Freud*, pp. 110–129.

18 (Harmondsworth, 1976), ch. 6.

19 Transcripts of Lacan's twenty-seven *Séminaires* are still slowly being published in a corresponding number of volumes.

20 Cf. Régis Debray, *Teachers, Writers, Celebrities: The Intellectuals of Modern France* (London, 1981).

21 Cf. Julia Kristeva, *Desire in Language* (Oxford, 1980), and Pierre Macherey's tentative use of Freud in *A Theory of Literary Production* (London, 1978).

22 E.g. in *Lenin and Philosophy* (London, 1977).

23 *Anti-Oedipus: Capitalism and Schizophrenia* (New York, 1977).

24 *Freud and Philosophy: An Essay on Interpretation* (New Haven, CT, 1977).

25 *Modern French Philosophy* (Cambridge, 1980), p. 3.

26 Cf. *Philosophy in France Today*, ed. Alan Montefiore (Cambridge, 1983), especially the editor's Introduction.

27 Jacques Derrida, 'Freud and the Scene of Writing', in *Writing and Difference* (London, 1978), p. 212. Derrida also 'read' Freud – and Lacan – inter alia in *La carte postale* (Paris, 1980).

28 *The Standard Edition of the Complete Psychological Works of Sigmund Freud*, ed. and trans. James Strachey et al., 24 vols (London, 1953–1974) (hereafter *SE*, cited by volume and page number), 14.32.

29 Cf. Samuel Weber, *The Legend of Freud* (Minneapolis, 1982).

30 Quoted by Clark, *Freud,* p. 355. Cf. Bruno Bettelheim, *Freud and Man's Soul* (New York, 1983) for the argument that Freud aimed at individual self-knowledge, not general science.

31 Frank J. Sulloway, *Freud, Biologist of the Mind* (London, 1979) was perhaps the most controversial of the revisionists.

32 *SE*, 13.162 (anthropology, mythology, religion); 21.213–14 (art, literature, aesthetics).

33 *SE*, 1.170.

34 *SE*, 4.261ff.

35 15 Oct. 1897, *SE*, 1.265.

36 24 Jan. 1897, *SE*, 1.242–243. Cf. 17 Jan., 1.242, on hysteria and the medieval theory of possession.

37 Freud's learning, and the scope of the comparisons he was always drawing in order to clarify his arguments, are well brought out by Peter Gay in *Freud, Jews and Other Germans* (Oxford, 1979), and by the 'List of analogies' in *SE*, 24.179ff.

38 *Minutes of the Vienna Psychoanalytical Society*, ed. Herman Nunberg and Ernst Federn, 3 vols (New York, 1962–1974).

39 E. H. Gombrich, 'The Symbol of the Veil: Psychological Reflections on Schiller's Poetry', in Horden, *Freud*, pp. 75–109.

40 Cf. Ernest Jones, *Sigmund Freud: Life and Work* (London, 1953–1957), 3.402ff., a tactful summary; *SE*, 18.176.

41 *SE*, 9.

42 No attempt is made in what follows to give a proper digest of Freud's theories. It will be enough to refer to what is still the best short account: Richard Wollheim, *Freud*, Modern Masters (London, 1971); and to the best long account: Philip Rieff, *Freud: The Mind of the Moralist*, 3rd edn (Chicago, 1979). The most intelligent, and intelligible, philosophical exploration is that by Paul Ricoeur, *Freud and Philosophy: An Essay on Interpretation* (New Haven, CT, 1970).

43 *SE*, 9.

44 *SE*, 9.204.

45 *SE*, 21.122.

46 *SE*, 20.47.

47 *SE*, 11, 12.

48 *SE*, 1.253.

49 *SE*, 22.187ff, 132.

50 Cf. *SE*, 4.241, and Rieff, *Freud*, p. 103.

51 It would be of interest to explore the similarities between Freud's view of primitive mentality and that of his contemporary, the sociologist Lucien Lévy-Bruhl (1857–1939), whose work Freud apparently did not know. Cf. Lévy-Bruhl's *Les fonctions mentales dans les sociétés inférieures* (Paris, 1910).

52 Cf. Ricoeur, 'Psychoanalysis and the Work of Art', in *Psychiatry and the Humanities*, vol. I, ed. Joseph H. Smith (New Haven, CT, 1976).

53 Cf. Stephen Jay Gould, *Ontogeny and Phylogeny* (Cambridge, MA, 1977).

54 Jones, *Freud*, 3.330ff.

55 *A Psycho-Analytic Dialogue: The Letters of Sigmund Freud and Karl Abraham 1907–1926*, ed. Hilda C. Abraham and Ernst L. Freud (London, 1965), pp. 261–262.

56 An extreme interpretation of Freud as a Lamarckian is Sulloway, *Freud*.

57 *SE*, 1.184; *The Origins of Psycho-Analysis*, ed. Marie Bonaparte, Anna Freud and Ernst Kris (London, 1954), p. 72 – a letter not included in *SE*, 1.

58 *SE*, 17.119.

59 *SE*, 16.370–371.

60 *SE*, 23.240. Cf. SE, 7.225, 13.188, 19.37–38, 23.101; Sulloway, *Freud*, ch. 10.

61 Reported by Abram Kardiner. Quoted by Clark, *Freud*, p. 216. Cf. *SE*, 17.72, 21.171.

62 *SE*, 18.252.

63 *SE*, 23.199. 'Made in Germany' is in English in the original.

64 Cf. *SE*, 3.135–6, and the 22nd and 23rd *Introductory Lectures*.

65 Cf. *SE*, 14.53, 126.

66 *SE*, 9.152.

67 Cf. Ricoeur, 'Psychoanalysis and the Work of Art'.
68 *Écrits*, p. 163.
69 *SE*, 1.242 (Letter 56 to Fliess); cf. 3.20.
70 *SE*, 19.72. Cf. 11.50, 13.64–65.
71 Cf. *SE*, 21.43–44.
72 See Richard Wollheim, *On Art and the Mind* (London, 1973), p. 219. 'Dostoevsky and Parricide' (1928), in *SE*, 21, was Freud's only substantial essay on art after *Leonardo da Vinci* (1910).
73 Cf. Ricoeur, 'Psychoanalysis and the Work of Art', and *Freud and Philosophy*, pp. 163ff. Attempts have been made to extrapolate from Freud's theory of jokes to a general psychoanalysis of art. Cf. E. H. Gombrich, 'Verbal Wit as a Paradigm of Art', in his *Tributes* (Oxford, 1984); Jack Spector, *The Aesthetics of Freud* (London, 1972).
74 Jones, *Freud*, 3.441. Cf. *SE*, 6.227–228.
75 *SE*, 13.186, my italics.
76 *SE*, 13.188–189.
77 Quoted by Walter H. Sokel, 'Freud and the Magic of Kafka's Writing', in *The World of Franz Kafka*, ed. J. P. Stern (London, 1980), p. 146.
78 See *The History of Childhood: The Evolution of Parent–Child Relationships as a Factor in History*, ed. Lloyd DeMause (New York, 1974). Cf. David E. Stannard, *Shrinking History: On Freud and the Failure of Psychohistory* (New York, 1980).
79 Cf. Spector, *The Aesthetics of Freud*, ch. 4. On Stokes see Roger Scruton, *The Aesthetics of Architecture* (London, 1979), ch. 6, and Wollheim, *On Art and the Mind*, ch. 15.
80 Cf. Yannis Gabriel, *Freud and Society* (London, 1983); *Philosophical Essay on Freud*, ed. Richard Wollheim and James Hopkins (Cambridge, 1982).
81 On Kohut see Ernest S. Wolf, 'Psychoanalytic Psychology of the Self and Literature', *New Literary History*, 12 (1980).
82 Henri F. Ellenberger, *The Discovery of the Unconscious: The History and Evolution of Dynamic Psychiatry* (London, 1970), esp. pp. 534ff. Cf. Sulloway, *Freud*, and Hannah S. Decker, *Freud in Germany: Revolution and Reaction in Science 1893–1907* (New York, 1977).
83 'Psychology and Art Today', in *The English Auden*, ed. Edward Mendelson (London, 1977), p. 339.
84 See Bryan Magee, *The Philosophy of Schopenhauer* (Oxford, 1983). Cf. Erich Heller, 'Observations about Psychoanalysis and Modern Literature', in his *In the Age of Prose* (Cambridge, 1984).
85 *Psychoanalysis, Creativity and Literature: An Anglo-French Enquiry*, ed. Alan Roland (New York, 1978); Philip Rieff, *The Triumph of the Therapeutic* (New York, 1968).
86 Cf. Stannard, and B. A. Farrell, *The Standing of Psychoanalysis* (Oxford, 1981). Sebastiano Timpanaro, *The Freudian Slip* (London, 1976) is the most convincing single-handed refutation of one particular aspect of Freudian theory. J. M. Masson, *Freud: The Assault on Truth: Freud's Suppression of the Seduction Theory* (London, 1984) is a blatant *ad hominem* attack.
87 Emile Durkheim, *The Rules of Sociological Method*, ed. Steven Lukes (London, 1982), p. 129.
88 Cf. Meredith Anne Skura, *The Literary Use of the Psychoanalytic Process* (New Haven, CT, 1981); Peter Gay, *Art and Act: On Causes in History – Manet, Gropius, Mondrian* (New York, 1976).
89 Rieff, *Freud*, p. x; Karl R. Popper, *Realism and the Aim of Science* (London, 1983), p. 172.

POSTSCRIPT

This paper was written as an introduction to a collection of studies entitled *Freud and the Humanities*. The collection was about the influence of Freud and psychoanalysis outside the profession, on the arts and humanities and on the various disciplines by which they might be studied. There were thus chapters on, for example, the psychoanalysis of creativity, Freud and literary biography, psychoanalysis and anthropology, and psychoanalysis and the study of the ancient world; some at least of the lecturers were very big names whose writings in their respective fields endure (Richard Ellmann, E. H. Gombrich, Hugh Lloyd-Jones). My task as I saw it was threefold. First, it was to discuss in general terms the place within Freud's output of 'non-clinical' psychoanalysis: the analysis of religion, art, literature, culture; the life of the group and not just the individual, the whole life course of the historical individual and not just the neurotic patient. Second, it was to show how an investigation into Freud's influence might be undertaken: an investigation not mainly in terms of analytical schools, with its heroes, rebels, outcasts and heretics but, rather, one that would take seriously Auden's elegiac distillation in 1939: 'if often he was wrong and, at times, absurd, / to us he is no more a person/ now but a whole climate of opinion'. But, thirdly and lastly, my task was to complicate that investigation – by recalling the 'prehistory' of Freud's ideas, the influences on the influencer, the 'deep time' of subjects that he made his own and virtually claimed to have invented (as in a small way with the paper on perceptions of infant sexuality also reproduced here).

The resultant paper is a period piece. When I wrote, the prestige of Freudianism as a type of psychotherapy and as a means of diagnosing the wider phenomena of human culture was in evident decline, yet Freud still seemed to offer a body of ideas to be reckoned with. The contributors to the volume ranged in attitude from cautious admiration, despite the key figure's evident flaws, to a grudging concession of his continued relevance. How times change. Freud is not only no more a person now – there is not even much of a climate of opinion. History, the social sciences, religious studies, art history, literary studies, group psychology, biography – at least in the Anglophone world: all have very largely turned away from the psychoanalytic approach. The erstwhile master of suspicion is nowadays deeply suspect. It is a fair bet that there are more Marxists (self-conscious or unwitting) in the world today than there are Freudians. Possibly more Nietzscheans too (to recall the third member of the old triumvirate). To notice only, by way of example, the state of play in 'continental' European, but especially French, philosophy. (There is no point in looking to the Anglophone philosophical world, in which only Richard Wollheim among modern masters showed any deep interest in Freud.) So far as I know, Jacques Derrida (d. 2004), probably the most famous and widely influential philosopher in the late twentieth-century world, did not much engage with Freud after *The Post Card* (*La carte postale*, 1980) apart from the somewhat retrospective *Resistances of Psychoanalysis* (*Résistances – de la psychanalyse*, 1996) in which he grouped discussions of his affiliations with Freud, Lacan, and Foucault. The fierce critic of French psychoanalysis Gilles Deleuze did not mention Freud much after *A Thousand Plateaus* (*Mille plateaux*, 1980), the second volume of *Capitalism and Schizophrenia*. Freud dominated French intellectual culture through Lacan. He perhaps remains most fully present in the writings of the later writings of those often grouped together as psychoanalytic feminists such as Irigaray and Kristeva. Yet with them, too, the wave seems to have crested years ago. We are left with the pseudo-Lacanian posturing of Slavoj Žižek (and Clint Burnham's explicitly Žižekian *Does the Internet Have an Unconscious?* 2018). The adepts who gather in London in 2019 for the grand congress of the International Psychoanalytical Association will not be able to feel they are anywhere near the cynosure of European thought and culture.

Which is simply to say that Freud and psychoanalysis now belongs in the history of cultures of healing and of ideas in the way that Hippocrates and Galen do. What sort of history? There remains, rightly, space for intellectual and personal biography, using the full range of editions and archives now accessible, whether broadly admiring (Roudinesco, 2016; Whitebook, 2017) or 'debunking' (Crews, 2017). Freud's analyses of culture retain their advocates (Todd Dufresne, *The Late Sigmund Freud*, 2017). Yet in my paper I called for a type of history of Freudianism which was not fulfilled by narratives of individual analysts and schools and institutions of professional formation. That type of wider, yet fine-grained cultural history is still, surprisingly, quite rare. The magisterial, massive (and quirky) *Freud in Cambridge* – which he never visited – by John Forrester and Laura Cameron (2017) points out the continuing prevalence of the 'great man model' and the 'bureaucratic transplant' models of the history of psychoanalysis, in contrast to their approach (very congenial to me), which stresses a 'flurry of activity in loose networks' (p. 2). The other books I should most want to take into account if I were writing the paper now would include further exemplars of that wide-angled view, among them: the second edition of Sherry Turkle's *Psychoanalytic Politics* (1992), the original of which was used extensively above, and which takes the story forward into the years following Lacan's death in 1981; Elisabeth Roudinesco's books on Lacan and especially her *Jacques Lacan & Co.: A History of Psychoanalysis in France, 1925–1985* (1990; *La bataille de cent ans: histoire de la psychanalyse en France*, 2 vols, 1986); and Dagmar Herzog, *Cold War Freud: Psychoanalysis in an Age of Catastrophes* (2017), which sees this second golden age in which Freudianism 'came to inflect virtually all other thought systems' as ending in the 1970s or '80s.

There would be plenty to read; but it would be centred on Europe and North America. My impression is that the cultural history of psychoanalysis in Latin America, under a number of repressive regimes, following the major diaspora of Jewish analysts, is still relatively under-explored. (See Aline Rubin et al. in the journal *Psychoanalysis and History*, 18.1 (2016), 93–118, for Brazil and for wider bibliography.)

The 'prehistory' of Freud's ideas also needs more attention. There is nothing to replace Ellenberger's *Discovery of the Unconscious*, cited in the chapter above. See e.g., on a narrower front, Angus Nicholls and Martin Liebscher (eds), *Thinking the Unconscious: Nineteenth-Century German Thought* (2010).

19

PANDAEMONIUM

[Afterword to *Demons and Illness from Antiquity to the Early-Modern Period*]

It is a daunting task that this collection of essays[1] has set itself: to write, if only partially, the history of demons in relation to health, a subject necessarily involving aspects of theology, medicine, natural science more widely, magic, and witchcraft (among other scholarly minefields). We might think of seeking momentary relief from the complexities of the topic with people who seem to have achieved enviable clarity. The *Four Tantras* (*rGyud bzhi*) remains a foundational text of Tibetan medicine. The tantras are believed by some to reflect, in translation from the Sanskrit, the authentic teachings of the Buddha 'Master of Remedies', but more probably they represent a quite original piece of systematizing by a medieval author, such as the twelfth-century Yuthog the Younger. Part of the text considers the 404 specific illnesses to which anyone might succumb, regardless of age or sex. There are 101 light illnesses, which do not necessarily require treatment by a doctor; 101 serious illnesses, for which medicines are indispensable; 101 illnesses caused by the intervention of spirits and demons, which require not only medical treatment but also religious rituals performed by monks to appease these malignant forces; and, lastly, 101 untreatable illnesses, which are caused by karmic predestination and thus cannot be cured by doctors or by monks.[2]

So far so clear. Yet even this neat classification raises questions. What is the precise meaning of the term *gdon* usually translated as 'demon'? What difference would it make to our initial reaction to the text if it had been translated only as 'spirit', or as 'minor deity'? What here are the differences between medicine and monastic ritual, how are the two to be combined in treating spirit-based ailments, and what marks out these 101 ailments as requiring such a two-pronged response? In the New Age, or the post-new age, Tibetan medicine may seem more familiar to many in Europe than the (now ethically suspect) European 'classical heritage' – Graeco-Roman or Judaeo-Christian. And yet it is hard to discuss demons and disease without using Judaeo-Christian vocabulary, and thereby perhaps prejudicing all attempts at comparison.

The present little afterword to a rich collection of scholarly papers is headed 'Pandaemonium' because it looks back at all the demons encountered in previous pages and tries to draw some lessons from their attested activities that might be used to stimulate further research.

What might a historical pandaemonium – a genuinely rounded, comparative view of demons in the context of health and healing – look like? Under what headings might it be organized?

Geography

That could be the first such heading. It is no adverse reflection on a group of papers that spans at least two millennia and some half-dozen cultural traditions to say that the next task is to go global – and go later. Global, so that Tibetan demons, if that is what we should call them, are considered alongside Greek ones (Tibetan medicine owing so much to contact with the Greek world from the seventh century onwards) and alongside possible equivalents from Asia, Africa and the Americas. Later, so that we can begin to question and if necessary rephrase the Eurocentric narrative of 'disenchantment', the presumed decline of widespread acceptance of demons and of the need for demonology. It may well be that Europe's intellectuals lost their fear of demons in the earlier eighteenth century, but they did not all deny the existence of such beings; and they were, on a global scale, unusual.[3] In February 2005, thanks to Channel 4, I watched a purported exorcism on live television. There was a panel of experts to witness it and reflect on what they had seen: a psychiatrist, a religious person of some kind, an anthropologist, and so on. Cutting-edge neuro-imaging technology was primed to reveal the brain activity associated with the exorcism. The possessed person described the main symptom of his condition: an irresistible urge to push the foot on the accelerator pedal to the floor when driving and thus go much too quickly. The exorcist passed his hands over the victim's head and, if I recall correctly, the driver professed himself cured of his demonic speeding. Before we smile too readily and too knowingly, we should reflect on the number of cultures across the twenty-first-century globe in which such a performance would be viewed with great interest and seriousness. (I shall give two examples in a moment.)

Philology

Yet if we are to go global, we need next a pandaemonic philology, an attention to the precise words in question, their usual linguistic contexts and their meanings and overtones. It may not be enough to say in effect: 'In this culture in this period there are representations of beings the term or terms for which can be roughly translated as demons.' What are the obstacles to easy translation? J. H. Hexter once divided historians into lumpers and splitters. Comparative history requires a certain amount of lumping if it is to be more than a catalogue of cultural particularities. But how much? Perhaps we need to be clear first about what we are lumping. To use only the basic English terms, in this collection we have some spirits, angels, ghosts, demons, and others. Some cultures, such as Pharaonic Egypt, seem to have no overall category that we can translate as 'demon'. Others, from pre-classical Mesopotamia to early modern England, have highly variable, complex and much-debated taxonomies. For Konstantopoulos, the term demon 'ill applies' to *udug* and *lama*.[4] Some contributors mention, but do not follow through on, the possibility of using a neutral designation such as 'personified harmful forces', 'evil celestial beings', or 'chaotic natural forces' so as to facilitate broad comparisons. In this collection, we are operating within the very broad but still recognizable line of cultural descent from the ancient Near East, through the classical world, to the European and Middle Eastern cultures of the three Abrahamic religions. That does not mean, even within any one strand of that line of descent, that demons are simply demons (several contributors stress the diversity of views of demons found in their sources). To take one outlying example from an area not considered above: how much more are Anglo-Saxon elves than demons in local costume?[5] If we go global, the problems of translatability become even more acute.

Cosmology

One way to facilitate comparison is to place 'demons' whatever their local designation within their respective cosmologies and see what position they occupy. This is what the editors refer to at the outset as the necessity of demons. In almost all the cultures examined above, their position in the hierarchy is intermediate. They are lesser, or less than, deities, but are not objects of cult – with the cult of the devil in the supposed witches' sabbath being a possible exception. They are somehow above humanity. But we should be chary of describing them with that tired concept of liminality. They occupy a middle position, which is not the same thing at all. That relative position in the hierarchy offers a way of comparing across cultures. Apart from avoiding liminality, we should also be chary of assuming that demons are 'supernatural'. Most of the origin myths or creation narratives cited above have them as fully part of the created order. They are to that extent represented as natural beings.

Ontology

Are demons real (as well as natural)? It is apparently a naive question – but not the less worth asking for that. Put it another way: how close are the close encounters we can detect in the surviving evidence with demons or something like demons? There are ethnographic reports aplenty of the demeanour and behaviour of those possessed by a spirit, or of spirit mediums such as shamans. These are the contemporary equivalents of the possessed people mentioned above. Their experiences hardly fit with the narrative of disenchantment. There are perhaps even more accounts of peoples for whom the ancestors are as detectible as living relatives or for whom other spirits are real presences. Among the Buryats of Mongolia and China, for instance, the flickering of the oil lamps burning during a shamanic ceremony not only indicates the displeasure of the spirits who are feasting next to the Buryats, but is actually caused by it. Each spirit feasting at the table is, however, visible only to the shaman, since it is a 'thing of the air'.[6] Rather more unusual is an anthropologist who reports having seen a spirit. Edith Turner participated in the Ihamba tooth ritual of the Ndembu of Zambia in the mid-1980s. The sufferer here has been bitten by the tooth of a dead hunter. The tooth travels along the victim's veins, biting and causing a unique disease. The tooth is also a spirit, and is removed by the application of cupping horns after a long ritual involving singing, clapping, drumming and quaffing a (seemingly psychotropic) herbal preparation.

> Suddenly Meru [the patient] raised her arm, stretched it in liberation, and I *saw* with my own eyes a giant thing emerging out of the flesh of her back. The thing was a large grey blob about six inches across, a deep gray opaque thing emerging as a sphere. I was amazed – delighted. I still laugh with glee at the realization of having seen it, the ihamba, and so big![7]

Close encounters with individual spirits in the past are harder to find [although Jean Bodin, the French political philosopher (1530–1596), did claim that 'a friend', but fairly clearly himself, had a demon who touched one or other ear according to the rightness or wrongness of what he had just said.[8]] Gideon Bohak quotes a Talmudic recipe for a powder including ground afterbirth of a black female cat that, once put in the eye, enables the user to see demons.[9] But I think that is the closest we can get in this collection to an actual sighting. Nor do we hear much directly from individuals suffering from demonic interference or invasion. To take an example not discussed above: John Chrysostom (future bishop and saint), as a newly appointed deacon of the Church in Antioch, wrote at some point in the early 380s a long letter of consolation to an ascetic called Stageirios. This man thought himself vexed by a demon causing symptoms resembling those of epileptic fits. He was experiencing *athumia* – literally lack of spirit (ironically), depression – and he was near to succumbing to suicidal impulses. He did not think these were directly caused by the demon; rather, the demon was strengthened by the despair that led to ideas of suicide. In his letter Chrysostom never denies the 'madness of the demon' as one underlying cause of the *athumia*, but he focuses very much on what we might now describe as psychotherapy for this disease of the soul. He entirely marginalizes the demon, and indeed the epilepsy.[10] There is some analogy here with Arnald of Villanova, discussed above by Giralt, who thought that necromancers, spirit conjurors, were (diabolically?) deluded and were really exhibiting the symptoms of melancholy.[11] And of course in any of the periods covered above, there will have been demon-deniers, who claim that though demons exist, in some particular context they are not fully operative. Epilepsy is often a litmus of the extent to which disease aetiology is viewed naturalistically in any given period.[12]

The question of the ontology of demons could be pushed further. I am struck by the number of occasions on which demons appear in the foregoing chapters as figures that fit into a narrative, indeed that may be required by a narrative, whether Babylonian or Christian. Demons are good to tell with. Does that also apply to an incantation that addresses demons? Do we perhaps need to develop a rhetorical analysis of demonic invocations or adjurations? A psychological need for demon figures was recognized by some at the time. Demons, as the editors note in their introduction, are good to blame.[13] And that is because they are seen as personal. Does that make them less real on some occasions? When are they clearly personifications or figures of speech? There is still much to be said for the view that 'evil spirits are often no more than the evil itself conceived as substantial and equipped with power'. E. R. Dodds, who first developed the analogy between demons and germs explored by Bohak, quoted this dictum of Henri Frankfort and reminded us that the Greeks spoke of famine and pestilence as gods.[14] Put it another way: perhaps we need a literary history of demons before we tackle the question of where and how far people 'really' believe in demons.

Physiology

To the extent that demons are perceived as really existing, what is their physiology? Many are aery, intangible, but others are bestial, and procreate (Bohak), and fart. Some have claws (Verderame). What parts of the human body can they therefore affect? Often the mind only, according to several contributors (Crosignani, Bhogal), but the body directly also (Bailey).

Demography

How many demons? We have several differing answers to that question from the cultures surveyed above. Do demons operate as individuals or in small groups, or in 'gangs' (as in Pharaonic Egypt) or in tribes or clans (as in early Islam).[15] That is, how far does their presumed organization reflect or invert contemporary social structures? In pre-classical Mesopotamia or the late antique Mediterranean, they seem to be figures of chaos. Are they ever seen as more threatening because orderly? Are they more numerous in some periods than in others? Dodds attached the term 'age of anxiety', borrowed from his friend, the poet W. H. Auden, to late antiquity, the second to fourth centuries of the Common Era. Demons seem more prominent then. Some have seen the fourteenth century as a new phase in thinking about demons and the devil in medieval Christendom. Others would nominate the age of the witch craze as a period of heightened diabolism, in which the self-styled expert demonologist attains a high degree of prominence. Can such changes over the *longue durée* really be measured?

Ecology

Where are the characteristic haunts of demons? Tombs, pagan temples (under newly established Christianity), water, woodland, fields, bathhouses, ruins, sorb bushes . . . vulnerable because badly behaved young people at a dance, babies. All this needs proper classification and extension into fresh periods and cultures. The demonic aspects of toilets would make a good subject for comparative study, ranging from the Babylonian 'privy demon' Šulak, whose successor appears in the Talmud, to the lavatorial etiquette of twentieth-century Turks who will say *destur*, excuse me, to the demon in the toilet bowl before urinating on its head.[16]

Regimen

There is much in the chapters above about amulets and other apotropaic devices. Can homes be protected systematically against demonic assault? Can the known haunts of demons be avoided? Can the anxiety that demons might provoke be minimized by finding modes of accommodation? To put such questions is to ask in effect if there is an equivalent for the demonic environment of medical diet or regimen. Some prescriptive texts suggest as much: Peter of Spain's *Poor People's Treasure* (of medicine) for instance. 'If you place buckthorn in the house all demons will flee.'[17] Archaeology may help, where it can provenance apotropaic objects. It can lend support to the notion that 'the measures taken to cope with the unseen menace of demons constituted a domestic activity as familiar as cooking, working, playing games or bringing up children'.[18] A palatial house in late antique Butrint, Albania, across the straits from Corfu, has for instance revealed mosaics full of apotropaic designs and yielded finds such as a small copper amulet with an image of Solomon, master of demons, slaying the female monster Gyllou (among other names) who visited parturient women and sought to strangle their newborn.[19]

People learn to live with demons, to incorporate them into their lives at various points on the spectrum between the literal and the symbolic. Historians of cultures of healing need to do the same.

Notes

1 *Demons and Illness from Antiquity to the Early-Modern Period*, ed. Siam Bhayro and Catherine Rider (Leiden, 2017).

2 Patrizia Bassini, 'Harmony and Hierarchy in Tibetan Healing Practice', in *The Body in Balance: Humoral Medicines in Practice*, ed. P. Horden and E. Hsu (New York, 2013), p. 237.

3 Euan Cameron, *Enchanted Europe: Superstition, Reason, and Religion, 1250–1750* (Oxford, 2010), p. 311.

4 Gina Konstantopoulos, 'Shifting Alignments: The Dichotomy of Benevolent and Malevolent Demons in Mesopotamia', in Bhayro and Rider, *Demons and Illness*, pp. 19–38, at p. 23.

5 Alaric Hall, *Elves in Anglo-Saxon England: Matters of Belief, Health, Gender and Identity* (Woodbridge, 2007).

6 Katherine Swancutt, *Fortune and the Cursed: The Sliding Scale of Time in Mongolian Divination* (New York, 2012), pp. 74–75.

7 Edith Turner, with William Blodgett, Singleton Turner, and Fideli Benwa, *Experiencing Ritual: A New Interpretation of African Healing* (Philadelphia, 1992), pp. 2, 149.

8 Jean Bodin, *De la demonomanie des sorciers*, book I (Paris, 1580 edn), fol. 11v, a reference I owe to Ian Maclean and Sir Noel Malcolm.

9 'Conceptualizing Demons in Late Antique Judaism', in Bhayro and Rider, *Demons and Illness*, pp. 111–133, at p. 122.

10 Jessica Wright, 'Between Despondency and the Demon: Diagnosing and Treating Spiritual Disorders in John Chrysostom's *Letter to Stageirios*', *Journal of Late Antiquity*, 8.2 (2015), pp. 352–367, with further literature.

11 Sebastià Giralt, 'The Melancholy of the Necromancer in Arnau de Vilanova's Epistle against Demonic Magic', in Bhayro and Rider, *Demons and Illness*, pp. 271–290.

12 M. Carolina Escobar-Vargas, 'Demons in Lapidaries? The Evidence of the Madrid MS Escorial, h.I.15', in Bhayro and Rider, *Demons and Illness*, pp. 256–270.

13 Ibid. pp. 1–16.

14 *The Greeks and the Irrational* (Berkeley, CA, 1951), p. 41. G. Bohak, 'Conceptualizing Demons in Late Antique Judaism', in Bhayro and Rider, *Demons and Illness*, pp. 119–133.

15 M. W. Dols, *Majnūn: The Madman in Medieval Islamic Society* (Oxford, 1992), pp. 214–215.

16 Orhan M. Oztürk, with Fuat A. Göksel, 'Folk Treatment of Mental Illness in Turkey', in *Magic, Faith and Healing: Studies in Primitive Psychiatry Today*, ed. Ari Kiev (London, 1964), p. 351.

17 *Obras médicas de Pedro Hispano*, ed. Maria Helena da Rocha Pereira (Coimbra, 1973), p. 237. See also Catherine Rider, *Magic and Impotence in the Middle Ages* (Oxford, 2006), pp. 166–167. I owe these references to Catherine Rider.

18 J. Russell, 'The Archaeological Context of Magic in the Early Byzantine Period', in *Byzantine Magic*, ed. H. Maguire (Washington, DC, 1995), p. 50.

19 John Mitchell, 'Keeping the Demons out of the House: The Archaeology of Apotropaic Strategy and Practice in Late Antique Butrint and Antigoneia', in *Objects in Context, Objects in Use*, ed. L. Lavan, E. Swift and T. Putzeys (Leiden, 2007), pp. 273–310.

INDEX